FIRST EDITION

PDR®

Guide to
Pediatric & Adolescent
Mental Health

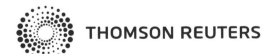

THOMSON REUTERS

PDR® Guide to Pediatric & Adolescent Mental Health

FIRST EDITION

Senior Director, Editorial & Publishing: Bette LaGow
Manager, Clinical Services: Nermin Shenouda, PharmD
Drug Information Specialists: Anila Patel, PharmD;
  Christine Sunwoo, PharmD; Greg Tallis, RPh
Manager, Editorial Services: Lori Murray
Project Editors: Sabina Borza, Kathleen Engel
Associate Editor: Jennifer Reed
Senior Director, Client Services: Stephanie Struble
Project Manager: Christina Klinger
Manager, Production Purchasing: Thomas Westburgh
Manager, Art Department: Livio Udina
Electronic Publishing Designers: Deana DiVizio,
  Carrie Spinelli Faeth

PHYSICIANS' DESK REFERENCE

Executive Vice President, PDR: Thomas Rice
Vice President, Product Management: Cy Caine
Vice President, Publishing & Operations: Valerie Berger
Vice President, Clinical Relations: Mukesh Mehta, RPh
Vice President, Strategy & Business Development: Ray Zoeller
Vice President, Finance: Donna Santarpia
Vice President, Manufacturing: Brian Holland
Senior Director, Copy Sales: Bill Gaffney
Senior Product Manager: Richard Buchwald

ISBN: 978-1-56363-729-2

Contents

Contributing Authors

Harris B. Stratyner, PhD, CASAC, is a licensed doctor of psychology and a credentialed alcoholism and substance abuse counselor, as well as an internationally recognized expert on addiction, with a particular specialty in co-occurring disorders. He is currently the Vice President and New York Regional Director of Caron Treatment Center and Clinical Associate Professor of Psychiatry at Mount Sinai School of Medicine. Dr. Stratyner is perhaps best known for his unique approach of "carefrontation" with addicted individuals and patients with psychiatric diagnoses. He is a frequent lecturer at major rehabilitation and psychiatric facilities and has had his own radio show for over 20 years.

Michael S. Behar, MD, is board-certified in Child, Adolescent and Adult Psychiatry. He is in private practice in New York City and Westchester County, NY, specializing in the treatment of anxiety and mood disorders in children and adolescents with expertise in psychotherapy, cognitive behavioral therapy, hypnotherapy, and psychopharmacology. Dr. Behar is also a senior psychiatric consultant for the Jewish Board of Family and Children's Services of New York City.

Acknowledgements

I want to thank my wife, Lynn, and daughter, Alex, for their loving support throughout my career of serving those with psychiatric and substance abuse issues.

Harris Stratyner

I would like to thank my wife, Lynne, for her loving support and encouragement and my son, Andrew, for his courage and fortitude.

Michael Behar

Last but certainly not least, we both want to thank Bette LaGow, who graciously guided us through writing this book and did it with gentle expertise.

Foreword

Health professionals who care for children and teens are faced with numerous challenges—from making correct diagnoses to determining the proper treatment regimens. And those professionals working in a more supportive role, such as school nurses or guidance counselors, need to have a solid understanding of childhood mental health issues to help kids within the academic setting. Concerned parents, as well, can only benefit from informing themselves as much as possible about the complex issues surrounding their children's mental health and well-being if a disorder or an addiction has been recognized. *PDR® Guide to Pediatric & Adolescent Mental Health* addresses this important subject with clarity and expertise.

Since the onset of addiction and mental illness are commonplace in youth, there is an urgent need to make early diagnoses to ensure that successful treatment can lead to lifelong health; this book can help. In addition to its extensive descriptions of legal, illegal, and over-the-counter psychoactive drugs, it provides both comprehensive descriptions of the criteria for many diagnoses and clear descriptions of effective treatment options including cognitive therapy, pharmacologic treatment, or a combination of both.

Written by Dr. Michael Behar, an expert in child and adolescent psychiatry and psychopharmacology, and Dr. Harris Stratyner, who is internationally known for his work in addiction, this book covers not only the mental health conditions most commonly diagnosed in this patient population, but also the critical importance of engaging the younger generation and practical advice on how to do it.

All in all, *PDR Guide to Pediatric & Adolescent Mental Health* is a welcome addition for anyone concerned with the health of our youth.

David C. Lewis, MD
Professor Emeritus of Community Health and Medicine
Donald G. Millar Distinguished Professor Emeritus
of Alcohol and Addiction Studies
Brown University
Center for Alcohol and Addiction Studies
Providence, RI

How to Use This Book

This first edition of the *PDR® Guide to Pediatric & Adolescent Mental Health* marks the collaboration of respected authors Harris B. Stratyner, PhD, CASAC, and Michael S. Behar, MD, and the clinical experts at *Physicians' Desk Reference®*—making it one of the most comprehensive mental health references to cover treatment issues specific to younger patients. The book is organized into three sections:

Section 1 includes overviews of the most common mental health conditions seen in children and adolescents. These chapters discuss prevalence and risk factors, symptoms and diagnosis, treatment issues, and instructive case studies. A chapter on helping addicted teenagers is also included. An important feature of these chapters is the discussion of how conditions present differently in a younger patient.

Section 2 covers street drugs, including more than 100 profiles on commonly abused substances. The section is divided into four parts:

Part 1: Commercial products, including alcohol, nitrites, and inhaled substances such as aerosol propellants and gases.

Part 2: Over-the-counter drugs, including commonly used antihistamines and cough medicines.

Part 3: Commonly abused prescription drugs, including benzodiazepines and other central nervous system depressants, barbiturates, stimulants, narcotic analgesics, and anabolic steroids. Some of the drugs discussed in this category may no longer be commercially available in the U.S. However, they are included because it may still be possible to obtain them from foreign countries or illegal sources.

Part 4: Illegal drugs, including cannabis, cocaine, heroin, and hallucinogens such as LSD.

Each street drug profile is listed alphabetically by generic name and includes brand names (if available) as well as common street names. Also included is the Drug Enforcement Administration (DEA) classification, which is based on the Controlled Substances Act of 1970. **Class I** drugs are illegal, have a high potential for abuse, and have no accepted medical use in the U.S. Drugs in the remaining classes are legal and have a currently accepted medical or research use, along with the following designations: **Class II** drugs have a high potential for abuse; **Class III** drugs have some potential for abuse; **Class IV** drugs have a relatively low potential for abuse; and **Class V** drugs have the lowest potential for abuse. Please note that while diligent efforts have been made to provide the most current information, the data on street drugs are constantly changing in all of the aspects discussed.

This section does not include information on drug screening, due to numerous variations in laboratory testing methods and collection procedures. For specific information, contact the Substance Abuse and Mental Health Services Administration at 800-967-5752 or *www.workplace.samhsa.gov*; and the DEA at 202-307-1000 or *www.dea.gov*.

Section 3 features profiles of drugs commonly prescribed to treat mental health disorders. The profiles are arranged alphabetically by brand name and, when available, include information on approved uses, warnings and precautions, reasons to avoid the drug, recommended dosages, common side effects (occurring in ≥3% of patients), precautions during pregnancy and breastfeeding, and storage information.

The drug information in this section contains FDA-approved prescribing information as published in the *Physicians' Desk Reference* or supplied by the manufacturer. This information is drawn from the *PDR* database, which is compiled and updated on a regular basis by a staff of experienced pharmacists. While diligent efforts have been made to ensure the accuracy of each drug entry, it is essential to bear in mind that the information presented here is merely a synopsis of key points in the official drug labeling, and that the complete labeling contains additional precautionary information that may be of significance in specific cases. If an entry leaves any question unanswered, be sure to consult *Physicians' Desk Reference* or the manufacturer for additional information.

Publisher's Note
The publisher, Physicians' Desk Reference Inc. (PDR), and the authors of the *PDR Guide to Pediatric & Adolescent Mental Health* have made diligent efforts to confirm that the drug and treatment information set forth in this book are in accordance with current recommendations and practice at the time of publication. Reasonable steps have been taken to ensure the accuracy of the information presented. However, the authors and publisher cannot ensure the safety or efficacy of any product or service described in this publication. Individuals are advised to consult a physician or other appropriate healthcare professional before undertaking any treatment referred to in this publication. Professionals must use and apply their own clinical judgment, experience, and training and should not rely solely on the information contained in this publication before prescribing any medication or treatment. PDR and the authors assume no responsibility or liability for personal or other injury, loss, or damage that may result from the suggestions or information in this publication.

PREFACE

The field of psychiatry has advanced in ways I never could have imagined when, as an eager young psychiatry resident, I first set foot in a bustling city hospital psychiatric emergency room almost 30 years ago.

In those years, the field of psychiatry was in a state of transition, and the teaching of biological psychiatry, as it was called then, was in its infancy. I feel fortunate that my early clinical training was firmly grounded in psychodynamic theory and the teaching of psychotherapy, as psychiatry at that time was still primarily a profession engaged in "the talking cure," as psychotherapy was sometimes known. This knowledge has greatly enriched my understanding of my patients and has informed my psychopharmacology practice as well.

During my training, the available somatic treatments were relatively few and the medications used, although sometimes helpful, were more akin to a sledgehammer than a delicate instrument.

Just some of the incredible advances that make the field of psychiatry so exciting and rewarding today include decades of research into genetics, epidemiology, the refinement of diagnostic categories, and evidence-based treatments; the development of more accurate imaging techniques (CT scans, PET scans, MRI, etc.) that have ushered in the field of neuroimaging and greatly expanded our knowledge of the neurophysiological basis of psychiatric disorders; the discovery of an ever-expanding roster of effective and selective medications and a growing understanding of their putative mechanisms of action to guide our treatment choices; and finally, the isolation of specific genes implicated in disease formation and the prospect of being able to intervene at this level to prevent or cure illnesses.

As rewarding as the field of adult psychiatry is, working with children and adolescents offers the rare opportunity to intervene at critical stages of development, sometimes enabling the clinician to alter the course of an illness and to prevent the otherwise inevitable downward spiral into disease and dysfunction. To correctly diagnose and treat bipolar disorder in a 9-year-old boy; using the technique developed by Dr. Harris Stratyner called "carefrontation," to engage an otherwise disaffected adolescent girl who is addicted to alcohol and cocaine, and thereby keeping her in treatment that will prove lifesaving; to successfully treat the ADHD and learning disorder that had prevented an otherwise bright 7-year-old from learning and progressing—these are just some of the rewards and challenges that face those of us who dedicate ourselves to working with children, adolescents, and their families.

The first section of this book is the culmination of years of clinical work and close collaboration with my dear friend and esteemed colleague, Dr. Stratyner. It is also the result of many years of clinical and research work of many dedicated colleagues too numerous to list.

This book has been a labor of love for both of us and we hope it provides information that will prove helpful to you and to your patients in the vital work that you do in treating children and adolescents.

Michael Behar, MD

Mental Health Conditions in Children and Adolescents

ANXIETY

OVERVIEW

Anxiety is a normal and adaptive response to real and present danger. The physiological response to danger includes increase in heart and respiratory rate, narrowing of focus, and hypervigilance—the "fight or flight" response. Anxiety crosses the line into pathology when there is a disconnect between the degree of danger or threat and the individual's response, both cognitive and somatic.

Anxiety disorders are very common in childhood and adolescence with up to 20% prevalence rates in some community samples. Developmental factors have an important impact on the expression of the different anxiety disorders. Some anxiety disorders are more common in younger children, whereas others are not typically seen until adolescence.

Longitudinal studies have shown a clear connection between childhood anxiety disorders and later adult psychopathology. Adults who experienced clinically significant anxiety as children are more likely to suffer both anxiety and mood disorders. Further, family studies strongly suggest that depression and anxiety in a parent is a risk factor for childhood anxiety disorder in the offspring. On the other hand, many children and adolescents who develop early-onset anxiety will not go on to an anxiety disorder in adulthood.

There appears to be a very strong association between early-onset anxiety and development of depression in later childhood or adolescence. One study found that anxiety preceded pediatric depression in 67% of children comorbid for both. Some have even suggested that this may represent a developmental progression from anxiety to depression. Longitudinal studies seem to corroborate this finding as peak age of onset for any anxiety disorder is between 5 to 10 years of age and for depression 15 to 20 years. This begs the question as to whether timely and effective treatment of childhood anxiety disorders might prevent this progression to adolescent and young adult depression.

Prevalence rates vary depending on inclusion criteria chosen, degree of impairment required, etc. In the general population, subclinical anxiety symptoms (ie, symptoms that do not meet full *DSM-IV-TR* criteria for anxiety disorder) are common. Fear of harm to self or to attachment figures and excessive worry are often encountered in the pediatric population. One study showed that 7-year-olds with subclinical anxiety may demonstrate significant impairment in academic achievement. This suggests that anxiety disorder must be ruled out as a diagnosis in any child presenting with academic difficulties.

Left untreated, anxiety disorders in children can lead to depression, trouble with focus, attention and academic failure, lower self-esteem, and impaired social relationships. Untreated pediatric anxiety disorder can ultimately lead to higher risk of adult depression, substance use, acting out behaviors, as well as suicide.

PREVALENCE AND RISK FACTORS

Prevalence rates, age of onset, and risk factors vary depending on the specific anxiety disorder studied. Of the 20% of children seen in community samples with anxiety, up to half of them suffer clinically significant impairment in daily functioning.

Lifetime prevalence rates for separation anxiety disorder approach 3.5%. For overanxious disorder, rates between 1.3% and 2.9% are reported. These are the most common anxiety disorders in the youngest age group. Specific phobias carry prevalence rates that vary between 0.3% and 2.4%. Social anxiety disorder occurs between 0.6% and 3.5%.

Generalized anxiety disorder (GAD), panic disorder, and obsessive-compulsive disorder (OCD) are less common in the pediatric population as the age of onset for these conditions is in middle childhood and adolescence. In the pediatric population, panic disorder prevalence rates range from 0.03% to 1.6%; GAD rates are 0.08% to 2.4%; rates for OCD are 0.2% to 0.7%. Prevalence rates for these three disorders are higher in later childhood and adolescence. Overall, prevalence rates for any anxiety disorder are higher for girls for all but OCD. These reported sex differences are seen by age 6, during which there is a sharp rise in rates of anxiety disorders in girls.

Genetic factors play a role in the transmission of risk. A number of studies report that the risk of developing any anxiety disorder is up to five times greater in first-degree relatives of family members with a specific anxiety disorder.

Some have postulated that some of the genetic vulnerability for anxiety disorders may involve heritability of the somatic symptoms (eg, increase in heart rate, breathing rate, etc.) associated with anxiety. Family studies also support high heritability rates for anxiety. Offspring of parents with anxiety disorder have an increased risk of developing anxiety.

Another interesting finding is that parents with depression also seem to confer a high risk of anxiety to their children, further supporting the proposed relationship of shared heritability between anxiety and depression.

Modeling of anxious parents by offspring can also explain some of the increased risk for anxiety.

Early exposure to severe trauma, whether abuse or traumatic separation, may affect critical neural pathways and lead to increased risk of developing an anxiety disorder.

Various personality traits have been cited as potential risk factors for anxiety. Among these traits are behavior inhibition and sensitivity to anxiety (the "fear of fear" reaction often seen in panic disorder) to name but a few.

PRESENTATION AND DIAGNOSIS

The *DSM-IV-TR* recognizes a number of anxiety disorders that are also seen in children and adolescents:

- Generalized anxiety disorder (GAD)
- Specific phobia
- Social anxiety disorder
- Separation anxiety disorder (SAD)
- Panic disorder (PD)
- Post traumatic stress disorder (PTSD)
- Obsessive-compulsive disorder (OCD) (See the chapter on OCD for detailed information on this condition.)

Each of the anxiety disorders has in common developmentally inappropriate levels of fear and anxiety.

Generalized Anxiety Disorder

In *DSM-III*, overanxious disorder was included as a distinct entity affecting children. In *DSM-IV-TR*, it has been subsumed under GAD. One of the primary symptoms of GAD is excessive worry that the child has trouble controlling. Associated features include:

- Restlessness
- Fatigue
- Difficulty concentrating
- Irritability
- Muscle tension
- Sleep difficulty

Adult criteria require at least three of six symptoms listed above. In children, only one or more symptoms are required.

Among the many anxiety disorders commonly affecting children and adolescents, GAD has the earliest age of onset. The median age of onset for GAD is 6 years. GAD is also the most common anxiety disorder seen in childhood.

Specific Phobia

Specific phobia has an age of onset immediately following GAD. Developmentally, younger children tend to be concrete in their thinking. It is this characteristic that lends itself to the development of specific phobias, such as fears of the dark, of monsters, of dogs, etc. Specific phobia is characterized by excessive and unrealistic fear that is persistent and interferes with functioning. The fear is triggered by either exposure to or anticipation of the feared object or situation. The anxiety can reach panic proportions. Although adult criteria specify that the individual recognizes the unrealistic and excessive nature of the fear, this is not necessarily the case with children, especially younger children.

As with all phobias, the feared situation or object is often avoided. In order to reach the threshold of a disorder, both the avoidant behavior and the degree of anxiety must cause functional impairment. This is to distinguish phobic disorder from transitory developmental fears which are normal and of no clinical consequence.

Genetic factors appear to play an important role in the development of specific phobias. Lifetime prevalence rates are estimated to be around 2.5%. Many children with specific phobia have more than one phobia, and the disorder is often comorbid with separation anxiety disorder (SAD).

Social Anxiety Disorder

Social anxiety disorder is the next anxiety disorder to appear in children, with a mean age of onset of 7.5 years. It is characterized by excessive and persistent fear in social settings. The child fears being judged harshly or feeling humiliated. When exposed to a feared social setting, the anxiety may approach panic levels. In general, social situations are avoided and there is a constriction of the child's activities.

Prevalence rates for social anxiety approach 5% in the 12 to 18 year age group, although rates are slightly higher in girls. Rates are significantly higher in adolescents compared with the pediatric population. In this population, the anxiety typically occurs in relation to school and is often disabling.

Epidemiologic data show that social anxiety disorder is often comorbid with depression as well as GAD, specific phobia, and ADHD.

Although *DSM-IV-TR* continues to classify selective mutism as a distinct entity, more recent evidence seems to support the conclusion that it is really a severe and early onset form of social anxiety disorder.

As with other anxiety disorders, genetics seem to play a role in transmission of the disorder.

Separation Anxiety Disorder

Separation anxiety disorder (SAD) has a mean age of onset of 8 years. It is characterized by excessive anxiety related to separation from an attachment figure. The anxiety must be developmentally inappropriate to be considered a disorder.

In order to meet criteria for SAD, at least three of the following symptoms must be present:
- Repeated and excessive anxiety experienced upon separation from home or an attachment figure
- Persistent worry about harm to an attachment figure

- Fear about becoming lost
- Extreme hesitancy or outright refusal to go to school
- Excessive and recurrent fear about being alone
- Fear or refusal to go to sleep without an attachment figure
- Somatic symptoms (stomachaches, headaches, dizziness, etc.) following separation

Symptoms must be present for at least four weeks and cause impairment. Prevalence rates for SAD vary between 3% and 5% and are higher during childhood than during adolescence. In a recent study, it was shown that offspring of parents with panic disorder and/or major depression were more likely to suffer from SAD.

Panic Disorder
Mean age of onset for panic disorder (PD) is 13.5 years; PD is relatively rare in the pediatric population. Studies using community samples have cited prevalence rates under 1%, whereas rates in pediatric and adolescent clinic samples approach 10%.

PD is characterized by panic attacks that are spontaneous—that is, they are not apparently triggered by external cues. A panic attack is an episode of intense fear and anxiety during which at least four of the following physiological symptoms must be present:

- Palpitations
- Experience of shortness of breath
- Shaky feeling
- Sweating
- Chest pains
- Nausea
- Dizziness or lightheadedness

Other related symptoms include:

- Feelings of unreality (derealization)
- Feeling of being detached from self (depersonalization)

In addition to the physiological symptoms listed above, cognitive symptoms must follow the somatic ones by at least 1 month. These cognitive symptoms include:

- Frequent and continuing worry about having another panic attack
- Recurrent fear about suffering some catastrophic event (eg, heart attack, stroke, dying, becoming paralyzed, etc.)

For children and adolescents, it is the physiological symptoms that are reported far more often than the cognitive, although older adolescents show both.

Comorbidity is high for PD. It is estimated that between 50% and 90% of children and adolescents with PD have another disorder. Comorbid

CASE STUDY

Kelly was a 16-year-old junior in high school when she was referred by her pediatrician for unexplained "anxiety attacks."

She was first evaluated medically, as her initial symptoms were difficulty breathing and palpitations during gym. The school nurse found Kelly's pulse and blood pressure elevated, and sent Kelly to the local ER for further evaluation. Full medical workup included thyroid studies, EKG, urine for toxicology, etc. BP was initially elevated but returned to normal limits after orally administered clonazepam (Klonopin). Except for BP, all medical findings were within normal limits, and Kelly was diagnosed with "anxiety." She was told to follow up with her primary care physician, who referred her for a psychiatric evaluation.

Kelly is the youngest of three children in an intact upper-middle class family. Parents are supportive and loving and Kelly has a "close relationship" with both. Kelly is an excellent student and is outgoing and popular. In grade school, she had some separation difficulties and used to miss days of school due to vague somatic symptoms.

Kelly presented as verbal and articulate. She expressed feeling stress preparing for the SATs and was anxious to get accepted to her father's Ivy League alma mater. Kelly admitted that she always had concerns about her parents' well-being and engaged in bedtime rituals over the years to "protect" them. She had several episodes lately during which she awoke in the middle of the night in a state of panic and could feel her heart pounding and her breathing labored. Now afraid of having another episode, she was fearful of going to sleep. For about 2 months prior to her visit to the ER, she had begun to have acute panic attacks during the day. Several occurred at home, one occurred while at the mall, as well as the recent episode at school. She began to avoid going out in crowds for fear of having another "attack." She had become less enthusiastic and admitted to an overall constriction in her activities and in her outlook.

Kelly was diagnosed with panic disorder with agoraphobia. She and her parents were given information about the panic attacks. Kelly was started on Zoloft (sertraline) 25mg, which was slowly titrated to 100mg.

Kelly also engaged in a course of panic-control therapy. She was taught progressive muscle relaxation and breathing retraining. Cognitive restructuring, with developing positive self-statements, identifying overestimation of negative outcomes, reducing catastrophizing, etc., was employed, followed by graded exposure techniques. Over the course of the 12-week CBT, Kelly began to experience fewer and less intense panic episodes, and after 3 months was free of any panic attacks. Booster sessions were scheduled to help Kelly stay symptom-free, and there has been no recurrence of symptoms 6 months later, even after tapering off the Zoloft.

conditions include other anxiety disorders, depression, and oppositional defiant disorder (ODD).

Post-Traumatic Stress Disorder

DSM-IV-TR defines PTSD as symptoms arising from exposure to a traumatic event. The traumatic event consists of actual or threatened death or serious injury to self or another. In the course of the event, the child responds with intense fear or feelings of helplessness. In addition, the child continues to re-experience the trauma in any of the following ways:

• Recurring and intrusive thoughts, images, or perceptions of the trauma
• Recurring dreams or nightmares
• Flashbacks; intense feelings of reliving the traumatic event
• Intense distress with exposure to reminders of the event

Avoidance phenomena are also a component of PTSD. This can consist of avoiding situations, thoughts, or feelings associated with the trauma.

Other symptoms include a general numbing of feelings, a sense of foreshortened future, lack of interest in life, etc.

DSM-IV-TR stipulates that these symptoms must be present for at least one month.

COMORBID CONDITIONS

Comorbidity is common in pediatric anxiety disorder and one of the most common comorbidities is a second anxiety disorder. More than half of children with anxiety will have at least one other anxiety disorder.

Comorbid depression is frequently seen in childhood anxiety disorders. Children with anxiety and comorbid depression often have more severe symptoms of anxiety than anxious children without depression.

ADHD is another disorder commonly seen co-occurring with childhood anxiety.

One can often see comorbid substance abuse disorder with adolescent anxiety disorder and it could be seen conceptually as a form of self-medicating.

ISSUES UNIQUE TO PEDIATRIC AND ADOLESCENT ANXIETY DISORDERS

Developmental issues play an important part in the clinical presentation of anxiety disorders.

Young children do not yet have the capacity for the more abstract thinking and reasoning seen in adolescence. Their thinking tends to be more concrete and influenced by their general emotional state. It is partly for this reason that specific phobias are seen more frequently during early and middle childhood. This may also be why children generally experience more somatic symptoms of anxiety (eg, stomachaches, headaches, fatigue, etc.) than do older children and adolescents. Children are also more dependent on parents and other attachment figures and SAD is also seen more frequently during this period.

With the gradual development of higher-order cognitive functioning and abstract thinking, adolescence is usually the period during which panic disorder emerges.

Although younger children can develop panic disorder, it is during adolescence when the cognitive symptoms of PD become more predominant over the somatic.

TREATMENT OF ANXIETY DISORDERS
Nonpharmacologic Treatment

Among the recognized nonpharmacologic treatments for pediatric anxiety disorder, behavior therapy, cognitive behavior therapy (CBT), and psychotherapy have convincing evidence of efficacy in this age group.

Current research into anxiety disorders has found it useful to group GAD, SAD, and social anxiety disorder together for the purposes of identifying effective treatment strategies.

OCD, panic disorder and PTSD have treatment recommendations that involve special modifications to standard CBT protocols.

To date, CBT is considered the treatment of choice for childhood SAD, social anxiety, and GAD. CBT techniques for these three disorders include teaching children to recognize signs of anxiety; teaching and practicing relaxation techniques (breathing and muscle relaxation); helping the child to observe and modify the negative self-talk that perpetuates the anxiety; helping the child to acquire problem-solving skills necessary to deal with the anxiety; and using exposure techniques.

Since parents can sometimes foster and maintain a child's anxiety symptoms, family therapy, parent education and/or family CBT are often recommended for those children whose parents also suffer from anxiety. Children without anxious parents seem to respond well to individual child-focused CBT.

Individual psychotherapy has also been used for a variety of anxiety disorders in children and adolescents. In individual psychotherapy, the child is given help in mastering issues of separation, is encouraged to improve autonomy and age-appropriate independent functioning, and is aided in improving self-esteem among other things. As in CBT, parent involvement is often helpful and recommended.

Anecdotal case studies suggest the usefulness of individual psychotherapy for the treatment of various pediatric anxiety disorders.

The nonpharmacological treatment of choice for panic disorder is panic-control therapy, which involves standard CBT techniques together with an exposure component.

The elements of CBT utilized in PD include education about panic; use of relaxation techniques (breathing retraining, progressive muscle relaxation); and cognitive restructuring, including the use of positive statements, recognizing risk-overestimation and predicting negative outcomes, as well as reducing "catastrophizing."

After these techniques have been mastered, exposure to a series of gradually increasing levels of anxiety triggers begins. With each exposure, use of cognitive restructuring and relaxation techniques are employed to help the child deal with the anxiety and ultimately master the panic.

Recommended nonpharmacologic treatment for PTSD involves CBT together with trauma-focused psychotherapy.

Pharmacologic Treatment
There are a number of effective medications for the treatment of pediatric anxiety disorders. With the exception of use in OCD, none of the pharmacologic treatments is approved by the FDA for use in children, and as such are considered off-label in this age group.

Because of the similarity in symptoms, genetics, and response to treatment, social anxiety, SAD, and GAD are usually grouped together for the purposes of evaluating effective treatment strategies.

Over 30 years ago, the tricyclic antidepressants (TCAs) were found effective for the treatment of anxiety disorder in adults. Tofranil (imipramine) has evidence for efficacy in pediatric anxiety disorder. Because of their side effect profile and cardiac safety concerns, the TCAs are no longer considered first-line treatment.

The selective serotonin reuptake inhibitors (SSRIs), and Prozac (fluoxetine HCl) in particular, have been found effective in one 12-week controlled study looking at children with GAD and social anxiety.

Another study used Luvox (fluvoxamine HCl) for children with GAD, SAD, and social anxiety and also found it safe and effective.

Recent concerns about potential risk of suicidal ideation with SSRIs used in children and adolescents has led to recommendations for closer monitoring during the first few months of treatment.

There are no data supporting the use of other medications in pediatric anxiety disorders. Buspar (buspirone) has been found effective in adult anxiety disorder. Results in children, however, are inconclusive.

Although no controlled randomized studies exist for pediatric panic disorder, there is evidence for the efficacy of the SSRIs. The benzodiazepines are useful and effective in adults with PD, but little data support their use in children.

Evidence for potential usefulness of the antihypertensive drugs Catapres (clonidine) and Inderal (propranolol) has been demonstrated in a small open-label study of pediatric PTSD.

Propranolol was found helpful in decreasing symptoms of intrusive thoughts and arousal. It has been shown that clonidine may also help reduce the hyperarousal seen in PTSD.

Some evidence also exists supporting the use of SSRIs for pediatric PTSD symptoms with comorbid depression.

SUMMARY

Pediatric anxiety disorders include generalized anxiety disorder, social anxiety disorder, specific phobia, separation anxiety disorder, panic disorder, post-traumatic stress disorder, and obsessive compulsive disorder.

Although anxiety and fear can be an adaptive and normal response, anxiety that begins to interfere with functioning can be debilitating and derail the course of normal development, affecting the child across multiple spheres.

Comorbidity is the rule in pediatric anxiety disorder and depression, as well as other anxiety disorders that are often seen together. It has been suggested that pediatric anxiety disorder may be the first stage in a developmental progression to pediatric depression.

Of all the recommended treatments for anxiety in youth, CBT remains the treatment of choice. Specialized CBT treatment protocols have been developed to address the unique nature of different anxiety disorders.

Studies have also shown effectiveness of SSRIs to treat the symptoms of pediatric anxiety disorder. With the exception of OCD, the SSRIs remain off-label treatments for anxiety disorders in children. As in other areas of child and adolescent psychiatry, further randomized controlled studies are needed.

ATTENTION-DEFICIT/HYPERACTIVITY DISORDER (ADHD)

OVERVIEW

ADHD is the most common neurobiological disorder in childhood. It is estimated that between 5% and 12% of children and adolescents have significant symptoms of this disorder. Although once felt to be a temporary condition that children "outgrow," it is now recognized that ADHD is often a chronic condition that can continue into adulthood. Up to 75% of children with ADHD will continue to have significant symptoms into adolescence; up to 50% will have signs of the disorder as adults.

With this in mind, any treatment recommendation must consider the possibility that it may need to extend through adolescence—and possibly into adulthood.

ADHD can affect a child in multiple spheres, including academic performance, peer interactions, and family relationships, and can have far-reaching consequences. If left untreated, ADHD can lead to dire outcomes, such as school failure, low self-esteem and depression, poor employment history, failed relationships, increased risk of motor vehicle accidents, increased risk of substance abuse, and involvement with the legal and criminal justice system.

PREVALENCE AND RISK FACTORS

ADHD is two and a half times more likely to occur in boys than in girls. Studies of twins show that ADHD is a highly heritable disorder involving multiple genes. A 2005 review of 20 twin studies that were conducted in the U.S., Australia, Scandinavia, and the E.U. calculated that the mean heritability estimate for ADHD was 76%, making ADHD one of the most heritable disorders. As with many disorders, environmental factors also have a role in affecting the expression of symptoms. Environmental factors implicated in the expression of ADHD seem to include prenatal exposure to nicotine and alcohol, which, in turn is associated with low birth weight. In one study, ADHD children were more than twice as likely to have been exposed to cigarettes, and two and a half times more likely to have had prenatal exposure to alcohol than the control group (which had no exposure). Postnatal exposure to family adversity (eg, marital stress, parental psychopathology, single-parent household) also seems to confer increased risk.

PRESENTATION AND DIAGNOSIS

The traditional diagnosis of ADHD involves a triad of symptoms, consisting of developmentally inappropriate levels of inattention, overactivity, and impulsivity. These symptoms must be pervasive, cause functional impairment, and cannot be more appropriately attributable to another disorder.

There are three subtypes of ADHD:
1) Combined type—the most common, affecting between 50% and 70% of ADHD children
2) Inattentive type—affecting between 20% and 30% of ADHD children
3) Hyperactive/impulsive type—accounting for <15% of cases

Examples of inattentive-type ADHD symptoms include:
• Makes careless mistakes
• Difficulty with sustained attention
• Does not seem to listen
• Has difficulty getting and staying organized
• Is easily distracted
• Is forgetful

Examples of hyperactive/impulsive-type ADHD symptoms include:
• Runs or climbs in inappropriate settings
• Fidgets; is restless
• Frequently gets out of seat
• Is often on the go
• Blurts out answers
• Has trouble waiting turn

   Associated features include risk-taking behaviors, low frustration tolerance, moodiness, and mood lability.

   Another way to conceptualize ADHD is to view it as a disorder of executive function, which involves working memory and response inhibition. Executive function is involved in planning, organizing, self-monitoring, affect (or emotion) regulation, etc.

   Deficits in executive function can lead to some of the major problems of ADHD such as impulsivity, acting before thinking, emotional lability, poor organization and lack of planning, minimizing consequences of actions, etc.

COMORBID CONDITIONS

Comorbid conditions—those disorders that can occur with another disorder—are important to identify, since the existence of unidentified comorbidities can often lead to treatment failures.

   Opposition defiant disorder (ODD) is probably the most common comorbid disorder seen with ADHD. Up to 60% of children with ADHD also have symptoms of ODD.

Anxiety disorders are seen in up to one-third of ADHD children. This can be a potential problem with some common medications used to treat ADHD, as one possible side effect of stimulant medications is increased anxiety.

Learning disorders are seen in between 25% and 35% of children diagnosed with ADHD, especially those with primarily inattentive type. Special classroom placement and specialized teaching techniques are most helpful for these children. Unrecognized learning disorders will often lead to treatment failure. If only the inattention is treated, the child with ADHD and a comorbid learning disorder will likely continue to experience academic failure.

Bipolar disorder and ADHD are often seen together, and it is estimated that between 25% and 90% of bipolar children also have ADHD. It must also be noted that there are many overlapping symptoms among the two conditions, making it difficult to distinguish between them. Symptoms of euphoria and decreased need for sleep are seen primarily in bipolar disorder and are helpful in distinguishing it from ADHD.

Major depression can also be seen with ADHD, but depressive symptoms can also be seen secondary to academic failure and peer and family problems common to children with ADHD.

Substance abuse is a common outcome of untreated ADHD during adolescence, as the adolescent with ADHD is often highly impulsive, risk-taking, minimizes consequences of actions, and is often thrill-seeking.

ISSUES UNIQUE TO PEDIATRIC AND ADOLESCENT ADHD

The need to keep a developmental perspective is vital in work with children and adolescents, as the central nervous system develops rapidly during this time. The presentation of many psychiatric disorders during childhood and adolescence may differ from how they present in adults. ADHD is no exception.

In pediatric ADHD, gross motor overactivity is a common feature. Children with ADHD cannot remain seated, are often in constant motion, often run and climb in inappropriate situations, blurt out answers, etc. An adolescent with ADHD may display less gross motor overactivity, but instead more subtle signs of motor activity, such as fidgeting and restlessness. Other features of adolescent ADHD can be increased risk-taking behaviors, increased incidence of drug use, reckless driving, etc. By adulthood, signs of motor overactivity may be hardly visible. Rather, signs of ADHD in an adult may include failure to pay attention to detail, verbal intrusiveness, interpersonal difficulties, reckless driving, poor work performance, impulsivity, etc.

Hepatic function is also different in children and consequently, medications may be metabolized at a faster rate. This can alter dosing strength as well as frequency of dosing.

TREATMENT OF ADHD
Nonpharmacologic Treatment

Although many nonpharmacological treatments of ADHD have been touted as useful, only a handful have documented evidence of true efficacy. Recent conceptual understanding of ADHD as a deficit in self-regulation and response inhibition has led to more effective treatment options. Treatments that address these deficits seem to be most helpful.

One of the mainstays of treatment for ADHD children involves use of behavior therapy. Behavior therapy involves identifying target behaviors and employing consequences for both positive and negative behaviors. Consequences for behaviors—both positive reinforcers as well as negative contingencies (punishments)—are used to shape more age-appropriate behaviors. These techniques can be taught to parents and to teachers in both individual and group settings. Parents use these techniques both at home and in other settings to enforce pro-social behaviors. Teachers and support staff can use behavior therapy to reduce frequency of disruptive behaviors, increase incidence of on-task behaviors, and more. There is abundant evidence that these techniques are very useful for ADHD as well as other disruptive behavior disorders. Behavior management techniques do not generalize to other situations, however, and the behavior improvements do not usually continue after the contingencies are lifted. In this respect, behavior management can be seen as akin to prosthetic devices—useful and effective only when in use. Nonetheless, by reducing disruptive behaviors, behavior therapy can reduce the negative spiral of worsening behavior, academic failure, negative self-view, and instead provide more positive experiences in school and with family that can promote further growth and development.

Since children with ADHD are often more immature than their peers, they tend to get ostracized and teased. In addition, their impulsivity and aggressive behaviors are often seen as annoying. This often leads to unsatisfactory peer interactions, which, in turn, often results in the child ultimately gravitating to other ostracized, acting-out peers. This frequently leads to even more aberrant behaviors. Social skills training attempts to help the child who is hampered by disruptive behaviors to deal more effectively with social situations and eventually have more successful and rewarding contact with peers. Social skills training is often best taught in a group setting, but can also be carried out individually. Skills taught include conflict resolution, controlling anger and impulsivity, and learning how to enter social situations as well as how to make conversation. After mastering these techniques in the group, the ultimate goal is to generalize these social skills to the child's everyday life.

Cognitive behavior therapy (CBT) techniques can also be incorporated into a multimodal treatment plan and can be helpful in guiding the child with ADHD to alter faulty percerptions, better recognize the consequences of their actions, and improve impulse control. Helping the child

CASE STUDY

Kevin was 7 years old when first referred by his school because of aggressive, disruptive, and "out of control" behavior. He is often involved in fights—especially during lunch and recess. He blurts out answers, turns around in his seat, and is frequently out of his seat. At home he is bossy and demanding and needs repeated reminders to do things. He is in constant motion and can only sit when playing video games or watching his favorite wrestling show on TV. His mother reluctantly acknowledged that she sometimes resorts to corporal punishment in an attempt to control Kevin's behavior.

Although on grade level for math, Kevin is 2 years below expected level for reading. Kevin does not like to read and often refuses to do his homework.

Past history is significant for the fact that Kevin was born with positive toxicology for cocaine. He was irritable as an infant and slept poorly. His parents fought often and his father left when Kevin was 2. His mother describes Kevin's father as "just like Kevin—impatient, irritable, and hyper." The father could not keep a job and was often getting into altercations with his supervisors. Additionally, he dropped out of college and began to abuse alcohol and cocaine. The mother's family history is significant for depression and anxiety.

Kevin was evaluated using Conners' teacher and parent behavior rating scales (testing instruments that use observer ratings and self-report ratings to help assess attention-deficit/hyperactivity disorder [ADHD] and evaluate problem behavior in children and adolescents). The scales revealed developmentally significant levels of ADHD symptoms.

Kevin was also referred for educational testing and both dyslexia and an auditory processing problem were discovered. Recommendations were made for medication, special education placement, as well as remediation for reading. His mother was engaged in parent and family counseling and guidance was provided in behavior management techniques as well as education about ADHD. Kevin was started on Adderall. Kevin's hyperactive and inattentive symptoms improved, and with remediation and special academic accommodations, his reading scores slowly improved over the course of the academic year.

to think before acting is an important step in this process. These techniques are often taught to parents and teachers and can be incorporated into a broader treatment strategy that includes behavior management, medication, educational interventions, etc.

Pharmacologic Treatment
The pharmacologic treatment of ADHD is divided into two broad categories: stimulant medications and nonstimulant medications.

Stimulants

The stimulants were the first compounds used to treat the symptoms of ADHD and remain the most effective medication treatments available. There are two different psycho-stimulants: methylphenidate (eg, Ritalin and similar compounds), and amphetamine salts (eg, Adderall and similar compounds). Both work by raising the concentrations of two neurotransmitters critical in the neurophysiology of ADHD: dopamine (DA) and norepinephrine (NE). Many studies seem to indicate that stimulant medications improve both overactive, impulsive behaviors as well as the cognitive symptoms of inattention and distractibility. Increase in focus and attention often leads to improved school performance and corresponding elevation in self-esteem and reduction in depressive symptoms. Reduction in hyperactive/impulsive symptoms yields corresponding improvements in peer relationships and fewer conflicts in family interactions.

These improvements are often seen in a dose-dependent fashion. In each of the two classes of stimulants, there are immediate-release and slow- or extended-release preparations. The slow- or extended-release medications are often preferred, as they allow once-daily dosing and avoid the peaks and troughs often seen in multiple-dose schedules. If one stimulant doesn't work, a different stimulant or a stimulant of the same class utilizing a different delivery system may be more helpful, or cause fewer side effects.

Drugs in the methylphenidate class include Concerta, Daytrana Patch, Metadate CD, Metadate ER, Methylin, Methylin ER, Ritalin, Ritalin LA, Ritalin SR (methylphenidate CII); and Focalin and Focalin XR (dexmethylphenidate HCl CII).

Drugs in the amphetamine class include Adderall and Adderall XR (amphetamine and dextroamphetamine mixture CII); Desoxyn (methamphetamine HCl CII); DextroStat and Dexedrine (dextroamphetamine CII); and Vyvanse (lisdexamfetamine dimesylate CII).

Side effects of the stimulant medications include delayed sleep onset, reduction in appetite, slight elevation in pulse and blood pressure, development or exacerbation of tics, and anxiety. About 10 years ago, reports of several sudden deaths of children who were on Ritalin and clonidine (a nonstimulant sometimes used to reduce impulsivity in ADHD) raised concerns about possible cardiac effects of stimulants. In each case, an underlying cardiac structural defect was found. Since then, there has been no clear causal link between stimulant medications and risk of sudden death. After careful review of the available data, the American Academy of Pediatrics determined that the stimulants were safe and effective for the majority of children with ADHD. However, EKGs are recommended prior to treatment for any child with cardiac symptoms (eg, chest pains, shortness of breath on exertion) or a family history of cardiac disease.

Concerns about possible abuse or the use of stimulant medications by someone for whom they are not prescribed must also be noted. There have also been concerns raised about possible use in childhood leading to later drug abuse. Current evidence clearly indicates that proper treatment of ADHD in childhood leads to lower rates of substance use disorders in adolescence.

The National Institute of Mental Health Multimodal Treatment Study of Childhood ADHD (known as the MTA study) was developed to determine the effectiveness of treatments for ADHD. Children between the ages of 7 and 10 years were divided into four groups: stimulant medication alone; behavior therapy alone; combination stimulant medication treatment and behavior therapy; and community comparison (control group). The data were compiled from six sites in the U.S. and Canada. Treatments were given over a 14-month period. The overall findings revealed that stimulant medication treatment and combined treatment were better than behavior therapy alone and the control group. Stimulant medication treatment alone and combined treatment were roughly comparable, showing the superiority of stimulant medication for the treatment of ADHD.

Nonstimulants

Among the many nonstimulant medications used for ADHD, only Strattera (atomoxetine HCl) is currently approved by the FDA for use in childhood ADHD. All other nonstimulants (as well as the antidepressants and antihypertensives discussed below) are considered off-label for use in ADHD. Strattera is a norepinephrine reuptake inhibitor that increases the presynaptic concentration of norepinephrine. Strattera is found to be effective for the core symptoms of ADHD, but the response is generally less robust than is seen with stimulants. Since elevations in norepinephrine levels may also improve mood as well as symptoms of anxiety, Strattera may be particularly well suited for children and adolescents with ADHD and comorbid depression and anxiety. The therapeutic effects of Strattera last all day, which is not the case with stimulants. This makes Strattera potentially useful for children whose symptoms continue to cause problems into the evening hours.

Antidepressants

Several different antidepressants have been found useful to treat symptoms of ADHD. All these drugs are considered off-label. The first compounds used were the tricyclic antidepressants such as Tofranil (imipramine HCl), Norpramin (desipramine HCl), and Pamelor (nortriptyline HCl). These compounds elevate norepinephrine. They may be particularly well-suited for children with comorbid depression, anxiety, and tic disorder. Their side effect profiles, and the potential risk of cardiac conduction delays (eg, bundle branch block, which can be fatal), has limited their use.

Wellbutrin (buproprion HCl) is a unique antidepressant that has dual-receptor site action, elevating both norepinephrine and dopamine. This profile would suggest benefit for the core symptoms of ADHD, and some studies have indicated usefulness for comorbid depression, substance use disorder, and ADHD.

Antihypertensives

Catapres (clonidine HCl) and Tenex (guanfacine HCl) have been used off-label in combination with stimulant medications to help reduce aggression and impulsivity. Catapres has also been used to help promote sleep when insomnia is a side effect of stimulant treatment. Blood pressure must be monitored and rebound hypertension can occur with abrupt discontinuation of Catapres. Depression can also occur.

Please see Section 3 for more information on psychotropic drugs.

SUMMARY

ADHD is one of the most common disorders in childhood. Its symptoms may change over time, but signs of the disorder often persist into adolescence and adulthood. There is a strong genetic component, but environmental factors also affect the clinical expression. ADHD affects many important aspects of a child's life—social, academic, family—and if left untreated, can lead to serious consequences, such as academic failure, impaired peer interactions, disruption of family interactions, depression, externalizing behaviors, substance use disorders, as well as possible criminal involvement. Effective treatments include behavior therapy, various academic accommodations, special classroom placement, as well as medication. Proper treatment often needs to continue through the years and can often prevent the more ominous outcomes commonly seen in untreated individuals.

BIPOLAR DISORDER

OVERVIEW

Until relatively recently, pediatric bipolar disorder was felt to be exceedingly rare. Over the last 30 years, however, advances and refinements in the diagnosis of adult bipolar disorder, the awareness of subtypes of the disorder as well as conceptualization of mood-spectrum phenomena have led to a rapidly expanding body of research into mood disorders in children and adolescents. Longitudinal, retrospective, and epidemiological studies have provided compelling evidence of the existence of prepubertal bipolar disorder. Although most experts agree about the presence of pediatric bipolar disorder, there remains much controversy over the inclusion criteria for diagnosis (strict adherence to *DSM-IV-TR* criteria with minor modifications for age and developmental level vs implementation of much broader inclusion criteria).

Pediatric bipolar disorder continues to be misdiagnosed and improperly treated. Many bipolar children do not receive proper diagnosis and appropriate treatment until years after the emergence of their first mood symptoms. This unnecessary delay can prove extremely detrimental in terms of severe disruption in family, academic, and social functioning. There is growing evidence that it can also render the course of illness more severe and resistant to standard treatments. Untreated or improperly treated bipolar disorder in youth can also lead to alarmingly high rates of both attempted and completed suicides. In addition, very early-onset depression is often the initial presentation of bipolar disorder. If these children are mistakenly diagnosed with major depression and treated with an antidepressant, there is a very high risk of precipitating a manic episode. For this reason, the level of suspicion for bipolar disorder must be very high in any child or adolescent who initially presents with symptoms of major depression, especially if there is a strong family history of mood disorder.

Rates of externalizing disorders such as ADHD and conduct disorder as well as substance abuse disorders are also very high in bipolar youth and these comorbidities can cause more serious impairment and disability.

The clinical picture of pediatric bipolar disorder, especially in younger children, is often very different than the clearly delineated mood episodes seen in older adolescents and adults. Rapid cycling (at least four mood episodes per year), ultra-rapid cycling (more than four but less than 365 cycles per year), and ultra-ultra-rapid cycling (more than 365 cycles/mood episodes per year, often multiple cycles per day) is often the rule and there is sometimes no clear change from baseline as the baseline is labile moods and chronic mixed-mood states (depressed and manic/hypomanic symptoms occurring together). Psychotic symptoms are also more common in pediatric and adolescent bipolar disorder. There is also some evidence that early-onset bipolar disorder may have a more chronic course and be less responsive to standard treatments.

Estimates of bipolar disorder in the general population are given as approximately 1%. Studies of bipolar children have cited similar estimates. When broader mood spectrum criteria are used, estimates of between 4% and 13% are seen.

Numerous studies have indicated a genetic basis of pediatric bipolar disorder and it is common to find evidence of multigenerational mood disorder in the families of bipolar children. Risk of a child developing bipolar disorder can be as high as 30% when one parent is bipolar. This risk goes up to between 50% and 75% when both parents are diagnosed.

PREVALENCE AND RISK FACTORS

The rate of newly diagnosed cases of pediatric bipolar disorder has been growing rapidly over the past 10 years. One study showed the number of pediatric admissions for bipolar disorder increased by a factor of six over the period from 1996 to 2004. Some outpatient studies have shown an even larger explosion in initial diagnosis of early-onset bipolar disorder.

Prevalence rates for full-symptom bipolar disorder in children and adolescents have been estimated to be approximately 1%. Since many children with bipolar disorder—especially prepubertal bipolar disorder—have atypical presentations and do not meet full *DSM-IV-TR* criteria (thus, they might be diagnosed with bipolar, NOS; see page 22), the 1% prevalence rate quoted above does not take these children into account. When the atypical, mood spectrum presentations are counted, prevalence rates are estimated to be between 4% to as high as 13%.

Retrospective studies of adult bipolar patients have shown that approximately 20% of these bipolar adults had onset of first symptoms prior to age 19.

Genetic factors play an important role in the development of bipolar disorder. Estimates of the heritability of bipolar disorder have been cited as being between 40% and 70%. The concordance rate for monozygotic (identical) twins has been given as 67%.

A meta-analysis of bipolar adults found that almost half of the off-spring of bipolar adults met criteria for at least one psychiatric illness—especially a mood disorder such as major depression or bipolar disorder. The risk of a child developing bipolar disorder has been estimated to be up to 27% if one parent is bipolar, and up to 70% if both parents have bipolar disorder. These alarmingly high heritability rates underscore the vital importance of screening the children of parents who are diagnosed with bipolar disorder.

Neuroimaging studies have suggested that part of the genetic impact in bipolar disorder may come from inherited differences in vital brain circuits that mediate affect regulation. Abnormalities in these prefrontal-cortical limbic circuits are believed to be central to the neuropathology of mood disorders.

Genetic factors alone, however, do not account for the development of bipolar disorder. As with other disorders that have a strong genetic component, it is the genetic vulnerability interacting with environmental stressors that result in the expression of illness. Postulated environmental factors include prenatal and perinatal insults (maternal infections, difficult delivery, etc.), as well as stressful and chaotic family interactions. Inherited traits such as emotional lability and susceptibility to stress are core features of bipolar disorder. When these traits are combined with the turbulent environment commonly encountered in families with bipolar parents, a toxic outcome is often the result.

Environmental factors can also have a big impact on treatment outcome. One study found that bipolar children living with intact biological families are two times more likely to recover from a mood episode than children who live in less ideal circumstances.

PRESENTATION AND DIAGNOSIS

The hallmark feature of bipolar disorder is a manic episode (for bipolar I) or a hypomanic episode (for bipolar II). A manic episode is described as the following:

- A distinct period of persistently and abnormally elevated (elated) and/or irritable mood. This mood state must be a significant change from the child's usual mood and must last for at least 1 week (or of any duration if hospitalization is required).

- During the mood episode, the child must show at least three of the following (four if only irritability is present):
  - Grandiosity or inflated sense of self
  - Decreased need for sleep
  - Racing thoughts/flight of ideas
  - Pressured speech
  - Hypersexuality
  - Increase in goal-directed activity
  - Involvement in reckless, daredevil acts
  - Distractibility

The mood episode must cause marked disturbance in normal functioning; not be part of a mixed manic episode; and not be due to the effects of drugs, medication, or another medical condition.

A mixed episode is a mood state characterized by co-occurrence of both mania and major depression lasting at least 1 week. A hypomanic episode is similar to a manic episode except for the severity of symptoms and duration of the episode. Although symptoms of a hypomanic episode represent a change from baseline functioning, the symptoms do not cause serious impairment, there is no need for hospitalization, and psychotic symptoms are not present.

The main subtypes of bipolar disorder are:

• *Bipolar I Disorder*—characterized by at least one manic episode or a mixed episode.

• *Bipolar II Disorder*—characterized by at least one episode of major depression and hypomania. No manic or mixed episodes can be present.

• *Cyclothymic Disorder*—*DSM-IV-TR* reduces the duration criteria for child and adolescent cyclothymia to a period of a year or more (2 years for an adult) of hypomanic and depressive symptoms that do not meet full criteria for bipolar I or II, but the symptoms nevertheless cause significant impairment in functioning.

• *Bipolar Disorder Not Otherwise Specified (NOS)*—includes mood disorders with features of bipolar disorder that do not meet criteria for any specific bipolar disorder due to not meeting minimum duration criteria, not meeting minimum number of required symptoms, or due to presence of other atypical features. Prepubertal bipolar disorder often falls into this category.

Some of the controversy regarding bipolar disorder in youth, particularly prepubertal (so-called early-onset) bipolar disorder, is due to lack of agreement regarding the degree of adherence to *DSM-IV-TR* adult criteria for bipolar disorder. Although some have suggested that the spectrum of mood disorders in children can include extreme irritability and unrelenting rage episodes without elated mood, grandiosity, or decreased need for sleep, others have urged a more conservative approach. In addition, many experts in the field of pediatric bipolar disorder have pointed out that some of the symptoms of bipolar disorder in children are not mania-specific, that is, they are also present in a wide variety of other disorders commonly seen in children. These nonspecific symptoms include irritability, rapid speech, distractibility, and increased energy. Irritability can be seen in pediatric depression as well as oppositional defiant disorder. All four symptoms are a common feature of ADHD. To further complicate the clinical picture, ADHD is very often comorbid with prepubertal bipolar disorder and estimates suggest that up to 90% of bipolar children also meet criteria for ADHD.

In an ongoing study of bipolar children at the National Institute of Mental Health (NIMH) by Dr. Barbara Geller and colleagues, four key symptoms were found to best differentiate bipolar children from non-bipolar children with ADHD: elated mood, grandiosity, racing thoughts, and decreased need for sleep. Other symptoms—hypersexuality, uncharacteristic silliness, dangerous daredevil behaviors, unusually uninhibited social behavior—only partially distinguish bipolar children from non-bipolar ADHD children.

What was also revealed in this study and corroborated by many who regularly work with prepubertal bipolar children is the fact that many of these children show an atypical clinical course. Rather than discrete mood episodes, many early-onset bipolar children demonstrate continuously shifting moods several times per day as well as mixed-mood states. These rapidly shifting moods often alternate from depressed to manic to irritable. One often sees more than one mood state simultaneously. This atypical clinical course and presentation is what seems to characterize early-onset bipolar disorder. Psychotic symptoms and suicidality are also seen frequently in pediatric bipolar disorder.

Older children and adolescents generally present with a more classical presentation of discrete mood episodes more closely akin to that seen in adults, although atypical presentations are also seen.

COMORBID CONDITIONS

ADHD is one of the most common comorbidities in pediatric bipolar disorder. Up to 90% of bipolar children may also meet *DSM-IV-TR* criteria for ADHD. As stated previously, the two disorders share a number of symptoms, including overactivity, increased energy, distractibility, irritability, and rapid speech. After careful evaluation of available data using validated rating scales that reliably discriminate between the two disorders, Biederman and colleagues concluded that despite symptom overlap, bipolar disorder and ADHD are often comorbid but remain distinct clinical entities.

Oppositional defiant disorder is also often seen in pediatric bipolar disorder as are other externalizing disorders.

Rates of substance abuse disorders are also very high in bipolar youth. A number of symptoms of bipolar disorder—impulsivity, involvement in risk-taking behaviors, impaired judgment, as well as "self-medicating" to intensify and prolong the "high" of mania—might also lead to much higher abuse of substances in bipolar youth. One study found that comorbid conduct disorder led to the highest rates of substance abuse in adolescents with bipolar disorder. An NIMH study concluded that bipolar disorder carried the highest risk of substance abuse disorder of any Axis I disorder.

Since continued substance abuse can lead to worsening mood symptoms, rapid cycling, intensification of depressed or manic mood states, noncompliance with drug treatment as well as interference with the therapeutic effect of medications, every effort must be made to concurrently treat both the mood disorder as well as the substance abuse disorder. Certain treatment failure will result if this is not done.

Other common co-occurring disorders seen in bipolar youth include obsessive-compulsive disorder, panic disorder, and other anxiety disorders. It is often because of these anxiety disorders that bipolar adolescents self-medicate with alcohol, benzodiazepines, marijuana, etc.

ISSUES UNIQUE TO PEDIATRIC AND ADOLESCENT BIPOLAR DISORDER

Although adolescents with bipolar disorder can present with symptoms and a clinical course that are typically seen in uncomplicated adult bipolar disorder (discrete mood episodes with full criteria being met for duration and number of symptoms, relatively good response to standard treatments, etc.), early-onset bipolar disorder is more likely to present with atypical features. Mixed-mood states, rapid cycling or even continuous cycling, no apparent symptom-free periods, and psychotic symptoms are just some of the atypical features that distinguish prepubertal bipolar disorder from adult bipolar disorder. Because of these atypical features, bipolar children are often diagnosed with either bipolar disorder NOS or bipolar II disorder. Longitudinal studies have shown that the clinical course of bipolar disorder in children is often more chronic, shows frequent relapses, and is less responsive to standard treatments. In this respect it resembles the more complicated presentations of adult bipolar disorder.

Developmental issues also alter the way various bipolar symptoms can be expressed. One example might be the fact that children do not generally have access to credit cards so they will not have the opportunity to accumulate mounting debt the way a bipolar adolescent or adult can. Similarly, they cannot enter into a series of failed marriages or run several businesses into the ground. Grandiosity in a bipolar child might be expressed by the child stopping a class and insisting that she can teach better than the teacher. Another example is a child who steals from a toy store and becomes furious when caught, screaming that he is the owner of the store and demands that the security guard who is restraining him be arrested.

Whether early-onset bipolar disorder is the same disorder seen in adults awaits the results of ongoing longitudinal studies.

TREATMENT OF BIPOLAR DISORDER
Nonpharmacologic Treatment

It is important to note that the issue of pharmacologic vs nonpharmacologic treatment in bipolar disorder is not an either-or proposition. Both are vital to the success of managing the symptoms of bipolar disorder and to preventing the more serious consequences of inadequate treatment.

We need to underline the importance of psychotherapy as an integral part of an overall treatment strategy that includes medication, individual and family therapy, school intervention, as well as other possible ancillary treatments (eg, treatment of comorbid substance abuse, learning disorders, ADHD, conduct disorder, etc.).

Although research into effective nonpharmacologic treatments is ongoing, current evidence seems to support the usefulness of a number of nonsomatic treatments for bipolar youth.

As in depression, the use of cognitive behavior therapy (CBT) techniques for bipolar children has growing support. These techniques can be taught in group settings with multiple families taking part, or in individual family therapy sessions. They can also be taught to the child in individual sessions along with collateral parent sessions and/or family meetings. It is of vital importance to include parents in the treatment, as the symptoms of the bipolar child have huge impact on family functioning and can affect all family members.

The general goals of treatment are to provide education to both the child and parents about bipolar disorder, to help the child and parents better manage symptoms of the disorder, to improve the child's coping skills, and to improve the child's relationships.

Education about bipolar disorder is an important foundation upon which to build the other treatment layers. With more knowledge, parents are less likely to blame the child for symptoms of the illness and are better prepared for the hard work of properly managing a bipolar child.

As in the CBT treatment protocol for OCD, the child with bipolar disorder is given a "toolbox" that is used to help the child better cope with symptoms, emotions, and impulses. The child is encouraged to come up with various ways he or she can deal with stressful situations or emotions. Techniques such as personal time-out, relaxation breathing, getting a snack, spending time with a pet, punching a pillow or soft doll, etc., are used. The child is also asked to externalize the illness—to see bipolar disorder as the problem and not to blame or demonize himself.

Cognitive distortions are also identified as a means of exploring the ways the child may misunderstand the intent of others and thereby cause undue conflict and anger.

Identifying emotions, being mindful of mood states, and understanding triggers that are likely to set off an episode are just some of the methods employed to help the child become more aware of internal and external factors that can affect mood and behavior.

CASE STUDY

Adam was diagnosed with ADHD when he was 5 years old. According to his mother, he had always been "a bundle of energy" and was often extremely active and could never sit still. He would run into the street, jump off furniture from dangerous heights, and fearlessly ride his bicycle heedless of obstacles or pedestrians. He was treated with Adderall with an ensuing reduction in overactive behaviors. Adam seemed to do well for a few years.

By the time he was 10, Adam began to require less and less sleep and would be up until late at night and wake up by 5 a.m. His mother sometimes found Adam building elaborate towers with his Lego blocks at 3 in the morning. Despite his lack of sleep, Adam was full of boundless energy during the day. After a week or so, he might "crash" and sleep for 14 hours. Adam's moods began to change during this time. Although he had always been a "sweet and affectionate" child, he was beginning to have sudden angry outbursts for no apparent reason. At other times, he would joke and laugh uproariously and his sense of humor was infectious. Adam was also becoming uncharacteristically challenging with his otherwise calm and patient father. Adam would proclaim with firm conviction that his father could not boss him because he was a "world-famous architect." His mother also discovered during this time that Adam had been going to various pornography websites and had taken the mother's credit card. Family history was positive for major depression in the maternal grandmother as well as bipolar disorder in a maternal female cousin. The cousin was on lithium and Seroquel and was reportedly stable on this combination.

Adam was seen during this time for an evaluation. He presented as a highly bright and articulate boy with a winning smile and quick wit. He engaged the clinician in a discussion of the books on the shelf and how he could be a psychiatrist himself. He acknowledged violent nightmares and his numerous fears of harm coming to his family. He also admitted that in the past he had been hearing a voice telling him to hurt himself, although he was able to resist this. He was no longer hearing the voice but had been frightened by it. He denied any acute suicidal plan or intent. It was not felt that Adam required acute hospi-

CASE STUDY *(Continued)*

talization, but his parents were informed about the nature of his past auditory hallucinations and were provided with instructions in the case of an emergency.

Adam was diagnosed with bipolar disorder NOS and was started on lithium since there was a family history of positive response. Blood work was obtained, including a CBC (complete blood count), T_3, T_4, TSH (thyroid function), BUN and creatinine (kidney function), electrolytes, fasting blood glucose, lead level, and lipids (cholesterol, triglycerides, etc.).

Adam's parents were provided with educational material about bipolar disorder as well as being engaged in parent sessions aimed at helping them with behavior management techniques, providing them with guidance in reducing conflicts, and with problem-solving skills.

Special accommodations were made at school and Adam was allowed extra time to hand in work as well as reduced course load. This was to reduce the stress that had been put upon Adam at his academically advanced, achievement-oriented private school.

Adam started individual counseling sessions aimed at educating him about his mood disorder, and he was also given help with stress-reduction techniques. He was also instructed to monitor the changing course of his moods with a mood chart, which he did with great care and detail. He was fascinated to learn about the neurobiological basis of his mood symptoms and took pride in learning whatever he could about bipolar disorder, about his family history, and about medications. By this means, he was able to feel in control of his previous out-of-control moods and behaviors.

Within 2 weeks the dose of lithium was titrated to a therapeutic level. After 4 weeks, Adam's moods began to stabilize but he reported return of vague, mumbling auditory hallucinations. Low-dose Abilify was added and within 1 week auditory hallucinations abated. Adam began to note the change in his moods as demonstrated by his mood charts and his parents observed a less chaotic course at home. Although there remained some periods of irritability and anxiety, both Adam and his parents felt a sense of calm that they had not experienced since the first appearance of Adam's mood symptoms a year earlier.

Problem-solving is also encouraged as a means of helping the child to stop, think, and plan before acting impulsively.

Further education about medications and side effects as well as the necessity of full compliance with medications is another important part of the discussion with both the family and the child. Emphasis on relapse prevention and understanding the factors that affect relapse—noncompliance with medication, lack of adequate sleep, undue stress, etc.—should be part of the discussion.

The use of mood charts can help a child recognize varying mood states as well as help the clinician and parents gauge response to treatment.

Interpersonal psychotherapy is also used and tailored to the developmental stage of the child. Generally, a more eclectic approach to psychotherapy is used with bipolar children and incorporates some of the techniques itemized above.

Since the symptoms of bipolar disorder rarely leave the educational realm unscathed, communication with school personnel and developing a plan to deal with behavior problems and academic issues is another component of the nonpharmacologic treatment plan.

Pharmacologic Treatment

The use of medication is an essential component of proper treatment of bipolar disorder in children and adolescents. Growing awareness that defects in critical brain pathways that regulate mood may form the putative basis of symptom formation in bipolar disorder helps our understanding of the central role that pharmacologic intervention can play. Furthermore, concern over the presumed toxic effects unleashed on brain cells by uncontrolled mood episodes gives added urgency to the need to effectively treat bipolar disorder in the young.

Most of the studies of medications for bipolar disorder come from the adult literature and only a handful of the medications used have FDA approval for use in children. Lithium, Abilify (aripiprazole), and Seroquel (quetiapine fumarate) have FDA approval for use in adolescent bipolar disorder.

Mood-Stabilizing Agents

Lithium has been used for decades in the treatment of bipolar disorder and it is still considered the gold standard. There is a very strong body of evidence showing the efficacy of lithium to treat bipolar disorder and it is FDA approved for adults in the treatment of acute mania, the depressed phase of bipolar illness, as well as for maintenance treatment. It is often noted that lithium is best-suited to treat uncomplicated, non-rapid-cycling bipolar disorder with a mood sequence of mania-depression-euthymia, but it can be helpful in some patients with mixed states and with more complicated presentations as well. Lithium also seems to possess antisuicidal as well as antidepressant properties.

Reports of the use of lithium in the pediatric population go back decades and an often-cited review article by Youngerman and Canino written 30 years ago documents this. There are numerous reports of lithium's effectiveness for treating bipolar illness in children and adolescents as well as treating manic-like symptoms in children with traumatic brain injuries and aggressive behaviors.

In depressed children with a family history positive for bipolar disorder, some experts have suggested that lithium be used instead of an antidepressant to prevent possible conversion to mania. This once again underlines the importance of considering bipolar illness in any child who presents with early-onset depression.

Although lithium has shown usefulness in treating bipolar disorder in the young, some have indicated that early-onset bipolar disorder may be less responsive to lithium than to other agents.

Lithium is generally well tolerated in children and adolescents but has a narrow therapeutic window. Doses below the window yield less efficacy and more risk of frequent relapses; above the window, side effects can become intolerable and serious neurotoxicity, renal damage, alterations in cardiac conduction, and even death are possible. Certain medications as well as state of hydration can also affect serum lithium concentrations, hence the patient's lithium levels need to be monitored. Because of this, families need to be aware of signs of toxicity.

Although generally safe in long-term use, studies of long-term use in children are needed. Lithium can cause hypothyroidism, which, if detected, must be treated.

Valproate (valproic acid) is the breakdown product of Depakote (sodium divalproex). It is approved for use in acute bipolar mania and maintenance treatment of adults with bipolar disorder. It has been used for many years in children and adolescents as an FDA-approved agent for seizure disorder, but is considered off-label for pediatric bipolar disorder. It has demonstrated clear efficacy in adolescent bipolar disorder and response rates of up to 50% in acute adolescent bipolar mania have been reported.

Data on use in children are more limited, but there is some evidence of effectiveness in this age group as well. Patients with either rapid cycling or with mixed/dysphoric mania seem to respond better to Depakote than to lithium. There have been rare instances of hepatotoxicity as well as blood count changes. For this reason, periodic blood monitoring must be performed when this drug is used.

There have been reports of polycystic ovary disease in some girls and young women who were treated with Depakote for seizure disorder. Some have suggested that this may be secondary to Depakote's tendency to cause weight gain and obesity, which, in turn, can result in elevated testosterone levels. Studies are needed to determine if girls and young women with bipolar disorder are also at risk.

Tegretol (carbamazepine) is approved for the treatment of acute mania in adults and has been used for years as an anticonvulsant. It has been prescribed in children and adolescents for various behavioral problems and aggression. Tegretol is reportedly more effective in treating mixed states as well as rapid cycling. In rare instances, Tegretol can cause hepatotoxicity as well as serious blood disorders. Tegretol induces both its own metabolism as well as the metabolism of other medications.

Trileptal (oxcarbazepine) is related structurally to Tegretol but has fewer side effects, has many fewer drug-drug interactions, and does not appear to cause the problems with liver function or blood count changes that Tegretol does. It is an anticonvulsant that does not have FDA-approval for bipolar disorder, but there is anecdotal evidence of its efficacy in treating the condition. Serum sodium levels must be monitored.

Lamictal (lamotrigine) is another anticonvulsant that has FDA-approval for treating bipolar depression in adults. It has also shown some effectiveness in treating mixed episodes and rapid cycling in adult bipolar disorder. Efficacy in children and adolescents has not been clearly established and will await further study. In very rare instances, Lamictal causes a potentially fatal autoimmune reaction, especially in the very young or if dosed too rapidly.

Antipsychotic/Mood-Stabilizing Agents

In addition to their proven antipsychotic effects, many of the antipsychotic medications have shown mood-stabilizing properties as well. A number of them have FDA approval for use in bipolar disorder in adults. The first to receive approval for this use was Thorazine (chlorpromazine), although other typical antipsychotic medications have also been used. Their burdensome side effects profile (tardive dyskinesia, dystonic reactions, akathisia, etc.) however, limit their use.

The atypical antipsychotic agents have added mightily to the psychopharmacology armamentarium. They have been found useful in a number of disorders beyond their antipsychotic effects and they all possess broad-spectrum properties. All of them have since been FDA-approved for use in adult bipolar disorder, and two of them have approval for use in battling bipolar depression.

Their side effects profile is more favorable compared with the older antipsychotic agents, but potential problems with weight gain (for all but two), potential for tardive dyskinesia (although the risk is lower than with typical antipsychotics), EKG changes, and metabolic abnormalities including diabetes and elevation of lipids (for all but two) must still be weighed against potential beneficial effects. Since these medications often must be administered chronically, weight gain and potential of developing glucose intolerance, diabetes, and hyperlipidemia can be particularly worrisome in children and adolescents.

Clozaril (clozapine) was the first atypical antipsychotic agent. Some studies have found it to possess antimanic effects. Potential for significant weight gain as well as risk of potentially fatal, precipitous drop in white blood cell count render this agent to second-tier status for pediatric bipolar disorder. EKG changes and arrhythmias have also been reported (QTc prolongation).

Zyprexa (olanzapine) has FDA approval for the treatment of acute mania and maintenance treatment of bipolar disorder in adults. When combined with Prozac (fluoxetine), it is FDA approved for bipolar depression as well. A number of case reports have shown efficacy for Zyprexa in bipolar adolescents. A small open-label study reported improvement in acute manic symptoms in three prepubertal children when Zyprexa was added to their ongoing mood stabilizer.

High incidence of significant weight gain, sedation, and metabolic changes (including development of diabetes) has limited use of Zyprexa in the young.

Risperdal (risperidone) is approved for the acute phase of bipolar disorder in adults. One retrospective study reviewing charts of a small group of outpatient children diagnosed with bipolar disorder and treated with Risperdal showed significant reduction in symptoms of mania, psychosis, and aggression. Limiting side effects include moderate weight gain, sedation, and risk of galactorrhea (development of breast milk secondary to elevation in serum prolactin levels).

Seroquel (quetiapine fumarate) has been FDA approved for the acute manic, depressed, and maintenance phases of bipolar disorder in adults. A number of case reports have also noted efficacy for Seroquel in adolescent and prepubertal bipolar disorder and onset of action is relatively rapid. Sedation and weight gain are potential problems.

Geodon (ziprasidone HCl) is FDA approved for acute mania in adults. There are some reports of its potential usefulness in child and adolescent bipolar disorder. In adults it has shown little evidence of causing weight gain or metabolic syndrome and this makes it a particularly attractive agent in treating patients with family history of diabetes, obesity, or dyslipidemia. Arrhythmias and potential for EKG changes (QTc prolongation) require that patients with family history of cardiac abnormalities obtain baseline and post-treatment EKGs.

Abilify (aripiprazole) is approved for treatment of acute bipolar mania in adults. As with most of the atypical antipsychotics, placebo-controlled studies in children and adolescents are needed to determine efficacy in this population. Despite the lack of available data, there is some evidence that Abilify may be helpful for pediatric bipolar disorder. Weight gain appears to be less of a problem with Abilify, although akathesia (motor restlessness) and insomnia are potential problems.

Although monotherapy is sometimes adequate to treat bipolar disorder, combination therapy is often required to treat the full spectrum of symptoms often encountered in children and adolescents with bipolar disorder. A mood stabilizer must be the foundation of the medication treatment. The goal is to stabilize the mood first. If residual symptoms persist after titrating to maximum dose, adding another mood stabilizing medication is often required. Further studies are required to aid in treatment choices in pediatric bipolar illness.

Even after combining two or even three different mood stabilizers, residual depression is often a problem. If left untreated, the depression can continue to cause significant morbidity. Antidepressants—selective serotonin reuptake inhibitors, tricyclic antidepressants, MAO inhibitors, etc. (see Section 3 for specific information on these agents)—are sometimes used for the depressed phase of bipolar disorder in adults. Many experts urge caution when prescribing an antidepressant in bipolar disorder, even when combined with a mood-stabilizing agent. The reason is the risk of causing manic-induction or precipitating rapid cycling, both of which might render the illness less responsive to standard treatments. This is even more imperative in children and adolescents who may be more sensitive to the destabilizing effects of the antidepressants and who are more prone to illness characterized by rapid or continuous cycling. I believe that the emergence of suicidal ideation in at least some children and adolescents treated with antidepressants might have been due to induction of dysphoric/mixed mania in an undiagnosed bipolar child or adolescent—a very high risk factor for suicide in the young.

Lamictal, Seroquel, and the Zyprexa/Prozac combination have FDA approval for bipolar depression in adults and carry little to no risk of inducing mania. Although not approved for use in pediatric bipolar disorder, these agents might be safer choices to treat residual bipolar depression in this age group.

If symptoms of ADHD are still evident after adequately controlling mood symptoms in a bipolar child with comorbid ADHD, careful addition of stimulant medication can be used. Although there have been reports of manic-induction with stimulants, others have reported good control of symptoms of both bipolar disorder and ADHD without destabilization of mood.

SUMMARY

Bipolar disorder in youth can be a devastating illness that causes major disruptions in all aspects of a child's life. Rapidly shifting moods, explosive rage episodes, extreme overactivity and impulsivity, psychotic symptoms with few if any periods of "normal" can wreak havoc on both child and family. Ultra-rapid cycling and mixed mood states with no euthymic periods are what often characterize prepubertal bipolar disorder. Although early-onset bipolar disorder is more widely recognized, many children still go untreated or improperly treated. Early-onset depression can sometimes be the first sign of childhood bipolar disorder and depression in the young should not be treated automatically as unipolar depression.

Untreated or improperly treated bipolar disorder in youth can lead to high rates of substance abuse, dangerously impulsive behaviors, academic failure, and alarmingly high rates of attempted and completed suicide.

Twin studies and family studies have established a clear genetic basis for the disorder. Environmental factors can have a large impact on the outcome of treatment as well. A multimodal treatment approach is essential. At minimum, medication, psychotherapy, and parent education will be required. Frequently, school interventions, special accommodations, family therapy, and even hospitalization will be needed.

Many medications have been found helpful for pediatric bipolar disorder, but continued research is necessary to firmly establish evidence-based treatment protocols in this age group. Longitudinal studies are also needed to determine the long-term outcome of early-onset bipolar disorder.

DEPRESSION

OVERVIEW

Pediatric and adolescent depression remains a serious public health challenge. Once thought to be rare, depression is seen in 2% of children and 4% to 8% of adolescents. By the end of adolescence, lifetime prevalence rates approach 20%.

Rates of suicide are alarmingly high in this age group, and Major Depressive Disorder (MDD) is a leading cause of suicide during adolescence. Adults who were depressed as adolescents have a fivefold risk of suicide. Left untreated, child and adolescent depression can be a deadly illness. This is all the more concerning given the recent downward trend in prescribing medication to depressed youths following FDA warnings about potential for suicidal ideation with SSRIs. Suicide rates had actually decreased during the period of more widespread use of antidepressant medication in children and adolescents, and seem to have risen during this recent period of reduced use.

During the prepubertal period, an equal number of boys and girls are affected by depression. By adolescence, the risk of depression is up to three times higher in girls. The reason for this dramatic increased risk in girls is believed to be due to a number of factors, including hormonal (increase in both estradiol and testosterone), an increase in anxiety symptoms in girls, as well as peer group pressure that girls seem to experience.

Pediatric depression can increase the risk for a number of other negative outcomes such as tobacco, drug, and alcohol abuse; personality disorders; conduct disorders; interpersonal difficulties; as well as academic and career underachievement.

PREVALENCE AND RISK FACTORS

Prevalence rates for pediatric and adolescent depression are reported to be up to 8.3%. Risk factors for depression in childhood include parental substance abuse, parental marital problems, family stress, and sexual abuse. Stressful life events in general may interact with genetic vulnerability via effects on increased stress hormone secretion, which, in turn, can have a cascade of negative effects on physical and mental health.

Other risk factors for depression in the young include tobacco use, drug and alcohol use, and lack of adequate adult supervision.

There seems to be a strong genetic component to MDD, and depression is often inherited together with anxiety disorder. Genetic predisposition and stressful life events seem to confer a high risk of early-onset depression. Parental depression is a very high risk factor for pediatric depression—both via genetic and environmental influences. The cognitive distortions frequently seen in child and adolescent depression are often the result of modeling of parental cognitive distortions.

Child abuse and neglect increase the risk of depression, as well as disruptive behaviors, PTSD, substance use disorders (SUD), and suicide.

As in adult MDD, depression in children and adolescents is recurrent, chronic, and often continues into adulthood.

PRESENTATION AND DIAGNOSIS

DSM-IV-TR makes little distinction between depression in adults and depression in children, except to note that irritable mood can be used in place of depressed mood to make the diagnosis of depression in children. Criteria for depression include:
• depressed mood
• decreased interest or pleasure in most activities
• decreased or increased appetite
• insomnia or hypersomnia
• psychomotor agitation or retardation
• loss of energy; feelings of guilt and worthlessness
• decreased ability to think or concentrate
• recurrent thoughts of death

Modifications need to be made when attempting to apply these criteria to children. For one, the symptoms do not need to be present and persistent for a full two weeks as they do in adults. Since children do not necessarily verbalize feelings, a depressed child may not directly voice feelings of worthlessness, guilt, or suicidal thoughts. Much of children's communication is via play—especially younger children. In order to detect these symptoms, close attention must be paid to a young child's play. Prominent and recurring themes in play can indicate the presence of suicidal and self-destructive thoughts as well as feelings of depression.

Children may also be more likely to display nonspecific symptoms of depression, such as increased acting out behaviors, aggression, and violent play. Decreased concentration and motivation, disturbed sleep, and low energy can affect academic performance and further increase depression. Somatic symptoms (eg, headaches, stomachaches, fatigue, lightheadedness, dizziness, etc., that are not attributable to an organic cause) are also common in pediatric depression and complaints of headaches, stomachaches are often heard in depressed children.

Depression in a child can often be the first sign of an underlying bipolar process. It is estimated that between 20% and 40% of children who are initially diagnosed with MDD will go on to develop bipolar disorder. This is especially important since medications used to treat MDD can make bipolar disorder worse and sometimes lead to a more virulent form of manic depressive illness. Strong family history of bipolar disorder in first-degree relatives or a multigenerational history of any mood disorder can increase the probability of bipolar disorder. Atypical depressive symptoms (increased sleep, increased appetite, extreme lethargy) can sometimes also increase the likelihood of a bipolar process. It should be clear that a level of suspicion for bipolar disorder should always be maintained when diagnosing pediatric depression.

MDD is a chronic and recurring disorder. Pediatric depressive episodes last, on average, eight months. The risk of recurrence is between 20% and 60% up to two years after remission. This number rises to 70% after five years.

COMORBID CONDITIONS

One of the most common comorbid disorders in pediatric depression is anxiety. As previously stated, there appear to be shared genetic risk factors for anxiety and depression, and early-onset anxiety in childhood often precedes pediatric depression.

ADHD is another disorder often occurring with depression, and is seen more often in preschool children with depression. In one study, 42% of preschool children also had symptoms of ADHD; 62% had Oppositional Defiant Disorder (ODD); and 41% had all three.

Undiagnosed and untreated comorbid disorders are often the cause for partial response or lack of response to standard treatment. Undiagnosed ADHD in a depressed child can lead to continued depression, as untreated ADHD often results in poor school performance, peer difficulties, family discord, and low self-esteem.

SUD can exacerbate comorbid depression as well as create symptoms that mimic those of MDD (ie, alcohol, benzodiazepines, barbiturates, opioids). Nicotine/tobacco use is often linked to onset of depression as animal studies have demonstrated that nicotine interferes with serotonin circuits in the brain. Serotonin neurotransmission is involved in mood regulation.

The externalizing disorders ODD and CD (conduct disorder) are often seen as comorbidities in depressed children.

ISSUES UNIQUE TO PEDIATRIC AND ADOLESCENT DEPRESSION

Although depressed children can display symptoms commonly seen in adult and adolescent MDD, the appearance of externalizing symptoms is more likely seen in pediatric depression. Aggression, oppositional behavior, irritability, tantrums, low frustration tolerance, and mood lability

CASE STUDY

Rebecca is a 14-year-old girl who was referred following an incident during which she came home intoxicated. She was taken to the emergency room where she was treated for acute alcohol intoxication and was referred for outpatient treatment.

Initially, Rebecca complained about her divorced parents and their "unfair" treatment of her. As the interview continued, she became tearful and admitted that she had become increasingly depressed over the past year since the death of her maternal grandmother, with whom she was very close. Rebecca had spent several years living with her grandmother during turbulent years in her parents' marriage. She viewed the grandmother as her "refuge from the insanity" of her parents.

Her mother was chronically depressed and had taken to abusing both alcohol and benzodiazepines. As a result, she was often emotionally unavailable. Rebecca perceived her father as harsh, demanding, and rejective; additionally, her father had had a number of extramarital affairs.

Rebecca had been an excellent student, was outgoing, and had many friends. After her grandmother's death, however, Rebecca began to have initial and middle insomnia, loss of appetite with a 10-pound weight loss, diminished interest in seeing friends, flagging motivation to do well in school, and failing grades. She began to cut classes, broke her curfew, and became sexually active—all very uncharacteristic behaviors.

During the interview, Rebecca admitted to passive suicidal ideation but denied any active plan or intent. She had begun to cut her arms superficially over the past three months. She also begun to drink during this time "to feel better" and, at other times, "to feel nothing." By this time, she had already had several blackouts after evenings of heavy drinking.

Rebecca was amenable to beginning psychotherapy and also began to attend ALATEEN. Her mother was referred for treatment of her depression and substance abuse. The father reluctantly agreed to collateral sessions but stopped coming after a month. Because of the severity of Rebecca's depressive symptoms, she was prescribed Prozac 10mg, which was titrated to 20mg. Her vegetative symptoms slowly diminished and she began to feel more positive and optimistic. She was eventually able to address both her intense anger and resentment toward her parents as well as mourn the death of her beloved grandmother. As these issues gradually resolved, Rebecca's acting out behaviors disappeared and she began to see her self-defeating behaviors as attempts to engage her distant and self-absorbed parents as well as to "pay them back." Her alcohol use was also seen in this context as well as an attempt to block her sadness.

By last report, she was doing well academically and had resumed her usual social activities and was able to abstain from any substance use.

are common to depression in childhood. Somatic complaints, although seen in adult MDD, are more frequently encountered in children.

The symptoms of childhood depression may not be as persistent when compared to adult depression. Depending on a child's age and cognitive and emotional development, feelings of sadness, anhedonia (an inability to experience pleasure), sense of hopelessness and worthlessness, and feelings of self-harm may go unexpressed verbally. Potentially the only clues to a depressive process may come from paying attention to a child's play, recognizing a change in functioning at school and with peers, or any change in sleep habits. A young child's lack of understanding of the permanence of death may also complicate the assessment of seriousness of suicidal behavior in younger children.

There is evidence that the genetics of early-onset recurrent depression may be different than adolescent onset MDD, which is more closely related to adult MDD. This may help explain why response rates to standard medication treatments are much less robust in childhood depression compared with adolescent and adult depression.

TREATMENT OF DEPRESSION
Nonpharmacologic Treatment
A number of nonpharmacologic treatments exist for MDD. Currently, only a few are supported by clinical evidence as being effective for childhood depression.

Cognitive Behavioral Therapy (CBT) has a growing body of evidence showing its effectiveness for children and adolescents. In CBT, skills are taught and then practiced. Faulty perceptions and automatic thoughts are identified and challenged with alternative ways of viewing the self, the world, the future (this is called cognitive restructuring). Other skills taught include monitoring of moods, thoughts, and behaviors; promoting involvement in activities likely to provide mastery and a feeling of accomplishment; creating a rewarding environment, etc.

CBT may be more helpful for mild to moderate cases of depression in children. Several studies have suggested that combination treatment with an SSRI, such as Prozac (fluoxetine HCl), added to CBT may be more helpful in more severe cases of MDD.

Interpersonal Psychotherapy (IPT) focuses primarily on areas of interpersonal conflict. Other areas of work include grief issues, major life transitions (eg, entry into school, moves, etc.), and conflictual relationships.

Current evidence supports the effectiveness of either CBT or IPT in adolescent MDD. Given the less-than-impressive data regarding the effectiveness of antidepressant medications in children, CBT and IPT are usually the treatments of first choice for less severe depression in children.

More severe pediatric depression will usually require use of medication—alone or in combination with CBT or IPT. School intervention may also be necessary. Educating teachers and guidance counselors about depression as well as recommending special accommodations (such as a reduced schedule and work load) is often helpful.

In addition to the above, certain lifestyle changes should also be part of the discussion in educating adolescents and their families. For instance, avoidance of unnecessary stress; avoidance of alcohol, drugs, and caffeine; implementing stress-reducing strategies such as yoga, relaxation breathing, exercise, and involvement in healthy, pleasurable activities; stressing the importance of adequate sleep, exercise, positive socialization, keeping usefully occupied, and avoiding isolation, etc. should all be a part of any attempt to treat depression.

Pharmacologic Treatment
There have been numerous trials studying the effectiveness of SSRIs in children and adolescents. To date, Prozac (fluoxetine HCl) is the only SSRI that is approved for use in pediatric MDD, and the only medication that has demonstrated clear efficacy in this age group. Evidence for effectiveness of other compounds is not as well documented, but there is some evidence for efficacy of some other SSRIs. Meanwhile, adolescents seem to show a more robust response to SSRIs—similar to that seen in adult populations.

In four randomized trials with Prozac, two of the studies failed to demonstrate significant difference between Prozac and placebo. One study showed significant improvement in the Prozac group, and the most recent study found that combined CBT and Prozac was most effective, although Prozac alone was also effective.

It is also important to note that children show an unusually high placebo response and this may explain why, in some studies, drug treatment was not distinguishable from placebo. Contributing to this may also be the fact that children are particularly responsive to the supportive aspects of any treatment. Some studies have shown that one-third of pediatric cases of depression show no clinical response to treatment with an SSRI. Some have pointed to this as proof of medications being "oversold" for use in children. Although continued research is needed in this area, many experts agree that drug therapy is often an essential and highly effective treatment for many young people with more severe depression.

Wellbutrin (buproprion HCl) has also been used off-label to treat pediatric depression. Wellbutrin increases presynaptic concentrations of both norepinephrine and, to a lesser extent, dopamine. This profile makes Wellbutrin potentially beneficial to children with depression and comorbid ADHD.

Other medications used off-label to treat pediatric depression include Effexor (venlafaxine), Lamictal (lamotrigine), and lithium carbonate (as an augmenting agent). Activation and conversion to mania can occur with exposure to SSRIs, especially in the prepubertal population. Since many children who later go on to develop bipolar disorder often initially show symptoms of MDD, the clinician must always be aware of the possibility of an underlying bipolar process before prescribing antidepressant medication.

The recent controversy regarding reports of an increase in suicidal ideation in children treated with SSRIs highlights the potential difficulty in correctly interpreting data from clinical trials. The FDA issued a Black Box Warning regarding the potential danger in prescribing SSRIs for children and adolescents. A year later, the FDA modified its warning in light of more recent analysis of available data, which found no clear causal link.

The widespread use of SSRIs to treat pediatric MDD corresponds with decreasing rates of suicide over the past two decades. The initial Black Box Warning appeared in 2004, and prescriptions for antidepressants for children and adolescents have decreased—while rates of suicidal behaviors have correspondingly increased.

Possible explanations for some of the increase in suicidal ideation seen with SSRIs include activation phenomena, akathesia (motor restlessness), and manic induction—all of which can cause suicidal ideation.

Most experts currently feel that there are no convincing data to indicate a clear connection between suicidal ideation and use of SSRIs in the majority of children treated. It is believed that the appropriate use of SSRIs in non-bipolar depressed children is a major reason for declining suicide rates in this age group.

With these concerns in mind, the FDA and The American Academy of Child & Adolescent Psychiatry Practice Parameters recommend that any child initiated on a trial of antidepressant medication be monitored at least once weekly for the first four weeks and then every two weeks after that.

Some animal studies have shown potential neurotoxic effects associated with depression and with stress in general. Proper and effective treatment of depression might prevent this and provide some neuroprotective effect.

When considering pharmacotherapy, the potential risks of treatments must be weighed against the potential effects of not treating.

In pharmacological treatment, once a clinical response is documented and possible side effects properly managed, continuation of medication should extend at least six to 12 months in order to prevent relapse.

SUMMARY

Depression is a potentially deadly illness that affects a growing number of children and adolescents. Signs and symptoms can be similar to those seen in adult MDD. Age and developmental level can significantly alter the clinical presentation. Conduct problems and aggression, irritability, somatic symptoms, and change in grades might be the only obvious signs of pediatric depression.

Since symptoms of depression can be the first signs of early-onset bipolar disorder, special care must be taken before diagnosing and treating MDD in the young.

If left untreated, MDD can have significant consequences, including conduct problems, impaired social functioning, academic underachievement, drug and alcohol abuse, and even suicide attempts and death.

Both genetic and environmental factors play a significant role in the development of MDD.

Several effective evidence-based treatments exist for pediatric depression. Among them are CBT, IPT, and pharmacotherapy.

Re-examination of the recent controversy over suicidal ideation and the use of SSRIs has shown no clear causal link for the majority of children and adolescents with depression. Since depression often has a protracted and relapsing course, any effective treatment must continue for at least six to 12 months.

Although evidence for effectiveness of pharmacotherapy in the pediatric population is conflicting, there can be no contesting the decrease in suicide rates in the young since the widespread introduction and use of SSRIs (especially Prozac) for depression in the young. Pharmacotherapy therefore must remain a first-line option in the treatment of pediatric depression.

OBSESSIVE-COMPULSIVE DISORDER

OVERVIEW

Compulsive behaviors are common and ubiquitous. Neatness, meticulousness, scrupulous attention to detail, and checking and rechecking are just some compulsive features that are seen in everyday life and can be adaptive and highly useful. At minimum, these are the traits most of us would certainly want in a neurosurgeon, a trial lawyer, or an architect, to name but a few.

Repetitive and ritualistic behaviors are commonly encountered across many phases of a child's development. Bedtime rituals, superstitious beliefs and routines, having to have things "just so" are often ways young children deal with anxiety, especially at bedtime or other times of separation. In the school-age child, strict adherence to elaborate rules of a game, use and repetition of "magical" numbers, and performing various rituals are also developmentally appropriate means to bind anxiety.

As with many such traits, it is the degree, frequency, and level of interference with functioning that make these traits no longer adaptive but hindrances and possible illness. Although once thought to be rare, obsessive-compulsive disorder (OCD) is now understood to affect many children and adolescents. When subclinical symptoms are included, prevalence rates can top 19%.

OCD is also known to be a chronic disorder, with symptoms typically waxing and waning over time. In addition, the type of symptoms may change over the course of the illness. Many adults with OCD had their onset of illness in childhood. Of these adults, about one-third to one-half had their first symptoms of OCD by age 15. The mean age of onset of OCD in pediatric samples is about 10 years, but there have been reports of clinically significant symptoms in children as young as 5 years old.

There is a genetic component to the disorder and it has been suggested that early-onset OCD may have a stronger familial component that later-onset OCD.

Symptoms commonly seen in pediatric OCD include contamination fears, compulsive checking, counting and ordering, having to have things "just right," having to create symmetry, etc. Ruminations can include obsessive doubting and mental rituals (such as praying, repetitive counting, etc.).

PREVALENCE AND RISK FACTORS

Prevalence rates for OCD are dependent on the level of impairment required. In community samples, prevalence rates for adolescent OCD range between 1% and 3.6%. Studies in prepubertal children are scarce, but prevalence rates are usually reported to be <1%. Since OCD symptoms are ego dystonic (that is, felt to be alien, distressing, not part of self), children and adolescents are often embarrassed by their symptoms and do not regularly report them unless they reach unbearable levels. This may also lead to under-reporting and undertreatment of the disorder in youth.

There appears to be a clear genetic component to OCD. Family genetic studies seem to confirm that offspring of OCD parents are at greater risk for developing the disorder. Twin studies also suggest heritability of some forms of OCD. In particular, the co-occurrence of OCD and tic disorder and Tourette's syndrome may be a more heritable disorder than OCD without comorbid tic disorder. There is further evidence that children with earlier age of onset may have a more familial illness in addition to having a higher rate of comorbidity with tic disorder and Tourette's syndrome.

Recent research has suggested that in a subgroup of children with OCD, infection by Group A beta hemolytic streptococcal infection can be the causative agent, so-called Pediatric Autoimmune Neuropsychiatric Disorder Associated with Streptococcal infections (PANDAS).

There is also evidence that family factors may play a part in the expression of symptoms of OCD. An example might be modeling of a parent's cognitive bias toward seeing danger in benign situations.

PRESENTATION AND DIAGNOSIS

There are a wide variety of symptoms displayed by children and adolescents with OCD. In addition to the variety of symptoms seen, the symptoms in any one individual can change over time.

The hallmark symptoms of OCD are compulsions and obsessions. *DSM-IV-TR* defines OCD as either obsessions or compulsions, where obsessions are defined as:

• Intrusive, unwanted and inappropriate thoughts, impulses, or images that are experienced repeatedly and persistently
• The thoughts, impulses, or images are not just intense worry about real-life events
• The child actively tries to block the disturbing thoughts, images, or impulses

• The child realizes that the thoughts, images, or impulses are generated by their own mind (this may not necessary be true in younger children)

Compulsions are defined as:
• Repetitive behaviors or mental rituals that the child feels compelled to repeat, usually in response to an obsession
• The behaviors or mental rituals are performed in order to prevent harm or danger, or to reduce distress and anxiety

Although *DSM-IV-TR* stipulates that the individual must realize that the obsessions and compulsions are excessive, this may not be the case for children. The symptoms must cause significant distress, or cause functional impairment.

In children and adolescents, the most common presentations of OCD are fear of contamination, compulsive washing, and attempts to avoid contaminated objects. The fears may be very specific, such as fear of contracting AIDS, fear of touching doorknobs, or a fear of objects that seem "dirty."

Another common symptom of childhood OCD is compulsive and repetitive checking. Children will repeatedly check to see that the doors are locked (sometimes a specific and rigidly adhered to number of times), or check to see if parents and siblings are safe, etc. Obsessive doubting can sometimes be a manifestation of ritualistic checking, and the child will feel compelled to make sure that they didn't run over a squirrel, or that they didn't say the wrong thing to a friend. The obsessive doubting can sometimes take the form of having to repeatedly "confess" perceived misdeeds or bad thoughts to parents. This can sometimes lead to compulsive praying, which can occupy several hours of mental activity and leave little time for normal daily activities.

Other commonly seen compulsions include counting rituals, touching, tapping, arranging, etc. Objects have to be counted or touched a certain number of times, or objects must be arranged and ordered in a specific pattern. If something gets in the way of the prescribed ritual, the child will have to start the ritual over from the beginning. Sometimes, these rituals can appear like complex motor tics.

Often, the obsessive worry is fueled by a grossly exaggerated perception of risk or danger. Performing the compulsive ritual eliminates the accompanying dread or fear.

In rare instances, children can have obsessions without compulsions. The intrusive thoughts are usually of a sexual or aggressive nature.

COMORBID CONDITIONS
The literature on pediatric OCD asserts that one-third to one-half of children with OCD will report a history of another anxiety disorder.

CASE STUDY

Eric was diagnosed with ADHD and tic disorder by his pediatrician at age 9 and was treated with Concerta (methylphenidate HCl) and Tenex (guanfacine) by a local neurologist. What Eric hadn't yet revealed to his mother or the neurologist was an ever-changing series of bedtime rituals that he felt compelled to perform. These symptoms had started the year preceding his ADHD diagnosis. Sometimes these rituals would consist of mentally counting a series of numbers. Other times, he would have to repeat certain words. The year before, his maternal grandmother was diagnosed with early stage Alzheimer's and was brought to live with Eric's family. Eric became fearful of touching his grandmother and feared that he would "catch an illness" from her. He began to avoid using the public bathroom at school. His mother became aware that there might be a problem when she noticed that Eric would cover his hand with a tissue before touching a doorknob. Eric was also engaging in repeated handwashing and this began to consume more and more of his time. It was at this point that his mother brought Eric in for an evaluation.

Eric's ADHD symptoms were under reasonable control with Concerta. Although there are reports of high doses of stimulant medication causing transient over-focusing, repetitive behaviors, or perseveration, Eric was on an appropriate dose of Concerta and his OCD symptoms preceded the initiation of stimulant medication.

Eric's parents were provided with education about the nature of OCD as well as the available treatment options, including ERP, medication, and combination treatment. They were concerned and caring and were not overly enmeshed in Eric's symptoms. Eric started a course of ERP but he was fearful of engaging in even imagined exposure to feared situations involving germs and contamination.

It was at this point that his parents agreed to an initial trial on Zoloft. After eight weeks, the intensity of his OCD symptoms began to wane and Eric was more amenable to re-introducing the ERP protocol. ERP proceeded with Eric's improved mastery over anxiety and he approached the "homework assignments" with enthusiasm. His parents noted that although Eric was still engaged in handwashing, he was able to stop after only two or three washings (rather than taking up to 30 minutes) and no longer feared touching doorknobs or using public restrooms.

Depressive disorders are also commonly seen co-occurring with pediatric OCD and rates of a comorbid mood disorder range from 20% to over 70%. Additionally, researchers have suggested that a subgroup of children with early-onset (prepubertal) OCD have high rates of tic and Tourette's disorders.

ISSUES UNIQUE TO PEDIATRIC AND ADOLESCENT OCD
Early-onset (prepubertal) OCD seems distinct from later-onset OCD. In addition to the high correlation between tic disorder and early-onset OCD, this subgroup of children shows a very high incidence of comorbid disruptive behavior disorder as well as male predominance. Later-onset OCD is present in a roughly equal male-to-female ratio.

Additionally, this subgroup seems to have a less impressive response to treatment with SSRIs than the later-onset group.

Unlike their adult counterparts, children with OCD do not necessarily perceive that their obsessions and compulsions are excessive or unreasonable.

TREATMENT OF OCD
Nonpharmacologic Treatment
In the past, standard psychotherapy and even psychoanalysis were treatments employed in an attempt to combat OCD in adults. For most patients suffering from OCD, these treatments were found to be woefully lacking. Over the past 15 years, the development of specialized cognitive behavior therapy (CBT) techniques has paved the way for proven and effective treatment of adult and pediatric OCD, and standardized treatment protocols have been developed and refined for use in the pediatric population.

The hallmark of the specialized CBT treatment for OCD involves the technique of exposure and response prevention (ERP). Although the introduction of the drug class known as selective serotonin reuptake inhibitors (SSRIs) has also improved treatment outcomes for both children and adults with OCD, the lack of durability of drug effect after medication has been withdrawn, frequent side effects, and continued residual symptoms have led many experts to agree that specialized ERP is the treatment of first choice (with and without medication) for pediatric OCD.

In CBT, obsessions are viewed as intrusive thoughts or images that trigger increasing anxiety and even panic. Compulsions are seen as behaviors or cognitions (for example, mental rituals) that are employed to reduce the anxiety. In standard ERP, the patient is systematically exposed to the fear that triggers the compulsive behavior. The response prevention component involves the patient being prohibited from engaging in the compulsive behavior(s). A so-called fear hierarchy is developed by the patient, beginning with least to most fear-inducing anxiety. In a step-by-step fashion, the patient is exposed gradually to more and more anxiety-inducing situations after each subsequent fear is conquered.

With children, the active cooperation of the parents and their involvement in the program is often necessary in order to prevent treatment failure, which is often seen in highly enmeshed families. In these families, parents often become unwittingly entangled in the child's symptoms and disengagement is often helpful.

The treatment approach is tailored to the developmental level of the child. Prepubertal children are given a "tool box" that they can use to "boss back" OCD. The child is given an appropriately worded explanation of OCD (eg, for younger children, OCD can be described as "brain hiccups") and is then encouraged to make OCD the problem – thus externalizing the disorder. The child is also asked to give OCD a derogatory name and to use this in doing battle with OCD. In addition to the CBT/ERP component, which typically can take between 10 to 15 sessions, children are also taught relaxation techniques and cognitive training. Other specialized techniques used in treating pediatric OCD involve the use of a "fear thermometer" (the fear hierarchy), "mapping" OCD (in which the child is encouraged to observe where OCD reigns supreme as well as areas of the child's life which are relatively free of OCD), and helping the child with constructive self-talk. After this foundation has been laid, the child is carefully guided through ERP.

Parents are included in sessions as needed and also educated about OCD as well as the techniques used. For some children, behavioral rewards for completing each assigned task and "homework" can also be useful.

For many children, use of CBT/ERP is highly effective in reducing the often debilitating symptoms of OCD. Unlike medication, the benefits of ERP often continue after treatment has ended, but booster treatments are sometimes necessary to maintain remission.

Pharmacologic Treatment
Tricyclic Antidepressants

With the introduction of the tricyclic antidepressant Anafranil (clomipramine) over 20 years ago, the successful pharmacologic treatment of OCD became possible.

There are ample placebo-controlled, double-blind studies documenting the effectiveness of Anafranil in the treatment of pediatric OCD. The mechanism of action that favored Anafranil over the other tricyclic antidepressants for OCD seems to be directly related to its potent serotonergic properties. Anafranil has been approved for use in OCD in children 10 years of age and older. As with all tricyclic antidepressants, burdensome side effects and potential cardiac effects make Anafranil a second-tier choice in pediatric OCD.

Selective Serotonin Reuptake Inhibitors (SSRIs)

There is convincing evidence for abnormalities in serotonergic (and possibly dopaminergic) transmission in the neurophysiology of OCD. With the understanding of the importance of Anafranil's potent serotonergic blockade in its effectiveness in treating OCD, the SSRIs were viewed as ideal compounds given their more favorable side effect profile.

Although all of the SSRIs have shown efficacy for OCD symptoms, only Zoloft (sertraline HCl) and Luvox (fluvoxamine maleate) are FDA-approved for use in children. Zoloft is approved for ages 6 years and up and Luvox for ages 8 years and up.

Prozac (fluoxetine HCl) has been used for over 20 years for both depression and OCD. One early double-blind, placebo-controlled study using Prozac in children 8 to 15 years of age reported a response of up to 45% in reducing OCD symptoms. Similar response rates have also been reported in pediatric age groups for Zoloft, Luvox, Paxil (paroxetine HCl), and Celexa (citalopram HBr).

In treatment-refractory cases, use of a low-dose atypical antipsychotic medication such as Risperdal (risperidone) has been cited as potentially beneficial (particularly in children with comorbid tic disorder), although its use is considered off-label. Concerns about possible metabolic side effects, increase in the hormone prolactin, as well as risk of developing tardive dyskinesia (a serious movement disorder) may limit its use to the more severe cases.

In the subgroup of children who developed OCD symptoms following a documented streptococcal infection, investigational trials of intravenous immunoglobulin, as well as trials of antibiotic therapy (penicillin) have been performed, but these methods are considered experimental.

For many children and adolescents, especially those with more severe symptoms or with comorbidities, combination treatment involving both ERP and an SSRI can be more helpful than either treatment alone.

SUMMARY

Obsessive-compulsive disorder is no longer considered uncommon in children and adolescents. The mean age of onset in pediatric samples is 10 years. There is a genetic component to OCD, especially in OCD that has its onset in childhood. OCD is frequently a chronic disorder and its symptoms are recurrent and often debilitating. Obsessive-compulsive traits are very frequently encountered in everyday life and can be adaptive and useful. OCD, on the other hand, is often distressing and can interfere with functioning at every level.

Rates of comorbidity are high in pediatric OCD. Comorbid disorders include tic disorder and mood disorders as well as another anxiety disorder.

Dysfunction in the serotonergic pathways is postulated to play a significant role in the neuropathology of OCD. Correspondingly, medications that have robust ability to increase levels of serotonin have been found to possess therapeutic effect.

The tricyclic antidepressant Anafranil, as well as all of the SSRIs, have proved useful pharmacologic agents in the treatment of pediatric OCD.

The development of specialized CBT protocols (namely ERP) to address the core symptoms of OCD has a strong body of evidence to support its usefulness for pediatric OCD. Many experts consider ERP to be the treatment of first choice for all but the most severe cases of pediatric OCD. Combination treatment using serotonergic agents in concert with ERP may be more effective for both children with comorbidities as well as those with more debilitating symptoms.

PERSONALITY DISORDERS

OVERVIEW

The Diagnostic and Statistical Manual of Mental Disorders, Fourth Edition, Text Revision, (2000) (*DSM-IV-TR*) is highly cautious about applying the diagnosis of a personality disorder to a child or even an adolescent given that their personalities are still emerging. With the exception of Antisocial Personality Disorder (which is only diagnosed in individuals 18 or older) a child or adolescent must continuously exhibit features for a minimum of one year to carry such a "label." However, clinicians can certainly identify personality features that qualify someone under the age of 18 to have a personality disorder (in the absence of a better explanation, such as their respective developmental stage or an Axis I psychiatric disorder, such as schizophrenia). Yet, the careful consideration with which this label is applied cannot be overemphasized—especially regarding someone so young (particularly a child), because we are dealing with a trait versus state diagnosis that can be extremely lasting and stigmatizing. This challenges those of us in the clinical trenches working with children and adolescents because early intervention is advantageous. In light of the scarcity of formal research studies on such disorders in children and adolescents, we will turn to what we do know about this diagnostic entity more broadly.

PREVALENCE

Epidemiological studies of personality disorders in the United States set the incidence between 10% and 13%, with some surveys placing the rate as high as 15%. Of course, there are extenuating circumstances that could potentially raise these figures, such as living in severe poverty, witnessing a traumatic event, or being the victim of physical or sexual abuse. Some personality disorders (such as borderline personality disorder, histrionic personality disorder, and dependent personality disorder) are more associated with females, while antisocial personality disorder is more frequently diagnosed in males (though *DSM-IV-TR* warns it is important not to get caught up in diagnosing an individual based upon stereotypes associated with a particular gender). It is equally important to realize that one's culture may dictate certain personality features that should not be considered abnormal. Certainly it is possible that specific personality disorders (eg, antisocial and borderline personality disorders) come to our attention at greater rates because of legal infractions, etc.

A more recent phenomenon is viewing someone with a personality disorder as having what this author has termed "enviable powers," such as the antisocial traits evidenced by the lead character in the detective show "Psych," who cons people into believing he is psychic when he is simply observant; or glorifying narcissism, because it has become associated with acquiring power, wealth, or fame. It should also be noted that it is possible to have more than one personality disorder, as well as having a personality disorder and an Axis I clinical syndrome such as a mood disorder or substance abuse/dependence disorder.

PRESENTATION AND DIAGNOSIS

When we speak of an individual's values, belief system, attitudes, the way they react emotionally, as well as their interpersonal relatedness, what motivates them, and how they respond to stimuli, we are really talking about one's personality. We expect these characteristics to be dependable; that is the person that we know. However, these unique traits do not necessarily cause disturbance and inability to effectively deal with life. When they do, one's "personality" is considered "disordered." We consistently see evidence of maladaptive coping strategies and that individual is usually miserable about their interactions with society.

DSM-IV-TR defines a personality disorder as "an enduring pattern of inner experience and behavior that deviates markedly from expectations of the individual's culture, is pervasive and inflexible, has an onset in adolescence or early adulthood, is stable over time, and leads to distress and impairment." It specifies that this perceived dysfunction must occur in at least two (or more) areas: "cognition," "affectivity," "interpersonal functioning," and "impulse control." Of note is the fact that most personality-disordered individuals find their personalities ego-syntonic. In other words, they see their personalities as harmonious with who they are and generally fault others for their failings.

The specific personality disorders are based on a system of grouping comparable characteristics, according to *DSM-IV-TR*:
• Cluster A (paranoid, schizoid, schizotypal, or the odd-eccentric cluster)
• Cluster B (antisocial, borderline, histrionic, narcissistic, or the dramatic-emotional cluster)
• Cluster C (avoidant, dependent, obsessive-compulsive, or the anxious-fearful emotional cluster)

It has been noted earlier that this type of cluster analysis does not prohibit an individual from having more than one personality disorder or traits from various clusters. It may be helpful to see personality disorders as running along a continuum—personality traits that range from normal to abnormal. (There are a number of dimensional approaches to viewing personality disorders, but they will not be elaborated on in this chapter.)

For ease of reference, we've drawn comparisons here to characters from popular culture. Not only does this allow for a quick identification, but it can help practitioners more readily explain characteristics of a disorder to patients or caregivers.

Paranoid Personality Disorder

A suspicious individual who may believe that other people wish to hurt them by cheating them or by lying to them or plotting against them. As a result, this type of person has difficulty formulating relationships characterized as being intimate. They may even have difficulty working with others. At times, they can become psychotic under extreme stress. It has been estimated that as many as 2.5% of the general population may qualify for this diagnosis. Think of Humphrey Bogart's character in *The Caine Mutiny* or elements of Richard Nixon's personality.

Schizoid Personality Disorder

A person who is seen as keeping to themselves; a complete loner if you will. Their isolative behavior usually applies to other family members as well. There is an inability to demonstrate emotional expression. They appear to be lost in their own thoughts and may fantasize a great deal. Estimates place schizoid personality disorder at 2% to 4% in the general population, and may be somewhat more common in males. Some would say William Hurt's character in *The Big Chill* had a schizoid personality.

Schizotypal Personality Disorder

Picture an individual who dresses in an odd manner and appears rather eccentric, with unusual speech patterns, and you most likely have someone with a schizotypal personality disorder. Social settings are unbearable to these individuals. A notion that they are psychic can often dominate what is best described as magical thinking. Often this person is suspicious and paranoid—evidencing thoughts of reference. Estimates place schizotypal personality disorder at 3% in the general population, and it may be more common in males. If you recall Robert De Niro's character in *Taxi Driver*, it will help you to envision this type of individual.

Antisocial Personality Disorder

In an extreme form, an individual with an antisocial personality disorder can be viewed as a sociopath or even a psychopath. These individuals will literally do whatever it takes to get their way—that can include stealing, deceiving, aggression, or being obsequious (syrupy sweet to con and swindle). A complete lack of empathy and remorse dominate this personality disorder. These are irresponsible, self-absorbed people who often end up in jail, in treatment for addiction, act out sexually, and even have been know to die in a violent manner or commit suicide. Estimates place antisocial personality disorder at 3% in the general population for men and 1% for women. Perhaps the best recent example of an antisocial personality disordered individual would be the character of Tony Soprano, in the television series "The Sopranos." Additionally, the character of Alex in *A Clockwork Orange* certainly had an antisocial personality disorder, as did Angelina Jolie's character, Lisa, in *Girl, Interrupted*, while Wynona Ryder's depiction of the lead character in the same film certainly portrayed the next personality disorder described: borderline personality disorder.

Borderline Personality Disorder

Individuals with borderline personality disorder can best be viewed as lacking any sense of constancy. This instability can be seen in their self-image (including sexual orientation), mood, relationships, and behaviors that are often impulsive (ie, dominated by sexual acting out, eating disorders, substance abuse, and engaging in risk-taking behaviors such as ignoring traffic regulations). There is often a total fear of being abandoned. Thinking is dominated by an all or nothing (black-and-white) logic. "I love you or I hate you" is the norm rather than the exception. Self-mutilating, parasuicidal behaviors such as cutting themselves or burning themselves with cigarettes as well as real attempts at suicide are not uncommon. While borderline individuals do often harm others emotionally with primitive defense mechanisms such as projective identification and splitting, they very rarely physically look to hurt others. In the movie *Fatal Attraction*, Glenn Close's character Alex can be seen as the embodiment of borderline personality disorder, although perhaps there were aspects to her personality that were exaggerated for theatrical reasons (such as boiling the pet rabbit). Borderline personality disorder is found in roughly 2% of the population; 75% of borderline individuals are women.

Histrionic Personality Disorder

It is helpful to think of Shakespeare's famous monologue, "All the world's a stage...," when one tries to define histrionic personality disorder. Individuals with this disorder crave attention and are willing to get it by utilizing extreme attention-seeking behavior. They are often seductive and utilize flirtation to draw others into their world. They are emotionally shallow and not truly capable of authenticity. They are people who try to be the center of attention and will do what they have to in order to accomplish this goal. They tend to shift their opinion like the wind, and usually can be heard emphatically quoting whomever they spoke with last. Histrionic personality disorder is found in approximately 2% to 3% of the general population. While this disorder has traditionally been associated with women more than men, this seems to be one of those examples where gender bias may be at play. Some have argued that Jackie Gleason's character in the television show "The Honeymooners" was histrionic, although this author would point to a clearer example embodied in the portrayal of Scarlett O'Hara in *Gone with the Wind*.

Narcissistic Personality Disorder

Individuals with narcissistic personality disorder are simply full of themselves. They go through life trying to impress others in the name of being viewed as "simply the best." It is not necessarily that they want to be successful, but instead need to be admired—constantly striving for fame. This behavior often leads to living in a fantasy world. They truly lack empathic understanding of others because they are so invested in themselves. It should be noted that if they do not reach their often unrealistic goals, they feel a sense of worthlessness. This leads them into conflict with others because they refuse to accept their own shortcomings. Narcissistic personality disorder affects less than 1% of the general population, and 75% of that 1% are males. Many clinicians point to the character Julian in the film *American Gigolo* as a good example of someone with narcissistic personality disorder, and the character of the news achorman played by Ted Knight in the classic television series "The Mary Tyler Moore Show" is another good example.

Avoidant Personality Disorder

Individuals with avoidant personality disorder have a profound sense of feeling inadequate, particularly when it comes to forming social relationships. This should not be confused with a lack of desire to form such relationships, but should be seen as a marked sensitivity to being shamed by others—they actually may come to believe that others are focusing on them so that they can pass judgment. This disorder is often tied to another personality disorder, namely, dependent personality disorder (see below), as well as having some symptoms of social phobia. If one thinks of the humor of Woody Allen, avoidant personality disorder often comes to mind. Additionally, if the Winnie the Pooh character Piglet were placed under pressure, that avoidant personality disorder could be evidenced. One can particularly see why it is so important to be careful when diagnosing children and adolescents when viewing the benchmarks of avoidant personality disorder, given the natural developmental insecurities and "drama" of youth. Roughly .05% to 1% of the general population has an avoidant personality disorder.

Dependent Personality Disorder

Individuals with dependent personality disorder struggle with being independent. They have a pathological need for others to take control. This would appear to stem from significant insecurity—a complete lack of self-confidence. They have extreme existential isolation, which propels them to be submissive and tolerate abusive relationships. There is a pervasive sense of learned helplessness. A modern television character that was initially portrayed as having a dependent personality was that of

Robert, the brother in "Everybody Loves Raymond." As the series progressed, Robert emerged from the submissive abuse of his mother and father and the need to cling to his brother's family. Reliable studies on the frequency in the general population are not available. Like histrionic personality disorder, dependent personality disorder may be more frequently diagnosed in women due to gender bias.

Obsessive-Compulsive Personality Disorder

Obsessive-compulsive personality disorder must be distinguished from Axis I Obsessive-Compulsive disorder, which is considered under the rubric of anxiety disorders and can be paralyzing. The former is characterized by obsessions and compulsions performed to reduce anxiety, whereas the latter is more focused on being a perfectionist. Perhaps it is helpful to think of Felix Unger in the "Odd Couple," and the lead character in the television series "Monk" as having obsessive-compulsive disorder. Obsessive-compulsive personality disorder is dominated by the sense that there is a right way to do things and think about things "period." Often others cannot be trusted to comply, and therefore cannot take part in a particular process. Ethical standards are "written in stone" and cannot be debated. The person with obsessive-compulsive personality disorder is often tight-fisted with money. They may not be able to discard things easily. Their primary focus is on work above all else. Approximately 1% of the general population has obsessive-compulsive personality disorder. Men outweigh women 2 to 1.

ETIOLOGY OF PERSONALITY DISORDERS

Although previously mentioned that one must be very cautious about diagnosing a personality disorder in childhood and even in adolescence because of developmental issues, childhood must be viewed as a starting point.

Perhaps the nature-nurture model best explains personality disorders. There is some evidence that certain personality characteristics are based on brain biology and genetic factors as well as interactions with the primary caregiver. Factors such as a traumatic brain injury in childhood, family history of a major mental illness and/or personality disorder, and inconsistent parenting due to abuse and addiction, are probable culprits. Carefully controlled empirical studies must occur in greater numbers to be able to quantify this more definitively.

COMORBID CONDITIONS

As we have seen, it is understandable that an Axis II personality disorder would raise an individual's vulnerability to other Axis II as well as Axis I syndromes. Increased susceptibility for anxiety, suicidality, mood-spectrum disorders, risk-taking behaviors, eating disorders, isolating, violence, criminality, and of course, substance abuse can increase exponentially.

At times it is difficult to clearly understand what is truly an Axis I clinical state or an Axis II trait. Perhaps it is best to view the two as having a "hand and glove" connection. Certainly, an individual's severe agoraphobia will only hamper treatment of that same individual's dependent personality disorder. Whereas an individual may be more prone to agoraphobia if they have a schizotypal personality disorder, etc.

It is helpful to try to view Axis I and II disorders as running along a continuum. For example, one of the latest theories is that borderline personality disorder is subsumed under the bipolar disorder spectrum.

Additionally, if one looks at the personality disorders that are listed under the three clusters, they will realize that they share many of the same traits—at times distinctions are hard to draw.

Lastly, a clinician would have to work with an individual for a rather long period of time to truly see the necessary sustained traits needed to warrant assigning a full-blown personality disorder versus a particular clinical state. Since this is often not the case, historical information is gathered and is usually replete with distortions from the identified patient or significant others with a stake in rewriting history.

ISSUES UNIQUE TO PEDIATRIC AND ADOLESCENT PERSONALITY DISORDERS

As previously noted, there is scant research on child and adolescent personality disorders; however, clinicians know that adolescents and even children do, at times, evidence sustained diagnostic traits that qualify as personality disorders. The intervening variables that confound formal studies of personality disorders in children and adolescents primarily revolve around distinguishing pathology in the context of normal developmental processes. Cognitive development, interacting with one's environment, particularly interacting with others, is a time of great experimentation and stress. The most salient issue related to child and adolescent personality disorders for the diagnostician is gathering collateral information systematically from multiple sources. Clinicians must utilize an armamentarium of clinical skills. The identified patient as well as nuclear and extended family members, friends, and educators must all be interviewed. The goal is to reveal those traits that have been sustained for at least one year, without a break in time, that cause significant issues in at least two or more areas related to perception and thought, affectivity, social relationships, and impulse control.

One of the greatest issues that we see in children with emerging personality disorders is anxiety, which can be accompanied by depression. Initially, this can be manifested in extreme fears of separation from the primary caregiver. Adolescents can also exhibit anxiety and depression, usually in the form of feeling inadequate about a specific task. While this does not have to lead to a personality disorder, certainly the chances that it will do so increase with environmental stress (eg, violence in the home, school, or social environment). Learning disorders, communication disorders, attention-deficit and disruptive behavior disorders, as well as mood, anxiety, sexual and gender identity, eating, substance-related, and adjustment disorders can all be associated with emerging personality disorders in childhood, as well as part of a comorbid condition in adolescence. Again, the reader is cautioned that extreme diagnostic care must be taken before labeling a child or adolescent with a personality disorder. It is important to rule out a differential diagnosis and not jump to the conclusion that a personality disorder is a better explanation or co-occurring.

TREATMENT OF PERSONALITY DISORDERS

Clearly, the most important objective in any clinical work with an individual is developing a therapeutic alliance. This is obviously not an easy task as one reviews all of the traits across the three clusters of personality disorders. Add to this the complicating developmental factors that children and adolescents present and the task can become quite daunting. Indeed, most young clinicians will tell you that these patients are their least favorite to treat. Often, the patient dictates the therapeutic modality.

Nonpharmacologic Treatment
Psychodynamic Insight-Oriented Therapy
This form of therapy requires the patient to be capable of being able to develop insight. If the individual is so defensive that they cannot be open to engaging in this process, it is of little benefit. One must be able to tolerate the frustrations that this process can raise. It is also quite time-consuming.

Cognitive Behavior Therapy
This methodology has gained a great deal of attention in the treatment of personality disorders. Cognitions, or thoughts, are challenged, followed by a process of restructuring these thoughts and developing new ways of thinking, which in turn results in developing new behaviors. This form of therapy is not interested in the "why" someone became a certain way, but is more concerned with correcting faulty cognitions. It is a faster method of therapy than those more psychodynamic insight-oriented processes.

Dialectical Behavior Therapy (DBT)
Perhaps one of the newest forms of therapy for personality disorders is DBT. This type of therapy is also cognitive in nature. The goal is to have the patient develop coping mechanisms, by utilizing the formation of a dialectic between the practitioner and the client such that a state of "mindfulness" can be accomplished, resulting in a genuine observation of the truth and a diminution of acting out behavior.

Pharmacologic Treatment

An individual's specific personality disorder may warrant adjunctive pharmacotherapy.

Antidepressants, particularly the selective serotonin reuptake inhibitors (SSRIs) such as Prozac (fluoxetine HCl), Paxil (paroxetine HCl), Zoloft (sertraline HCl), Celexa (citalopram HBr), and Lexapro (escitalopram oxalate), have been utilized effectively in conjunction with psychotherapy to help alleviate depression and anxiety. Seizure medications such as Tegretol (carbamazapine), Depakote (divalproex sodium), and Topamax (topiramate) have been used for treating emotional dysregulation in individuals with borderline and antisocial personality disorders, as have mood stabilizing drugs such as lithium. Those individuals with the possibility of losing touch with reality (eg, borderline or schizotypal personality disorders), can benefit, at times, from antipsychotic medications such as Zyprexa (olanzapine) and Risperdal (risperidone). Anxiolytics such as Xanax (alprazolam), Valium (diazepam), and Klonopin (clonazepam) can prove to be effective in treating much of the agitation that corresponds with many of the personality disorders.

Of course, being aware of dependency issues and the threat of lethal results when these drugs are combined with alcohol and other drugs is paramount. In general, it is important to understand the unique risks in prescribing medication to children and adolescents (just think about the recent controversy over the use of SSRIs). None of the medications noted above is FDA-approved for children and adolescents (with the exception of Prozac), although they are commonly prescribed. Healthcare providers must be cognizant of specific warnings and precautions relevant to this patient group when prescribing. That is why parents and caregivers should only go to psychiatrists and psychopharmacologists board certified for specializing in child and adolescent issues when addressing these conditions.

With regard to the specific modality of psychotherapy, individual as well as group therapy can be effective and should be used in combination whenever possible. Of course, this is warranted by the patient's level of functioning, which is dictated by their diagnosis. Additionally, family therapy and couples therapy should be considered when the counselor feels the timing is right. Self-help programs such as Alcoholics Anonymous, Gamblers Anonymous, etc. should also be encouraged depending on the patient's symptomatology. Unless an individual is truly a risk to themselves or others, inpatient treatment for personality disorders is generally not required.

SUMMARY

Personality disorders can occur in childhood and adolescence, but should only be diagnosed after careful consideration of patients who have character pathology lasting at least one year without interruption. These personality traits generally affect at least two areas of functioning: thinking, emotions, social functioning, and impulse control. While some personality disorders can get better as the individual ages (eg, borderline and antisocial personality disorders), others do not necessarily improve (eg, schizotypal and obsessive-compulsive personality disorder). Epidemiological studies, while scarce, point to a combination of biological and environmental factors. Personality disorders are difficult to treat, although it is important to address issues as soon as possible. A combination of psychotherapy and medication is often utilized.

ADDICTION

OVERVIEW

Statistics on alcohol, tobacco, and drug abuse are more complicated than they may initially appear. Different drugs (legal and illegal), age of user, gender issues, ethnicity, socioeconomic issues, co-occurring psychiatric issues, etc., make this a multivariate "nightmare." The National Institute on Drug Addiction (NIDA) has shown a consistent decline in substance use over the past several years, but the news is not so encouraging when one breaks down the demographics. For example, fewer 8th graders are using illicit drugs, but 12th graders are abusing prescription drugs such as Vicodin and Oxycontin at consistently dangerous levels.

In general, alcohol and tobacco are still the two substances that are used more than any others across all categories of teenagers. This may be related to their legal status. Not only are they easier to obtain, but being legal may convey a belief that they are "safer" than illicit drugs, contrary to reality. Alcohol and tobacco may also be used more often because teenagers are modeling the behavior of older siblings, parents, and other adults.

With regard to illicit substances, marijuana ranks number one across teenage demographics. This might also be due to modeling by older siblings, parents, and other baby-boomer generation adults.

Other commonly abused substances across all categories of adolescents include inhalants and prescription drugs. Perhaps the availability of inhalants has something to do with this phenomenon. Also, these chemical agents are constantly advertised and may work their way into the unconscious minds of youngsters who mistakenly associate the ads with some unspoken imprimatur to use them in what I refer to as "off-line" (for the sake of getting high despite their intended use). With regard to prescription substances, there is also the issue of ready availability in the medicine cabinet, and the sense that these medications are given out by physicians to parents, grandparents, etc., so how could they possibly be unsafe.

PREVALENCE AND RISK FACTORS

The presentation of an individual using a particular substance depends on the individual and the substance. Most of the time, specific drugs result in specific reactions. If one uses a narcotic such as heroin, he will generally have a feeling of peace and tranquility; however, he may also experience side effects such as nausea and respiratory depression; it all depends on the amount one takes, any interactions with other drugs, and the individual's own "biological idiosyncrasies." In essence, when you add in genetics or hereditary factors, the possibility of an allergic reaction, and other variables, it becomes a bit like playing with a chemistry set.

Drugs can be placed into specific categories: central nervous system depressants such as sedatives and anxiolytics (tranquilizers); stimulants; opiates and narcotics; psychedelics or hallucinogens; cannabinols; and inhalants; among others.

It is ironic that the most-abused central nervous system depressant is legal—alcohol. Sedatives such as alcohol diminish the speed of brain functioning, and can effect the development of executive functioning in burgeoning adolescents.

It should be noted that regardless of the type of substance or substances being abused, it will ultimately affect a number of areas of functioning, including physical, emotional, family relations, academic performance, and social interactions.

Sedatives and Anxiolytics

Sedatives and anxiolytics are used for insomnia and anxiety. Anxiolytics (tranquilizers) can also be utilized as muscle relaxants. Teenagers like the effects of sedative hypnotics and anti-anxiety drugs because they create a sense of euphoria and reduce tension. It is interesting to think about why a teenager might need to relax and to speculate how many teens have co-occurring disorders such as generalized anxiety disorder and panic attacks that they rarely speak about. One such drug that is very popular on the streets is Xanax (alprazolam). It is often referred to as "bars," "french fries," and "coffins." Anxiolytic agents are highly addictive because they have a fast onset and the effects only last a short period of time, requiring an increased dosage to derive the same effects as one develops physiological tolerance. Other central nervous system depressants include GHB (gamma-hydroxybutyric acid) and Rohypnol (flunitrazepam), which are not FDA-approved for use in the U.S.

Stimulants

Teenagers, and very often, teenage girls (in order to lose weight), are drawn to stimulants such as amphetamines. In general, both male and female adolescents who are looking for an increased ability to stay awake, pay attention, and concentrate, or who simply want to feel a sense of physical stamina, are drawn to these drugs. Again, this raises the question of co-occurring disorders, in this case, psychiatric diagnoses such as attention-deficit/hyperactivity disorder (ADHD). This is not to say that all adolescents who use stimulants should be thought of as having a dual diagnosis, but certainly as clinicians we must open our minds to the combinations and permutations that motivate youngsters to use cocaine, methamphetamines, etc.

It should also be noted that caffeine is a stimulant despite its legal status, and after nicotine, is the second most addictive substance. It can have dangerous effects on the cardiovascular system when used in excess. Given all of the new energy drinks that are loaded with caffeine, this becomes a real danger to adolescents and must be considered, particularly when combined with other drugs and alcohol.

Opiates and Narcotics

Opiates and narcotics are good examples of how teenagers are not only influenced by fads in clothing and music, but also in drugs of choice. Drugs such as heroin and morphine used to be very popular in the 1950s and early 1960s. The "beat" generation of writers, poets, and musicians were known for injecting heroin in order to feel a sense of euphoria that was believed to be more conducive to creativity. Teenagers who wanted to emulate these literary and musical giants would often follow suit, as would those unfortunate teenagers who got sent to war and became addicted.

With the emergence and prevalence of HIV/AIDS and the risk of transmission associated with injecting drugs, IV drug use has fallen out of favor over the last few decades. But heroin that can be snorted is on the rise and opiate painkillers are sitting in many medicine cabinets, causing an unwelcome resurgence in the use of these drugs.

Psychedelics and Hallucinogens

In the latter part of the 1960s and into the 1970s, hallucinogens were quite popular. More recent studies show that today's adolescents are less interested in these drugs. While you still hear of the occasional LSD trip and use of "'shrooms" (psilocybin) or PCP (also known as "angel dust"), they are simply not as popular. This is not to say that they may not come back into popularity as the social and political zeitgeist changes, but for now, we don't hear of the "good trip" or the "bad trip" quite so often. Perhaps this has to do with the fact that today's adolescents are inundated by computer and video games with vivid imagery, muting their interest in manipulating their mental imagery through peyote. Alternately, it may have something to do with teenagers being more interested in having control of things—and being in control—than earlier generations.

Cannabinols

It seems that the cannabinols, namely, marijuana and hashish, are still quite popular among teenagers, despite the National Institute on Drug Addiction citing various studies that show evidence of physical as well as psychological addiction over time. Additionally, marijuana has been shown to have negative effects on the brain, particularly with regard to memory, attention and learning, as well as the presence of many other

CASE STUDY

John was a 16-year-old student when he was first brought to my office by his mother for what was described as his use of her "tranquilizers and pain pills." He complained that he was constantly nervous and was simply looking for a way to "calm down." Upon drug screening, he was positive for Xanax and Oxycontin, which corresponded with what his mother related. No other drugs were found in his system, and he claimed that the only other substances he tried were alcohol and marijuana, but that the former made him sick to his stomach and the latter resulted in paranoid feelings.

John also liked to consume six to eight energy drinks a day. He said he needed these to stay awake in class. At times, John's speech was pressured, and his legs were in constant motion. When discussing his plans for the future, he would make grandiose, sweeping statements about becoming a senator, never taking into consideration that he had rather poor grades. Instead, he discussed that his "wisdom and good looks would serve him well." He also made references to feeling "sad and that only some people are able to understand me…" He denied any suicidal ideation, and assured me that he would never do anything to hurt himself.

Upon taking a thorough family history, it was discovered that John's father had been arrested on several occasions for drug possession (cocaine). There was also a history of bipolar disorder on his mother's side—his maternal grandmother had been on lithium for many years and was hospitalized twice.

John's father had recently started attending 12-step groups, and when I suggested that it would be wise to have John see a psychopharmacologist to rule out the possibility of bipolar disorder and/or ADHD, his father became irate and stated, "all those shrinks love to label kids and fill them with drugs that they can charge big money for, and I'm not going to have my kid taking anything." I tried to explain that if John were found to have a formal psychiatric diagnosis, he would not be placed on addictive substances but on regulated medications, but the father could not see the difference.

It was decided in light of the father's resistance and the mother's relative passivity, that we would begin by working on motivating John to stop consuming caffeine and encourage him to attend some 12-step adolescent groups, as well as see me weekly, and attend an adolescent after school program. He refused to attend the after school program, but agreed to everything else, including random observed drug screens at home.

After three months of weekly therapy sessions and some attendance at a few open 12-step meetings, all of John's urine screens were clean;

CASE STUDY *(Continued)*

however, his mood had become exceedingly labile and his anxiety had increased (even though he claimed to have completely stopped using caffeine). Finally, John's father was convinced that he might need to see a psychopharmacologist.

Upon referral and assessment, it was decided to first start John on a low dosage of a mood stabilizer (lithium). John was carefully monitored and the psychopharmacologist also took over his drug screens. John continued to attend weekly therapy and after six months there was a noticeable change in his mood, which was much more stable. His school work began to improve slowly, and I was able to begin to work on improving his sense of genuine self-worth by using cognitive restructuring (helping John to learn new ways of thinking about stressful situations), which in turn reinforced new behaviors and also reinforced the new thinking strategies.

John began to want to attend 12-step meetings on a regular basis, and by the time he was accepted to college, he was sober for two years. We made sure that he continued in therapy, by facilitating a referral to the college counseling department, and I continued to see John on college breaks. John's father was not able to get sober and his parents eventually separated.

While cases don't often go this smoothly, this case points to the importance of ruling out co-occurring disorders. It also points to the importance of working with patients where they are in the process—which can be thought of under the general heading of harm reduction, and will be elaborated on further in the next chapter.

chemicals that may be carcinogenic. Perhaps most disturbing is the effect marijuana has on an adolescent's level of motivation, sometimes impacting their goals for years to come.

Inhalants

Inhalants are chemicals often found in household cleaning products, but also include industrial solvents, nitrates, and gases. They are particularly abused by "'tweens" (youngsters between the ages of 10 to 14), but have also been know to be abused by some into their early 20s. Using inhalants is a dangerous practice that can result in brain damage, general nerve damage, and even immediate-onset cardiac arrest, as well as damage to the liver and kidneys.

By spraying aerosols over the nose and mouth ("sniffing"), placing a paper or plastic bag or rag over the mouth and nose ("huffing"), or snapping a capsule that releases a nitrate ("poppers"), youngsters are able to get a cheap high. Some examples of inhalants include: nail polish remover; glue; gasoline; magic markers; whipping cream cans that contain nitrous oxide ("whipped cream hits"); and amyl, butyl, or isobutyl nitrates, sometimes marketed as "rush," or "locker room," which are often utilized during sexual activity to intensify orgasm.

Other Drugs of Abuse

Other drugs of abuse include Ecstasy—a combination of stimulant and hallucinogen—ketamine, and dextromethorphan (found in many cough formulations), which result in a dissociative-like state. Steroids are often abused by young men to build muscles. Additionally, there is also abuse of psychoactive herbs such as *Salvia divinorum*.

ISSUES UNIQUE TO PEDIATRIC AND ADOLESCENT ADDICTION

Alcohol and drug abuse can be devastating to the "'tween" and adolescent, as well as to their family. It is often said that addiction is a family disease, and this is indeed true when it comes to the younger patient as well. Parents see the devastating impact on their children's school work, their socialization patterns, mood, sleep patterns, overall motivation, appetite, physical hygiene, and general familial relations.

Adolescence is a time of great stress. As this book goes to press, there are discussions of restarting a military draft, depleting supplies of money available for school loans, global warming, and the possibility of a devastating economic depression. Is it any wonder that today's youngster is scared of the future and wants to simply get high for a few hours or even stay high?

The competition and pressure to get into a good college is greater than ever. Today's teenager is growing up in a society of immediacy: Food has to be fast, communication is practically instantaneous, information is being shared at rapid rates—it is a full-time job just trying to keep up! I have referred to today's generation of teens as the "microwave generation." When does a teenager sleep? When does a teenager eat? With all the blogs out there, how does a teenager know what is actually reliable information?

Teens see the pressure their parents face as divorce rates are at an all-time high, and when parents do decide to stay together (and not "bail," in the teen vernacular), moms and dads are constantly working, having grown dependent on two incomes. And not just so they can have a boat or vacation home, but so they can pay the mortgage. Parents may tell their children to come to them any time with their problems, that they can tell them anything, but this is impossible because life is simply too busy.

Recently, Joseph Califano, the former Secretary of Health, Education and Welfare under President Carter, stressed the importance of families having dinner together. As the current Chairperson of the National Center on Addiction and Substance Abuse at Columbia University, Califano cited a recent survey that showed that the more frequently families dine together, the less likely adolescents are to have alcohol and drug addiction.

Of course, the fact that we need a research study to inform us to eat a meal as a family is a sad commentary on life in the 21st century. Nevertheless, it is an important finding. As a result of familial tumult, adolescents turn away from their families and toward friends or the Internet, where they learn newer and better ways to self-medicate instead of effective coping strategies or healthy ways to build their resilience to life's psychosocial and environmental stressors.

TREATMENT OF PEDIATRIC AND ADOLESCENT ADDICTION

Early intervention is critical. Parents must not be afraid to approach their children and adolescents about the dangers of tobacco, alcohol, and other drug abuse. This is particularly important for those families where there is a genetic predisposition to the disease of addiction. While there is no set rule on how soon is too soon, parents need to be positive role models, and when they do make a mistake, not try to sweep it under the rug. This must include not just "do as I say," but a general tone in the household that parents are approachable about all questions children and adolescents have whether they are related to smoking, drinking, using drugs, or use of the Internet. This latter point is vital in today's society.

Recent studies have shown that parents may not understand their children's activities on the Internet. Who better to show them than their children? Parents need to say to their adolescents that they want to know about their Internet activities and that they will be looking to them for guidance. This relates to a sense of what this author refers to as "structured or selective autonomy" in the adolescent. Rules must be established about Internet use. Parents today are no longer afforded the "luxury" of worrying solely about their preteen's and teenager's friends, but must also be concerned with their children's virtual friends. Parents must set rules that their children have to use their computers in active areas of the household and make the teens aware their Internet activity will be monitored. This can not be overemphasized.

Finding Help and Starting Treatment

Hopefully, parents can avoid the need to seek treatment for their children by taking preventative measures. But even the most well-intentioned parents could find themselves needing professional advice. Parents must understand that there are many types of treatment options available. One of the best things for them to do is speak with other parents about their experiences. There are myriad support groups that can be located through school counseling departments, community agencies, and the Internet (eg, the National Institute on Drug Abuse: *http://www.nida.nih.gov/* or The National Counsel on Alcoholism and Drug Dependence: *http://www.ncadd.org/*). Parents should always make sure they are dealing with licensed or credentialed professionals with extensive experience in not only alcohol counseling and drug treatment, but also in mental health and co-occurring disorder treatment.

Each child and adolescent is a unique individual and must be treated as such. There are so many different types of programs for treating substance abuse, as well as levels of treatment (ie, individual, group, out-patient, inpatient). The adolescent must be treated with respect and dignity; this is not a time for angry accusations. Often, defense mechanisms play a large part in how the identified patient reacts, and also how the parents and other siblings react. Denial, projection, and rationalization are very common among identified patients and family members, and must be dealt with in a firm but caring way (this will be discussed in great detail in the chapter on engaging cooperation from teen patients).

Perhaps the most important thing that parents must do first is take their child for what is referred to in the field as a comprehensive biopsychosocial evaluation. This would include the completion of a thorough anamnesis (a complete history recalled and recounted by the patient) that looks at addiction on both sides of the identified patient's family as well as psychiatric history. Collateral information is always important and should preferably (when possible) include parents, as well as brothers and sisters, grandparents, aunts and uncles, friends, teachers, etc. The information gathered should look at medical history, psychiatric history, drug and alcohol history, academic history, and social history.

Once this clinical information is developed, a picture will emerge that will dictate the level of care required—whether inpatient or outpatient detoxification is needed; inpatient versus outpatient rehabilitation; the focus of the treatment—addiction issues as well as mental health issues; the necessity of educational remediation; the necessity of psychopharmacology and, if so, for how long; and the length and intensity of the treatment.

Length of stay in treatment must be gauged carefully. It is important when determining length of stay to ensure that each patient's plan is individualized. Generally speaking, individuals begin to show signs of improvement as they complete 90 days in treatment, depending on their specific diagnosis(es). For example, if an individual is an alcohol abuser, but does not have any other complications, either physical or mental, their length of stay in an inpatient setting would be expected to be shorter when compared with a person with bipolar disorder and polysubstance abuse. Research studies have long shown both physiological as well as environmental issues as responsible for this time frame. With regard to environmental issues, a teenager may be the victim of physical or sexual abuse in their home, dealing with a parent's or parents' psychiatric or substance abuse issues, or dealing with a legal issue. Some residential programs will last up to 18 months and decrease in intensity (ie, supervision) as the individual becomes more responsible for his or her own sobriety.

Payment for treatment is also a consideration of length of stay no matter how offensive this may be to society's sensibilities.

Realities of Treatment

Regardless of the treatment program, there are always some "mainstays" for all addiction treatment. Teenagers who abuse substances, like their adult counterparts, are not always the most truthful, and should be breathalyzed and urine tested. They must learn to develop new and effective coping strategies that result in sober behaviors. If a teen is not motivated to engage in treatment, they must form a dialogue with the counselor that results in what Prochaska and colleagues have referred to as "readiness to change." It must also be understood that addiction is a disease—it is primary, progressive, chronic, and, if not treated, fatal. There is no cure; remission and relapse are always an issue. Therefore, relapse prevention strategies must be learned. Part of this process involves staying in the moment and developing a network of supportive, sober friends. This can often be accomplished by attending 12-step support groups as well as attending treatment, and should always be considered an important adjunct in treatment and discharge planning.

It should be noted that group therapy is generally the accepted form of therapy for addiction; although, more and more treatment programs are adding individual treatment as cases become exceedingly complicated and the group format is negatively impacted by the heterogeneity of the population. I have been a great proponent of what I term "functional homogeneity" versus "diagnostic heterogeneity." Simply stated, it is more important for a group of teens to function at the same level than it is for them to all carry the same or similar diagnosis(es). This can actually make the group a fertile ground for learning about others and developing and nurturing mutual respect.

HOW TO ENGAGE COOPERATION FROM TEEN PATIENTS IN TREATING ADDICTION

OVERVIEW

The impact of alcohol and illegal drug use on teens simply costs too much in terms of the actual loss of lives for society to ignore the problem. We cannot simply rationalize that it is part of normal developmental experimentation.

The previous chapter showed the critical importance of early intervention. The younger the preteen or adolescent, the greater the danger that a full-blown addiction will result. Counselors have a very difficult task in that they must be able to engage the patient while at the same time breaking through denial, projection, and rationalization. There is no one treatment style that will satisfy every individual's needs. One must consider the patient and how they came to enter treatment. Was he involved in a formal intervention (something popularized by reality television recently)? Did she come through the legal system (which may also speak to her personality)? Did his parents or school force the issue, or perhaps he came on his own?

Eric Erickson, in his psychosocial stages of development, stated that the first thing an infant must learn is "basic trust"—the development of trust leads to hope. Likewise, the addicted teen must learn to trust his or her therapist. Without trust, there is no chance or hope of recovery.

ESTABLISHING RAPPORT AND ENGENDERING COOPERATION

When a teen shows up at your door, regardless of whether you work in an outpatient or inpatient facility, be it primarily addiction or mental health (although one would hope that today's clinician has been trained in both), as the counselor, you have only one task at hand: you must engage that teen. While it is important to take a thorough history, and when the time is right, speak with collaterals, the most important task is enlisting the cooperation of that youngster. This does not mean you are there to entertain them, but it does mean that you have to make a connection.

Over the last 30 years, I have developed a style of therapy called "carefrontation.*'" Simply stated, it says that every individual must be treated with respect; no shame or blame should ever be involved. However, it also states that the patient must be held responsible for dealing with his or her illness. This pertains to either addiction or mental health issues.

As an example, consider a teen who abuses alcohol but has no other comorbidities (although there is no longer such a thing as "uncomplicated addiction"). It has been shown that addiction is a disease. Based upon this premise, the addicted person is not a client, but a patient. Someone who is ill should not be treated disrespectfully in the name of breaking through denial. Indeed, confrontation can raise someone's defenses and often leads to resistance. Even though the example here is "simple" alcohol abuse, there are always psychological aspects to every case. Why would one risk using a confrontational approach with someone who may be psychologically unstable? Empathy is always better.

The counselor must be caring and convey that he "hears" the patient, respects what they are saying, but at the same time know that the disease of addiction is complicated and often victimizes the person who has it, driving them to lie, to blame others, and to concoct explanations to hide behind.

The carefrontation model looks to empower patients by letting them know they can deal with their "illness" and rely on others to help (what Rotter and others have called "an internal and external locus of control"). They have the ability to choose to treat their illness by working in tandem with the counselor who will help them develop what Prochaska and colleagues referred to as "readiness to change"—a motivational model that leads to the patient taking "action" (stopping the active addiction) and ultimately going on to "maintaining" that behavior.

This method does not fly in the face of what has become a popular term, "tough love." What could be tougher than to deal with an addiction or co-occurring disorder? What could be more loving than to make sure you don't allow your teen to suffer in silence, but instead make sure they get the help they need by engaging them in a dialogue? If a teen is resistant, then the parents must make sure to understand that their first responsibility as parents is to help their child. Parents are not their son's and daughter's buddies; they are their parents first and foremost. But that does not mean that the adolescent should feel they cannot come to their parents with any problem they might be having. It is a parent's responsibility to watch out for their child's welfare, and it is the child's responsibility to yield their parent's direction. When this give and take breaks down, then the carefrontation model states that in order for parents to treat their teens with respect and dignity and not shame or blame them for an illness, they must not give up on them but do whatever they can to get them the help they need.

As the teen becomes trusting and comfortable with the counselor, they will begin to become more open and honest. Teens welcome direction and therapists must utilize this fact to help engage the teen patient. Addiction treatment for all individuals, including teens, must be multifaceted. This includes a comprehensive workup to establish a diagnosis(es), including getting the answers to the following questions:

- What is going on biologically?
- Are there any medical issues?
- What is happening psychologically?
- Is there a concomitant psychiatric clinical syndrome?
- Is there a personality issue?
- Has there been psychological damage in the form of physical, sexual, or verbal abuse?
- What is going on for the teen socially? Is she hanging out with a new peer group because she was rejected by another peer group? Did the rejection come about because the teen was doing alcohol and/or drugs, or did it come about because she was resisting, only ironically to lead her to use alcohol and drugs and hang out with a more drug-oriented peer group?

ISSUES UNIQUE TO PEDIATRIC AND ADOLESCENT PATIENTS

Perhaps there is no group of individuals more affected by concerns over being stigmatized than "'tweens" and teens. And with good reason. Regardless of the fact that addiction is a disease, because of the way individuals act under the influence, it is still seen as a moral failing associated with underachievement, lack of motivation, and general inability to control one's life. Why would a teen want to admit that they have a problem if it would embroil them in such controversy? Even if their peers use alcohol and drugs, if their own use results in being recommended for treatment, it elevates "recreational" use to a whole new level.

In my own experience, when I recommend attendance at 12-step meetings, an outpatient program, or inpatient treatment, my teen patients recoil. I hear things like, "losers," "weak," "never," "not into religion," "my parents don't have that kind of money," and finally, "I am not coming to see you anymore."

Thus, it is important that the counselor proceed slowly. Remember that teens are developing on so many levels, which while a good thing also makes treating them so unique. On one hand, we want to nurture their autonomy, see them blossom into the future leaders of the world. But on the other hand, as stated earlier, if a teen is using alcohol and drugs, affecting the development of their brains, robbing themselves of a future, how can we allow that to go on? So if they are seeing a counselor, we are *not* allowing it to go on. This may be viewed as "harm reduction," which has become a negative term. But the reality is that "harm reduction" embraces all treatment. Indeed, the greatest example of the harm reduction model is Alcoholics Anonymous, which embraces the credo of a "desire to stop drinking," knowing full well that as long as the alcoholic is willing to attend a meeting, there is a chance that they will stop drinking.

CASE STUDY

Joanne was 17 when she was asked to see me by her parents and school, after she got drunk at a school dance. She was very resistant to treatment and felt as though she were being singled out. Her parents were both recovering alcoholics, and despite their constant warnings to her about the dangers of addiction in the family, she ignored them.

When she was brought to my office, she was binge drinking vodka and beer on weekends. She was resistant to discussing amounts, and we didn't force the issue in the first session. By the third session she was willing to discuss not only the amount of alcohol she consumed on the weekends, but also the fact that she was smoking marijuana and had experimented with Ecstasy and cocaine.

We established a very clear understanding and a written contract was drawn up saying that she would see me weekly and would try going to an AA meeting. While she would not to commit to giving up alcohol, she did agree to not smoke marijuana or to use any other drugs. She also agreed to random drug screens.

Joanne had a strong desire to be a fashion designer and I saw that as an opportunity to introduce her to a female college student majoring in fashion who attended AA and had been sober for five years. Joanne was very open to this and began attending AA and slowly developing a network of sober friends through the self-help program, as well as at school.

By the time she began college, she had been abstinent for almost a year from all substances.

In preparing this chapter, I spoke with Joanne recently, who was gracious enough to relate what helped her to get sober:

"When my parents brought me to your office the fact that you didn't force rules down my throat really helped me relate to you. I mean I saw you as another authority figure at first, but then after awhile I felt like I could talk to you. You didn't threaten me and you showed me that you would keep your word and I could trust you. Also, you were willing to discuss facts about addiction with me and not try to intimidate me like the DARE program tried to do. I also liked it when you showed a real interest by introducing me to Grace (name has been changed), who brought me to some meetings and showed me that I could accomplish my goals."

Abstinence must always be the goal of addiction treatment, but when dealing with individuals, progress comes in steps. The counselor must contract with the teen patient. They must explain choices and agree to the goal of complete abstinence within appropriate timeframes. In my own practice, this is where the concept of "selective autonomy" comes into play. The adolescent is offered alternative treatment levels to choose from. This way they are an active partner in their treatment; their autonomy is not being thwarted, but their potential inability to set up their own treatment options is being addressed by a professional.

TREATMENT OF ADDICTION

There are so many different ways to treat addiction in "'tweens" and adolescents. However, there are some commonalities across all levels and styles of treatment.

It has already been noted that therapeutic alliance is the most important variable in treatment. Without a trusting relationship between the adolescent and treatment professional, there simply is no hope of a good outcome. The teen must come to know that their opinion is clearly heard and understood, but that does not mean it is the only opinion. I often like to say to all of my patients, but particularly teens, that I work for them, but they hired me because I have the expertise to help them make informed decisions. If they come back at me with, "my parents hired you…" I reinforce that they are my patient and that the process of therapy is between the two of us. The constant reinforcement of getting the teen to take ownership of the therapeutic process is vital.

Cognitive restructuring, which has already been discussed, is highly effective in helping teens look at things from a new perspective. It raises new concepts and ideas and helps the adolescent engage in an intellectual process that is very empowering—new thoughts lead to new behaviors which in turn reinforce new ways of thinking. Cognitive therapy does not mean that insight into certain behaviors is not also effective and necessary. However, the two are not mutually exclusive.

At times, depending on one's diagnosis(es), medication may be necessary, but this should not be rushed into or approached lightly. The identified patient must have a say in this process as well, or they will feel, and rightfully so, unheard. Often, it is a very valuable technique for the psychopharmacologist and the therapist to meet with the teen alone, and then with their parents, to discuss medication options. Indeed, that is why it is so important for nonmedical clinicians to have a working knowledge of the various medications that are available. This process always leads to a clearer treatment course that circumnavigates the defense mechanism of splitting that teenagers so often utilize.

When working with children and adolescents, it is important to look at systems. Of course, the family is one system, and all members of the family should be engaged in some process that allows them to discuss their feelings. Self-help programs can be quite effective in this area. The educational system is another area that is important to consider. It is very helpful for the counselor and the school guidance department to be in touch with one another.

If the adolescent requires inpatient care, it is vital that the outpatient therapist maintain an ongoing dialogue with the inpatient treatment team, so that there is no confusion upon discharge.

SUMMARY

Treating adolescent addiction is very complicated. It involves well-informed clinicians who are looking for reasons and ways to keep adolescents engaged in treatment, and not looking to kick them out for not being immediately ready to put down the drink or the drug. While the goal has to be complete abstinence, it takes time to get there.

Comprehensive assessment over time must occur, and can only occur if a trusting relationship is established between the counselor and the identified adolescent patient. Caring must be the foundation of this therapeutic alliance. I don't feel that "in your face therapy" works, and in a time when adolescents often have complicated diagnostic pictures, there simply is no place for this type of antiquated treatment method. Instead, empowering the patient to take responsibility for dealing with his or her illness must be the rule rather than the exception.

*Carefrontation was developed by Harris Stratyner, PhD, CASAC, during his many years as a practicing clinician.

Street Drug Profiles

Part 1.
Commercial Products

AEROSOLS AND GASES

COMMON STREET NAMES: Air blast, discorama, huff, laughing gas, moon gas, Oz, toncho, whippets
DEA CLASS: Not classified
PHARMACOLOGIC CLASS: Inhalants

Description: Except for medical anesthetics, aerosols and gases are not classified as drugs because they are not manufactured for pharmacologic use. Abused substances include household and commercial products such as butane lighters, propane tanks, and refrigerant gases; household aerosol propellants such as spray paints, hair or deodorant sprays, cooking oil, whipping cream, and fabric protectors; and medical anesthetic gases such as ether, chloroform, halothane, and nitrous oxide or "laughing gas." Most of these products produce short-term psychoactive effects similar to alcohol.

Method of use: Inhaled through the mouth or nose. In addition to inhaling directly from aerosol cans, users sniff the fumes from a plastic bag or through a cloth saturated with the substance (known as huffing). Users also inhale directly from balloons filled with nitrous oxide.

Duration of action: Onset is rapid but effects last only a short time. Inhaled nitrous oxide is rapidly eliminated by the lungs as unchanged gas.

Psychological effects: Aggressive behavior, apathy, delusions, distorted perception of reality, euphoria, hallucinations, impaired thinking and spatial judgment, loss of coordination, and loss of inhibition.

Physical effects: Depressed reflexes, dizziness, drowsiness, gait disturbance, head rush, headache, inattentiveness, limb spasm, loss of equilibrium and coordination, loss of sensation, nausea, rapid heartbeat followed by lethargy, slurred speech, vomiting, and wheezing. Long-term use may cause irreversible brain or nervous system damage, hearing loss, certain types of anemia, and bone marrow damage. Frequent use can cause tolerance and physical dependence. Serious burn injuries were reported because of the highly flammable nature of these products.

Overdose symptoms: Because these products are short-acting, users tend to inhale the fumes repeatedly for several hours, which increases the risk of overdosing. Symptoms may include impaired muscle tone, numbness and tingling in the extremities, respiratory depression, and heart and lung damage. Chronic exposure may induce heart failure and death within minutes of use, known as sudden sniffing death (SSD). High concentrations of inhalants can cause death from suffocation by displacing oxygen in the lungs. Nitrous oxide may cause sudden death by restricting oxygen to the brain. Death is usually related to asphyxia rather than a specific nitrous oxide level.

Withdrawal symptoms: Withdrawal symptoms may develop within several hours to a few days after the last use. Symptoms may include profuse sweating, rapid pulse, weight loss, disorientation, irritability, depression, sleeplessness, nausea, vomiting, physical agitation, anxiety, tremors, hallucinations, and seizures.

ALCOHOL

COMMON STREET NAMES: Booze, hooch
DEA CLASS: Not classified
PHARMACOLOGIC CLASS: CNS depressant

Description: Alcohol is a liquid made by yeast fermentation of carbohydrates such as grain or fruit. There are many varieties of alcohol, but ethanol (ethyl alcohol) is the type used to make alcoholic beverages and the one that is most commonly abused.

Method of use: Ingested

Duration of action: Onset and duration depend on various factors: the amount ingested, the type(s) of alcohol used, whether it was taken with or without food, and whether the individual is a chronic or occasional user.

Detection in blood screening: Alcohol use is best confirmed by breath or blood analysis. Blood alcohol content (BAC) helps determine the individual's intoxication level. BAC is influenced by the individual's weight, gender, height, tolerance, how quickly the alcohol was consumed, and whether it was taken with or without food. Most of the alcohol consumed is processed by the liver. A healthy liver metabolizes about 0.015 grams per deciliter per hour, which means that three-fourths of an ounce of pure alcohol is metabolized in 2 hours (this is equivalent to one 5-ounce glass of wine, one 12-ounce can of beer, or one 1.5-ounce shot of hard liquor). If the BAC is more than 100 milligrams per deciliter, the individual is considered intoxicated. Heavy drinkers have more active livers and may be able to metabolize up to three drinks an hour.

Psychological effects: Initial effects may include confusion, euphoria, and a false sense of well-being, which is replaced by anxiety, restlessness, mood changes, and depression as the BAC increases. Chronic use can cause psychological dependence.

Physical effects: Chronic alcohol abuse may cause anemia and other blood disorders, color-blindness, constipation, diarrhea, elevated blood pressure, inflammation of the pancreas, inflammation of the stomach lining, irregular heart rhythm, liver damage, low blood sugar, muscle weakness, and seizures. Chronic use can cause tolerance and physical dependence.

Overdose symptoms: The effects of alcohol intoxication vary among users. Some individuals may become intoxicated at a much lower BAC than others. The following data are based on clinical studies:

1. BAC of 0.02-0.03: Slight euphoria and loss of shyness.
2. BAC of 0.04-0.06: Sense of well-being, relaxation, lowered inhibitions, euphoria, and minor impairment of memory.
3. BAC of 0.07-0.09: Slight impairment of balance, speech, vision, reaction time, memory, and hearing. Loss of judgment and self-control are also noticeable at this stage.
4. BAC of 0.10-0.125: Significant impairment of balance, motor coordination, vision, speech, reaction time, and hearing. Euphoria is still apparent.
5. BAC of 0.13-0.15: Lack of physical control, blurred vision, and major loss of balance. Euphoria is reduced and replaced by anxiety and restlessness.
6. BAC of 0.16-0.20: Significant anxiety and restlessness, glossy eyes, and nausea. Pupils are slow to respond to stimuli.
7. BAC of 0.25: Significant anxiety and restlessness, nausea and vomiting, irregular "drunken" gait, loss of fine motor coordination, and mental confusion.
8. BAC of 0.30: Loss of consciousness.
9. BAC of 0.40 and up: Onset of stupor, coma, and possibly death due to respiratory depression.

Other symptoms of intoxication include constricted pupils, decreased heart rate, low blood pressure and respiration rate, diminished reflexes, and profuse sweating. Binge drinking is the most dangerous way to get severely intoxicated and is alarmingly prevalent among high school and college students. A binge is usually defined as having four or more drinks (for women) or five or more drinks (for men) in about 2 hours.

Withdrawal symptoms: Abruptly stopping use may cause strong alcohol cravings, nausea, excessive sweating, shakiness, depression, mood changes, headache, insomnia, unstable heart rate or blood pressure, tremors, anxiety or panic attacks, confusion and/or hallucinations (delirium tremens), and in extreme cases, seizures.

NITRITES (nonprescription products)

COMMON STREET NAMES: Ames, Amys, aroma of men, bolt, boppers, climax, hardware, pearls, poppers, quicksilver, rush, snappers, thrust, whiteout
DEA CLASS: Not classified
PHARMACOLOGIC CLASS: Inhalants

Description: Nitrites are volatile liquids that are readily absorbed from the lungs. Unlike other inhalants, they work primarily by dilating blood vessels and relaxing the muscles. Amyl nitrite and glyceryl trinitrate are used medically to treat acute chest pain (angina) and severe heart murmurs (see the prescription nitrites entry listed on page 484. Industrial nitrites that are reportedly abused are cyclohexyl nitrite, an ingredient found in room deodorizers, and butyl nitrite, which was used previously in the manufacturing of perfumes and antifreeze but is now considered illegal. Most of these products are used as sexual enhancers.

Method of use: Inhaled through the mouth or nose. In addition to inhaling directly from aerosol cans, users sniff the fumes from a plastic bag or through a cloth saturated with the substance (known as huffing).

Duration of action: Onset is rapid but effects last only a short time, usually 30 to 60 minutes.

Psychological effects: Loss of inhibition, distorted perception of reality, aggressive behavior, apathy, impaired judgment, euphoria, hallucinations, loss of coordination, and delusions.

Physical effects: Rapid heartbeat followed by lethargy, head rush, headaches, nausea, vomiting, slurred speech, loss of coordination, and wheezing. Frequent use can cause tolerance and physical dependence. Serious but reversible physical effects may include liver or kidney damage and blood oxygen depletion. Chronic use can cause serious damage to the heart and lungs and suppress the immune system, increasing the risk of infection. Prolonged use can also lead to poor muscle tone, muscle wasting, and numbness and tingling in the extremities.

Overdose symptoms: Because these products are short-acting, users tend to inhale the fumes repeatedly for several hours, which increases the risk of overdosing. Prolonged inhalation of nitrites may cause irregular and rapid heart rhythm, heart failure, and death within minutes of use.

Withdrawal symptoms: Abrupt discontinuation of use may cause sweating, rapid pulse, hand tremors, insomnia, nausea, vomiting, physical agitation, anxiety, hallucinations, and seizures.

Part 2.
Over-the-Counter Drugs

DEXTROMETHORPHAN
BRAND NAMES: Delsym, Robitussin DM, Benylin DM, Triaminic DM, Vicks 44 Cough Relief, and others
COMMON STREET NAMES: Robotripping, Robo, Triple C, Snurf
DEA CLASS: Not classified
PHARMACOLOGIC CLASS: Antitussive

Description: This medication is indicated for the temporary symptomatic relief of nonproductive cough occurring with colds and inhaled irritants. There are many cough and cold combination products that contain dextromethorphan as an active ingredient.

Method of use: Ingested

Duration of action: The antitussive effects last up to 6 hours.

Psychological effects of abuse: Subjective effects reported with abuse of dextromethorphan include euphoria, floating/flying sensation, hallucinations (auditory and visual), increased self-awareness, increased perception, increased sense of self, increased sociability, modification of sounds, and synesthesia (association of sounds with color). Other mental and emotional effects associated with dextromethorphan abuse include anxiety, panic, dysphoria, depression, fear of sleep, loss of memory, forgetfulness, stupor, confusion, restlessness, agitation, irritability, paranoia, and psychosis. May result in drug abuse or dependency, although this is very infrequent.

Physical effects of abuse: Euphoria and restlessness, persisting for 15 minutes to 2 hours, followed by depression, tiredness, and dizziness. Some other effects include nausea, vomiting, drowsiness, and fatigue (with chronic use).

Overdose symptoms: CNS effects are more prevalent and include shakiness and unsteady walk, blurred vision, coma, confusion, drowsiness or dizziness, respiratory depression, severe nausea and vomiting, unusual excitement, restlessness, irritability, and difficulty in urination.

Withdrawal symptoms: Abrupt discontinuation is not associated with physical withdrawal symptoms; however, intense cravings for the drug have been reported.

It should be noted that a pill sold over the Internet as an herbal supplement called "snurf" has been found to contain mostly dextromethorphan. It is marketed as having hallucinogenic properties.

DIMENHYDRINATE

BRAND NAME: Dramamine, Driminate
DEA CLASS: Not classified
PHARMACOLOGIC CLASS: Antihistamine

Description: Dimenhydrinate is primarily used in the prevention and treatment of vertigo, motion sickness, and nausea and vomiting during pregnancy.

Method of use: Ingested

Duration of action: The antiemetic effects last 3 to 6 hours.

Psychological effects of abuse: Abuse of dimenhydrinate has resulted in psychotic-like reactions, including delirium and hallucinations.

Physical effects of abuse: Hypertension, increased heart rate, and drying of mucous membranes. Dimenhydrinate may frequently be used by women with anorexia or bulimia, because of the drug's sedative, anorexic, and emetic properties.

Overdose symptoms: Overdose may result in CNS depression and/or stimulation and may resemble anticholinergic overdose. Effects may include fixed and dilated pupils, flushed face, dry mouth, excitation, hallucinations, and tonic-clonic seizures. In young children, CNS stimulation is the predominant overdose symptom.

Withdrawal symptoms: Withdrawal of the drug resulted in enhanced excitability, increased heart rate, hypertension, and mydriasis.

DIPHENHYDRAMINE

BRAND NAMES: Benadryl, Benylin Decongestant Cough, Diphenhist, Diphenyl, Nytol, and others
DEA CLASS: Not classified
PHARMACOLOGIC CLASS: Antihistamine

Description: Diphenhydramine is an antihistamine with many therapeutic applications. Some oral dosage forms are available without a prescription for use as an antitussive, a nighttime sleep aid, or to relieve allergy symptoms. There are many combination products that contain diphenhydramine as an active ingredient.

Method of use: Ingested

Duration of action: Effects have been noted to last 4 to 6 hours.

Psychological effects of abuse: Anticholinergic side effects such as insomnia, tremors, nervousness, psychomotor agitation, and dyskinesias. A combination of butorphanol and diphenhydramine is being increasingly used as a drug of abuse. Tolerance develops and progressively higher doses are needed to reach the desired state, which is described as "being on the nod."

Physical effects of abuse: Sedation and mild euphoria, irritability, palpitations, blurred vision, constipation, urinary retention, tachycardia, and dryness of the mouth, nose and throat.

Overdose symptoms: The following symptoms have been observed: **Mild/Moderate:** tachycardia, dry flushed skin, hallucinations, mydriasis, decreased bowel sounds, urinary retention. **Severe:** seizures, coma, electrocardiogram QRS-wave widening, dysrhythmias, torsades de pointes. **Rare:** rhabdomyolysis, renal failure.

Withdrawal symptoms: Chronic abuse has resulted in withdrawal symptoms, including recurrence of insomnia, increased daytime restlessness, irritability and excessive blinking

Part 3.
Prescription Drugs

ACETAMINOPHEN WITH CODEINE PHOSPHATE
BRAND NAME: Tylenol with Codeine
COMMON STREET NAMES: Dreamer, God's drug, mister blue
DEA CLASS: Class III (tablets) and Class V (suspensions and elixirs)
PHARMACOLOGIC CLASS: Antipyretic analgesic, narcotic analgesic

Description: This medication is a fixed-dose combination of acetaminophen, an antipyretic (fever-reducing) analgesic; and codeine, a narcotic analgesic. It is prescribed for the relief of mild to moderately severe pain.

Method of use: Ingested

Duration of action: The analgesic effects usually last 4 to 6 hours after ingestion.

Psychological effects of abuse: Euphoria alternating with depression, confusion, nervousness, and hallucinations. The psychological dependence associated with narcotic addiction is complex. Long after physical dependence has ended, the addict may continue to think and talk about the drug and feel unable to manage daily activities without it.

Physical effects of abuse: Light-headedness, dizziness, nausea, vomiting, constipation, stomach discomfort, shortness of breath, and elevated blood pressure. Physical dependence can occur after prolonged use. Chronic use of acetaminophen is associated with liver damage. Abusing codeine may lead to breathing difficulties followed by respiratory arrest.

Overdose symptoms: Tolerance develops rapidly, and the progressively higher doses needed are often in the toxic range. Acute acetaminophen overdose can potentially result in fatal liver toxicity. Early symptoms include nausea, vomiting, sweating, and weakness. Clinical and laboratory evidence of liver toxicity may not be apparent until 48 to 72 hours after ingestion.

Overdose symptoms related to codeine include cold and clammy skin, severe drowsiness, constricted pupils, severe weakness, low blood pressure, respiratory depression, and coma.

Withdrawal symptoms: Although withdrawal is painful physically and emotionally, it is rarely life-threatening if adequate hydration and nutritional support are maintained. Withdrawal symptoms are similar to those of morphine but are considerably less intense. Abruptly stopping use can cause excessive tearing, yawning, and sweating in about 12 to 14 hours after the last dose. Additional symptoms may include diminished appetite, irritability, tremor, seizures, and loss of consciousness.

Adderall *see Dextroamphetamine, page 98*

Adipex-P *see Phentermine, page 146*

ALPRAZOLAM
BRAND NAME: Xanax
COMMON STREET NAMES: Candy, downers, sleeping pills, tranks, xanies
DEA CLASS: Class IV
PHARMACOLOGIC CLASS: Benzodiazepine, antianxiety

Description: Alprazolam is used to treat anxiety disorders with or without depression, acute stress reactions such as anxiety prior to surgery, and panic attacks with or without irrational fear. Abuse of benzodiazepines is particularly high among heroin and cocaine users.

Method of use: Ingested

Duration of action: 6 to 12 hours, but may persist longer in obese individuals.

Psychological effects of abuse: Amnesia, depression, difficulty concentrating, diminished sexual desire, impaired judgment, reduced inhibition, pressured speech, and suicidal ideation. Paradoxical reactions may include aggressive and agitated behavior. Prolonged use leads to psychological dependence and may cause behavior problems such as extreme aggression and hostility.

Physical effects of abuse: Change in appetite, constipation, difficulty urinating, dizziness, impaired muscle coordination, irregular gait, lightheadedness, low blood pressure, menstrual irregularities, and slurred speech. Long-term use may cause physical dependence.

Overdose symptoms: The most severe signs of overdose are respiratory depression and loss of consciousness. Other symptoms may include confusion, rapid and slurred speech, extreme sleepiness, diminished reflexes, and loss of muscle coordination. Death from overdose of a single benzodiazepine is extremely rare. However, there is an increased risk of toxicity when benzodiazepines are combined with alcohol and/or other CNS depressants. Fatalities have been reported in individuals who have overdosed with a combination of a single benzodiazepine and alcohol.

Withdrawal symptoms: Abrupt termination following long-term use may precipitate withdrawal symptoms and require hospitalization. Symptoms may include abdominal and muscle cramps, depression, insomnia, sweating, vomiting, tremors, and seizures.

Alurate *see Aprobarbital, page 87*

Ambien *see Zolpidem, page 159*

AMOBARBITAL SODIUM
BRAND NAME: Amytal sodium
COMMON STREET NAMES: Blue heavens, dolls, downers, goofballs, M&Ms, rainbows, red and blues, red devils, yellows
DEA CLASS: Class II
PHARMACOLOGIC CLASS: Barbiturate, hypnotic, sedative, anticonvulsant

Description: Barbiturates depress the sensory cortex, decrease motor activity, alter brain function, and produce drowsiness, sedation, and hypnosis. Amobarbital is used for the short-term treatment of insomnia. It is also used as a sedating agent for reducing anxiety prior to surgery.

Method of use: Injected IV or IM

Duration of action: 6 to 8 hours following a standard therapeutic dose.

Psychological effects of abuse: Barbiturates can cause psychological dependence, especially following prolonged use of high doses. Principal psychological effects include confusion, alternating euphoria and depression, and memory loss.

Physical effects of abuse: The most frequent physical effects are due to CNS depression, including dizziness, headache, excessive sleepiness, drowsiness, and irregular gait. Other physical symptoms may include headache, stomach pain, and skin rash. Paradoxical excitement and irritability may also occur. In chronic users, blood disorders such as megaloblastic anemia may develop. Physical dependence is a significant risk, since it can develop after short-term use.

Overdose symptoms: Overdosing with amobarbital may result in severe CNS depression. Initial symptoms include eye gazing, contracted pupils, slurred speech, irregular gait, and interrupted breathing. More serious overdose may result in respiratory and cardiovascular depression, severely low blood pressure and body temperature, coma, and shock that can lead to death. Reddish, bleeding blisters ("barb-burns") may occur on the hands, buttocks, and back of knees in about 6 percent of users; however, barbiturate overdose is not the sole cause of such blisters. All harmful effects are enhanced when barbiturates are taken with alcohol and/or other CNS depressants.

Withdrawal symptoms: Amobarbital is one of the most commonly abused barbiturates. Symptoms are similar to those of alcohol withdrawal and characterized by severe apprehension, weakness, elevated anxiety, irritability, dizziness, headache, sleeplessness, muscle twitching, nausea and vomiting, distortion of visual perception, and rapid pulse. Severely low blood pressure and convulsions may develop after a day or two, which eventually leads to hallucinations, delirium, and continuous seizures, followed by coma and death.

AMOBARBITAL AND SECOBARBITAL

COMMON STREET NAMES: Dolls, downers, goofballs, M&Ms, rainbows, red and blues, red birds, red devils, yellows
DEA CLASS: Class II
PHARMACOLOGIC CLASS: Barbiturate

Not commercially available in the U.S.

Description: Barbiturates depress the sensory cortex, decrease motor activity, alter brain function, and produce drowsiness, sedation, and hypnosis. This drug combination is used as a sedative to relieve anxiety before surgery and as a supplemental agent for the short-term treatment of insomnia.

Method of use: Ingested

Duration of action: 6 to 8 hours following a standard therapeutic dose.

Psychological effects of abuse: Barbiturates may cause psychological dependence, especially following prolonged use of high doses. Psychological effects may include confusion, alternating euphoria and depression, and memory loss.

Physical effects of abuse: The most frequent physical effects are due to CNS depression, including dizziness, headache, excessive sleepiness, drowsiness, and irregular gait. Other symptoms may include headache, stomach pain, and skin rash. Paradoxical excitement and irritability may also occur. In chronic users, blood disorders such as megaloblastic anemia may develop. Physical dependence is a significant risk, since it can develop after short-term use.

Overdose symptoms: Overdosing with this drug may result in severe CNS depression. Initial symptoms include eye gazing, constricted pupils, slurred speech, irregular gait, and interrupted breathing. More serious overdose may result in respiratory and cardiovascular depression, severely low blood pressure and body temperature, coma, and shock that can lead to death. Reddish, bleeding blisters ("barb-burns") may occur on the hands, buttocks, and back of the knees in about 6 percent of users; however, barbiturate overdose is not the sole cause of such blisters. All harmful effects are enhanced when barbiturates are taken with alcohol and/or other CNS depressants.

Withdrawal symptoms: Amobarbital, one of the ingredients in Tuinal, is a commonly abused barbiturate. Symptoms are similar to those of alcohol withdrawal and characterized by severe apprehension, weakness, elevated anxiety, irritability, dizziness, headache, sleeplessness, muscle twitching, nausea and vomiting, distortion of visual perception, and rapid pulse. Severely low blood pressure and convulsions may develop after a day or two, which eventually leads to hallucinations, delirium, and continuous seizures, followed by coma and death.

Amytal *see Amobarbital, page 85*

Anadrol *see Oxymetholone, page 138*

Android *see Methyltestosterone, page 125*

Anolor *see Butalbital, page 89*

APROBARBITAL

COMMON STREET NAMES: Dolls, downers, goofballs, M&Ms, rainbows, red and blues, red devils, yellows

DEA CLASS: Class III

PHARMACOLOGIC CLASS: Barbiturate, hypnotic, sedative

Description: Aprobarbital is used for the short-term treatment of insomnia. It is also used as a sedating agent for reducing anxiety prior to surgery.

Method of use: Ingested

Duration of action: About 6 to 8 hours following a standard therapeutic dose.

Psychological effects of abuse: Barbiturates may cause psychological dependence, especially following prolonged use of high doses. Principal psychological effects may include confusion, alternating euphoria and depression, and memory loss.

Physical effects of abuse: The most frequent physical effects are due to CNS depression, including dizziness, headache, excessive sleepiness, drowsiness, and irregular gait. Other symptoms may include headache, stomach pain, and skin rash. Paradoxical excitement and irritability may also occur. In chronic users, blood disorders such as megaloblastic anemia may develop. Physical dependence is a significant risk, since it can develop after short-term use.

Overdose symptoms: Overdosing with aprobarbital can cause severe CNS depression. Initial symptoms may include eye gazing, contracted pupils, slurred speech, irregular gait, and interrupted breathing. More serious overdose may result in respiratory and cardiovascular depression, severely low blood pressure and body temperature, coma, and shock that can lead to death. Reddish, bleeding blisters ("barb-burns") may occur on the hands, buttocks, and back of knees in about 6 percent of users; however, barbiturate overdose is not the sole cause of such blisters. All harmful effects are enhanced when barbiturates are taken with alcohol and/or other CNS depressants.

Withdrawal symptoms: Aprobarbital is one of the most commonly abused barbiturates. Symptoms are similar to those of alcohol withdrawal and characterized by severe apprehension, weakness, elevated anxiety, irritability, dizziness, headache, sleeplessness, muscle twitching, nausea and vomiting, distortion of visual perception, and rapid pulse. Severely low blood pressure and convulsions may develop after a day or two, which eventually leads to hallucinations, delirium, and continuous seizures, followed by coma and death.

Aquachloral *see Chloral hydrate, page 92*

Astramorph PF *see Morphine, page 129*

Ativan *see Lorazepam, page 117*

Avinza *see Morphine, page 129*

BENZPHETAMINE HYDROCHLORIDE
BRAND NAME: Didrex
COMMON STREET NAMES: Chalk, crystal, crank, glass, meth, ice, speed
DEA CLASS: Class III
PHARMACOLOGIC CLASS: Amphetamine, CNS stimulant

Description: Benzphetamine is prescribed as a supplemental agent for weight loss. It is meant to be used along with caloric restriction, exercise, and behavior modification.

Method of use: Ingested and snorted

Duration of action: 8 to 24 hours

Psychological effects of abuse: Depression, hyperactivity, irritability, personality changes, and restlessness. Psychological dependence develops with chronic use.

Physical effects of abuse: Abdominal cramps, diarrhea, fatigue, insomnia, nausea, and vomiting. Long-term use may lead to physical dependence.

Overdose symptoms: Tolerance develops rapidly in chronic users, and progressively higher doses are needed to obtain the same effects as before. Overdose symptoms may include confusion, aggressiveness, hallucinations, panic state, severely elevated body temperature, tremors, rapid breathing, and muscle rigidity. Cardiovascular effects may include irregular heartbeat, severely low or high blood pressure, and circulatory collapse. The most severe symptom is psychosis that is clinically indistinguishable from schizophrenia. A fatal overdose is usually preceded by convulsions and coma.

Withdrawal symptoms: Benzphetamine is highly addictive, and physical dependence develops rapidly. Abrupt cessation of use may cause anxiety, extreme fatigue, paranoia, aggressive behavior, and strong drug cravings. Severe depression and suicidal ideation have also been reported.

Bontril *see Phendimetrazine, page 143*

BUTABARBITAL SODIUM
BRAND NAME: Butisol sodium
COMMON STREET NAMES: Barbs, downers, goofballs
DEA CLASS: Class III
PHARMACOLOGIC CLASS: Barbiturate, sedative, hypnotic

Description: Barbiturates depress the sensory cortex, decrease motor activity, alter brain function, and produce drowsiness, sedation, and hypnosis. Butabarbital is used primarily for daytime sedation.

Method of use: Ingested

Duration of action: Effects start within an hour and last for about 6 to 8 hours.

Psychological effects of abuse: Alternating euphoria and depression, confusion, and memory loss. Barbiturates may cause psychological dependence, especially following prolonged use of high doses.

Physical effects of abuse: Decreased blood pressure, unusual tiredness, nausea and vomiting, dizziness, drowsiness, heartburn, excessive sleepiness, shortness of breath, and dose-dependent respiratory depression. Prolonged use may cause tolerance and physical dependence.

Overdose symptoms: Unsteady gait, slurred speech, eye gazing, confusion, low blood pressure and body temperature, rapid heartbeat, and dose-dependent respiratory depression. All toxic effects are enhanced when butabarbital is taken with alcohol and/or other CNS depressant drugs.

Withdrawal symptoms: Symptoms are similar to those of alcohol withdrawal and characterized by severe apprehension, weakness, heightened anxiety, irritability, dizziness, headache, sleeplessness, muscle twitching, nausea and vomiting, distortion of visual perception, and rapid pulse. Severely low blood pressure and convulsions may develop after a day or two, which eventually leads to hallucinations, delirium, and continuous seizures, followed by coma and death.

BUTALBITAL COMBINATION PRODUCTS

GENERIC NAMES: Butalbital, aspirin, and caffeine (Fiorinal); butalbital, codeine phosphate, aspirin, and caffeine (Fiorinal with Codeine); Butalbital, codeine phosphate, acetominophen, and caffeine (Fioricet with Codeine) and butalbital, acetaminophen, and caffeine (Anolor, Esgic, Fioricet, Repan, Zebutal)

COMMON STREET NAMES: Barbs, downers, goofballs

DEA CLASS: Class III (Fiorinal, Fiornal with Codeine, Fioricet with codeine)

PHARMACOLOGIC CLASS: Barbiturate, sedative, hypnotic

Description: These products are used primarily to relieve muscle and tension headache.

Method of use: Ingested

Duration of action: Effects start within an hour and last for about 12 hours.

Psychological effects of abuse: Confusion, hallucinations, depression, and feelings of intoxication. Barbiturates may cause psychological dependence, especially following prolonged use of high doses.

Physical effects of abuse: Decreased blood pressure, unusual tiredness, nausea and vomiting, dizziness, drowsiness, heartburn, excessive sleepiness, shortness of breath, and dose-dependent respiratory depression. Prolonged use may cause tolerance and physical dependence.

Overdose symptoms: Symptoms may include unsteady gait, slurred speech, eye gazing, confusion, low blood pressure and body temperature, rapid heart rate, and dose-dependent respiratory depression. All toxic effects are enhanced when these products are taken with alcohol and/or other CNS depressants. In cases of serious overdose, respiratory depression may lead to Cheyne-Stokes respiration (abnormal breathing patterns characterized by alternating periods of shallow and deep breathing) as well as respiratory arrest and coma, followed by death. In extreme cases, electrical activities in the brain may cease and electroencephalogram (EEG) readings may be "flat," although this does not necessarily indicate clinical death and may be fully reversible.

Withdrawal symptoms: Symptoms are similar to those of alcohol withdrawal and characterized by severe apprehension, strong drug cravings, weakness, heightened anxiety, irritability, dizziness, headache, sleeplessness, muscle twitching, nausea and vomiting, distortion of visual perception, and rapid pulse. Severely low blood pressure and convulsions may develop after a day or two, which eventually leads to hallucinations, delirium, and continuous seizures, followed by coma and death.

Butisol sodium *see Butabarbital, page 89*

BUTORPHANOL TARTRATE
BRAND NAME: Stadol
COMMON STREET NAMES: Not known
DEA CLASS: Class IV
PHARMACOLOGIC CLASS: Narcotic analgesic

Description: Butorphanol is a mixed narcotic agonist/antagonist and produces generalized CNS depression. It is used to help manage moderate to severe pain, as a sedative prior to surgery, and as a supplemental agent during anesthesia.

Method of use: Injected IV or IM and sniffed via nasal spray

Duration of action: Depends on dose and method of use. The effects persist for about 3 to 4 hours after injection, and about 4 to 5 hours after nasal application.

Psychological effects of abuse: Anxiety, apathy, confusion, depression, euphoria, general sense of well-being, hallucinations, inability to concentrate, nightmares, paradoxical excitement, and psychological dependence (after prolonged use). The psychological dependence associated with narcotic addiction is complex. Long after physical dependence has ended, the addict may continue to think and talk about the drug and feel unable to manage daily activities without it.

Physical effects of abuse: Blurred vision, constipation, dizziness, drowsiness, constricted pupils, excessive sleepiness, excessive sweating, flu-like symptoms, headache, light-headedness, low blood pressure, nausea, respiratory depression, respiratory tract infection, shortness of breath, slow pulse, tremors, unpleasant taste, vomiting, and weakness. Prolonged use may cause tolerance and physical dependence. Signs of tolerance include euphoria, sedation, shorter duration of action, and weaker painkilling effect.

Overdose symptoms: Chronic use can lead to tolerance, with the user needing progressively higher doses to obtain the same effects as before. Signs of overdose include constricted pupils, cold and clammy skin, confusion, severe drowsiness, slow or labored breathing, CNS and cardiac depression, and convulsions.

Withdrawal symptoms: Abruptly stopping the drug after long-term use may precipitate withdrawal symptoms. Intensity of symptoms is directly related to total daily dose, frequency and duration of use, and health of the user. Withdrawal from narcotics is rarely life-threatening. Without medical intervention, most of the physical symptoms of butorphanol withdrawal disappear within 7 to 10 days. Early symptoms may include watery eyes, runny nose, repeated yawning, and excessive sweating. Later-stage symptoms may include nervousness, muscle twitching, drug cravings, restlessness, irritability, loss of appetite, chills alternating with flushing, nausea, vomiting, bone and muscle pain in the back and extremities, tremors, elevated heart rate and blood pressure, and severe depression.

CHLORAL HYDRATE

BRAND NAMES: Aquachloral, Somnote
COMMON STREET NAMES: Jellies, jellybeans, joy juice, knockout drops, Mickey, Mickey Finn, Peter, torpedo
DEA CLASS: Class IV
PHARMACOLOGIC CLASS: Sedative, hypnotic

Description: Chloral hydrate has properties similar to those of barbiturates. It is used for short-term sedation before diagnostic procedures, as a supplemental agent to manage pain following surgery, and for the short-term treatment of insomnia.

Method of use: Ingested or administered rectally

Duration of action: Chloral hydrate usually takes effect within 30 minutes and will induce sleep in about an hour following administration. The effects may last 4 to 8 hours.

Psychological effects of abuse: Confusion, disorientation, hallucinations, "hangover" effects, impaired judgment and concentration, nightmares, and paradoxical excitement.

Physical effects of abuse: Diarrhea, dizziness, headache, light-headedness, nausea, slow reflexes, stomach pain, unsteadiness, and vomiting.

Chronic use can lead to addiction, severe withdrawal symptoms, and possibly liver damage.

Overdose symptoms: Tolerance develops rapidly after prolonged use, and the progressively higher doses needed are often in the toxic range. Signs of overdose may include severe drowsiness, nausea, vomiting, severe stomach pain, slurred speech, irregular gait, difficulty swallowing, severe weakness, dilated pupils, shortness of breath or other breathing problems, low blood pressure, irregular heart rate, low body temperature, respiratory depression, convulsions, and coma.

Withdrawal symptoms: Abruptly stopping use may precipitate withdrawal symptoms such as anorexia, nausea, vomiting, muscle weakness, low blood pressure, tremors, and seizures.

CLORAZEPATE DIPOTASSIUM
BRAND NAME: Tranxene
COMMON STREET NAMES: Candy, downers, sleeping pills, tranks
DEA CLASS: Class IV
PHARMACOLOGIC CLASS: Benzodiazepine, sedative, anticonvulsant

Description: Clorazepate is used to treat anxiety disorders, alcohol withdrawal, and as a supplemental agent in certain types of seizure disorders. Abuse of benzodiazepines is particularly high among heroin and cocaine users.

Method of use: Ingested

Duration of action: 8 to 24 hours

Psychological effects of abuse: Confusion, depression, impaired judgment and thinking abilities, mild euphoria, pressured speech, reduced inhibition, and suicidal ideation. Prolonged use may cause psychological dependence.

Physical effects of abuse: Change in appetite, constipation, difficulty urinating, dizziness, drowsiness, dry mouth, impaired muscle coordination, insomnia, irregular gait, light-headedness, low blood pressure, menstrual irregularities, nausea, slurred speech, tremor, and vomiting. Long-term use may cause physical dependence.

Overdose symptoms: The most severe signs of overdose are respiratory depression and coma. Other symptoms may include confusion, diminished reflexes, paradoxical euphoria, extreme sleepiness, and impaired coordination. Death from overdose of a single benzodiazepine is extremely rare. However, there is an increased risk of toxicity when benzodiazepines are combined with alcohol and/or other CNS depressants.

Fatalities have been reported in individuals who have overdosed with a combination of a single benzodiazepine and alcohol.

Withdrawal symptoms: Abrupt termination following long-term use may precipitate withdrawal symptoms and require hospitalization. Symptoms may include abdominal and muscle cramps, depression, insomnia, sweating, vomiting, tremors, and seizures.

CHLORDIAZEPOXIDE

BRAND NAME: Librium
COMMON STREET NAMES: Candy, downers, sleeping pills, tranks
DEA CLASS: Class IV
PHARMACOLOGIC CLASS: Benzodiazepine, sedative, hypnotic

Description: Chlordiazepoxide is used to treat anxiety disorders with or without depression, alcohol withdrawal, and acute stress reactions such as anxiety prior to surgery. Abuse of benzodiazepines is particularly high among heroin and cocaine users.

Method of use: Ingested and injected IM or IV

Duration of action: 5 to 30 hours

Psycological effects of abuse: Confusion, depression, impaired judgment, mild euphoria, pressured speech, reduced inhibition, and suicidal ideation. Long-term use may cause psychological dependence.

Physical effects of abuse: Changes in appetite and body weight, dizziness, drowsiness, dry mouth, impaired muscle coordination, insomnia, irregular gait, light-headedness, low blood pressure, menstrual irregularities, nausea, slurred speech, and vomiting. Long-term use may cause physical dependence.

Overdose symptoms: The most severe signs of overdose are respiratory depression and coma. Other symptoms may include confusion, diminished reflexes, extreme sleepiness, unrealistic euphoria, and impaired muscle coordination. Death from overdose of a single benzodiazepine is extremely rare. However, there is an increased risk of toxicity when benzodiazepines are combined with alcohol and/or other CNS depressants. Fatalities have been reported in individuals who have overdosed with a combination of a single benzodiazepine and alcohol.

Withdrawal symptoms: Abrupt termination following long-term use may precipitate withdrawal symptoms and require hospitalization. Symptoms may include abdominal and muscle cramps, depression, insomnia, sweating, vomiting, tremors, and seizures.

CLONAZEPAM
BRAND NAME: Klonopin
COMMON STREET NAMES: Candy, downers, sleeping pills, tranks
DEA CLASS: Class IV
PHARMACOLOGIC CLASS: Benzodiazepine, anticonvulsant

Description: Clonazepam is used to treat panic disorder with or without irrational fears. It is also prescribed for certain types of seizures, either as monotherapy or an adjunct. Abuse of benzodiazepines is particularly high among heroin and cocaine users.

Method of use: Ingested

Duration of action: 18 to 50 hours

Psychological effects of abuse: Amnesia, confusion, depression, impaired judgment and thinking abilities, reduced inhibition, and suicidal ideation. Paradoxical effects include euphoria, hyperactivity, and extreme aggression. Prolonged use may cause psychological dependence.

Physical effects of abuse: Changes in sexual desire, constipation, decreased blood pressure, dizziness, drowsiness, fatigue, impaired physical capabilities, irregular gait, loss of muscle tone, sleepiness, slowed psychomotor performance, urinary retention, and visual disturbances. Prolonged use may cause physical dependence.

Overdose symptoms: The most severe signs of overdose are respiratory depression, loss of consciousness, and coma. Other symptoms may include confusion, diminished reflexes, slurred speech, impaired coordination, apnea, extreme sleepiness, loss of muscle tone, and severely low blood pressure. Death from overdose of a single benzodiazepine is extremely rare. However, there is an increased risk of toxicity when benzodiazepines are combined with alcohol and/or other CNS depressants. Fatalities have been reported in patients who have overdosed with a combination of a single benzodiazepine and alcohol.

Withdrawal symptoms: Abrupt termination following long-term use may precipitate withdrawal symptoms and require hospitalization. Symptoms may include abdominal and muscle cramps, depression, insomnia, sweating, vomiting, tremors, and seizures.

CODEINE PHOSPHATE AND CODEINE SULFATE
BRAND NAMES: Capital with Codeine, Tylenol with Codeine
COMMON STREET NAMES: Hillbilly heroin, killers, percs, poor man's heroin, schoolboy
DEA CLASS: Class II (single agent), Class III (combined with Tylenol), and Class V (cough suppressant products)
PHARMACOLOGIC CLASS: Narcotic analgesic, cough suppressant

Description: Codeine is produced by the chemical manipulation of morphine. However, codeine produces less analgesia and sedation than morphine, and is less likely to cause respiratory depression. Codeine is indicated for mild to moderate pain. In lower doses, it is used as a cough suppressant. Codeine is also indicated for the symptomatic relief of acute diarrhea.

Method of use: Ingested and injected IM or SC

Duration of action: Depends on the dose and method of use. In general, codeine's analgesic effects last 4 to 6 hours following administration.

Psychological effects of abuse: Confusion, false sense of well-being, inability to concentrate, and psychological dependence (after prolonged use). The psychological dependence associated with narcotic addiction is complex. Long after physical dependence has ended, the addict may continue to think and talk about the drug and feel unable to manage daily activities without it.

Physical effects of abuse: Blurred vision, change in heart rhythm, constipation, constriction of pupils, drowsiness, dry mouth, flushing of the face, low blood pressure, headache, nausea, respiratory depression, urinary urgency or retention, and vomiting. *High doses:* Lethargy, seizures, and coma may occur. Prolonged use can cause physical dependence, but codeine produces less euphoria and sedation than morphine.

Overdose symptoms: Tolerance can develop rapidly, and progressively higher doses are needed to obtain the same effects as before. Signs of overdose may include constipation, stomach cramps, nausea, vomiting, drowsiness, dizziness, slurred speech, extreme sleepiness, low body temperature, low blood pressure, swelling, cold and clammy skin, nonreactive pupils, pulmonary edema, CNS and respiratory depression, convulsions, and coma. Death may result from respiratory failure 2 to 4 hours postingestion. Risk of overdose increases significantly when the drug is taken with alcohol.

Withdrawal symptoms: Although withdrawal is painful physically and emotionally, it's rarely life-threatening if adequate hydration and nutritional support are maintained. The symptoms are similar to those of morphine withdrawal but are considerably less intense. Abruptly stopping use can cause excessive tearing, yawning, and sweating about 12 to 14 hours after the last dose. Additional symptoms may include diminished appetite, gooseflesh, irritability, tremors, seizures, and loss of consciousness.

Concerta *see Methylphenidate, page 124*

Dalmane *see Flurazepam, page 110*

Darvon *see Propoxyphene, page 148*

Daytrana *see Methylphenidate, page 124*

Delatestryl *see Testosterone, page 154*

Demerol *see Meperidine, page 118*

Desoxyn *see Methamphetamine, page 122*

Dexedrine *see Dextroamphetamine, page 98*

DEXMETHYLPHENIDATE HYDROCHLORIDE
BRAND NAME: Focalin, Focalin XR
COMMON STREET NAME: Working man's cocaine
DEA CLASS: Class II
PHARMACOLOGIC CLASS: CNS stimulant, nonamphetamine

Description: This drug has pharmacologic actions similar to those of dextroamphetamine. It is used to treat attention deficit hyperactivity disorder (ADHD) and excessive daytime sleepiness (narcolepsy). Severe complications can occur when dexmethylphenidate tablets are crushed and diluted in water for injection. The tablets contain insoluble fillers that can block small blood vessels, causing serious damage to the lungs and eye retina. In addition, there have been reports of fatalities among drug users who combined dexmethylphenidate with pentazocine, a narcotic analgesic.

Method of use: Ingested; tablets are also crushed and snorted or diluted in water and injected.

Duration of action: 4 to 5 hours following a standard therapeutic dose.

Psychological effects of abuse: Depression, nervousness, and psychotic behavior.

Physical effects of abuse: Abdominal cramps, chronic insomnia, diarrhea, loss of appetite, nausea, rapid heart rate, tiredness, vomiting, and weight loss. Severe blockage in the blood vessels of the lungs and eye retina can occur when the drug is injected.

Overdose symptoms: Signs of overdose may include excessive sweating and hyperactivity, vomiting, agitation, tremors, severely elevated body temperature and blood pressure, rapid heart rate, and hallucinations.

Withdrawal symptoms: Withdrawal reactions are less common than with other CNS stimulants. Symptoms may include severe fatigue, depression, nausea, vomiting, stomach cramps, insomnia, and nightmares.

DEXTROAMPHETAMINE

BRAND NAMES: Adderall, Dexedrine, DextroStat, Adderal XR
COMMON STREET NAMES: Bennies, black beauties, crosses, hearts, LA turn-around, speed, truck drivers, uppers
DEA CLASS: Class II
PHARMACOLOGIC CLASS: Amphetamine, CNS stimulant, anorexiant

Description: Dextroamphetamine has a marked CNS stimulant effect, particularly on the cerebral cortex. It is used to treat excessive daytime sleepiness (narcolepsy) and attention deficit hyperactivity disorder (ADHD).

Method of use: Ingested, snorted, smoked, and injected

Duration of action: About 4 hours for short-acting forms and 6 to 12 hours for long-acting forms.

Psychological effects of abuse: Aggression, confusion, depression, anxiety, delusions, agitation, paranoia, hallucinations, drug craving, and impulsive behavior. Tolerance and psychological dependence may develop after chronic use.

Physical effects of abuse: Blood-vessel inflammation in the brain, elevated blood pressure, fever, muscle pain, poor blood circulation, rapid heart rate, and weight loss.

Overdose symptoms: Overdose syndromes are characterized by circulatory collapse, seizures, irregular heart rate, significantly elevated body temperature, severe muscle weakness and pain, kidney and liver injuries, and coma. In some cases, severe psychosis was reported within 24 hours following IV administration.

Withdrawal symptoms: Abruptly stopping the drug after long-term use may cause extreme fatigue, overeating, depression, and stupor.

DIAZEPAM

BRAND NAME: Valium
COMMON STREET NAMES: Candy, downers, sleeping pills, tranks
DEA CLASS: Class IV
PHARMACOLOGIC CLASS: Benzodiazepine, sedative, antianxiety, anticonvulsant

Description: Diazepam is used to treat anxiety disorders with or without depression, acute stress reactions such as anxiety prior to surgery, panic attacks with or without irrational fear, alcohol withdrawal, and certain types of seizure disorders. Abuse of benzodiazepines is particularly high among heroin and cocaine users.

Method of use: Ingested and injected IM or IV

Duration of action: Effects can linger up to 4 days, but may persist longer in chronic users.

Psychological effects of abuse: Confusion, impaired judgment and thinking abilities, irritability, mild euphoria, pressured speech, reduced inhibition, and suicidal ideation. Long-term use may cause psychological dependence.

Physical effects of abuse: Changes in appetite and body weight, constipation, dizziness, impaired muscle coordination, low blood pressure, and vertigo. Long-term use may cause physical dependence.

Overdose symptoms: The most severe signs of overdose are respiratory depression and coma. Other symptoms may include confusion, diminished reflexes, unrealistic euphoria, extreme sleepiness, and impaired muscle coordination. Death from overdose of a single benzodiazepine is extremely rare. However, there is an increased risk of toxicity when benzodiazepines are combined with alcohol and/or other CNS depressants. Fatalities have been reported in individuals who have overdosed with a combination of a single benzodiazepine and alcohol.

Withdrawal symptoms: Abrupt termination following long-term use may precipitate withdrawal symptoms and require hospitalization. Symptoms may include abdominal and muscle cramps, depression, insomnia, sweating, vomiting, tremors, and seizures.

Didrex *see Benzphetamine, page 88*

DIETHYLPROPION HYDROCHLORIDE
BRAND NAMES: Tenuate
COMMON STREET NAMES: Bam, bambita, beans, black beauties, Christmas trees, dolls, jellybeans, little bomb
DEA CLASS: Class IV
PHARMACOLOGIC CLASS: CNS stimulant and indirect-acting sympathomimetic, anorexiant

Description: Diethylpropion is related to amphetamines both chemically and pharmacologically. It is used as a supplemental agent to help promote weight loss in conjunction with caloric restriction, exercise, and behavior modification.

Method of use: Ingestion

Duration of action: 6 to 8 hours

Psychological effects of abuse: Mental depression, restlessness, talkativeness, uncontrollable excitement, personality changes, and psychosis.

Physical effects of abuse: Constipation, dry mouth, nausea, vomiting, stomach cramps, dizziness, light-headedness, sleeplessness, headache, elevated blood pressure, rapid heartbeat, blurred vision, dilated pupils, and intermittent or painful urination.

Overdose symptoms: Signs of overdose include confusion, restlessness, rapid breathing, stomach cramps, exaggerated reflexes, extremely high fever, irregular heartbeat, elevated blood pressure, hallucinations, panic state, convulsions, and coma.

Withdrawal symptoms: Physical dependence is not common. However, abruptly stopping use can occasionally cause insomnia, tiredness, depression, stomach cramps, convulsions, and nightmares.

Dilaudid *see Hydromorphone, page 114*

Dolophine *see Methadone, page 121*

Dopram *see Doxapram, page 100*

Doral *see Quazepam, page 149*

DOXAPRAM HYDROCHLORIDE
BRAND NAME: Dopram
COMMON STREET NAMES: Not known
DEA CLASS: Not classified
PHARMACOLOGIC CLASS: CNS and respiratory stimulant, nonamphetamine

Description: This drug is used to manage respiratory depression due to anesthesia. It is also used to manage abnormally high levels of carbon monoxide in the blood secondary to chronic obstructive pulmonary disease (COPD). Doxapram may raise blood pressure and stimulate the nervous system.

Method of use: Ingested and injected IV

Duration of action: About 6 to 8 hours

Psychological effects of abuse: Confusion, delirium, and hallucinations.

Physical effects of abuse: Shortness of breath, coughing, respiratory problems such as hyperventilation, convulsions, headache, dizziness, hiccup, hyperactivity, sweating, flushing, fever, nausea, vomiting, diarrhea, excessive sweating, flushing, difficulty urinating, and sudden high or low blood pressure.

Overdose symptoms: Signs of overdose include anorexia, high fever, excessive sweating, flushing, muscle rigidity, delirium, hallucinations, seizures, coma, and respiratory failure.

Withdrawal symptoms: To date, there are no reports of withdrawal effects following a standard therapeutic dose.

DRONABINOL AND NABILONE

BRAND NAME: Marinol (dronabinol); also known as delta-9-tetrahydrocannabinol (THC)
COMMON STREET NAMES: Bud, endo, grass, herb, kind bud, Mary Jane, pot, shake, sinsemilla, weed
DEA CLASS: Class III
PHARMACOLOGIC CLASS: Antiemetic

Description: Dronabinol and nabilone are chemically related to THC, the active ingredient in marijuana. They are used to treat the nausea and vomiting associated with cancer chemotherapy and are prescribed only when other antiemetic drugs have failed to work. Dronabinol is also used to treat anorexia associated with weight loss in AIDS patients.

Method of use: Ingested

Duration of action: Onset of action occurs within 1 hour after ingestion and effects persist for 20 to 24 hours.

Psychological effects of abuse: Anxiety, confusion, depression, detachment from reality, hallucinations, memory loss, and mood changes.

Physical effects of abuse: Blurred vision, diarrhea, dizziness, drowsiness, dry eyes, dry mouth, feeling faint, headache, high blood pressure, increased appetite, irregular gait, rapid heartbeat, ringing in the ears, and vertigo. Chronic users may develop tolerance and physical dependence.

Overdose symptoms: Heavy users may develop tolerance rapidly and need progressively larger doses to obtain the same effects as before. Signs of overdose may include dizziness, drowsiness, slurred speech, irregular gait, decreased motor coordination and muscle strength, extreme tiredness or weakness, rapid heartbeat, high or low blood pressure, and rarely, psychosis.

Withdrawal symptoms: Abruptly stopping use may cause drug cravings, irritability, agitation, apprehension, insomnia, excessive sweating, aggressiveness, and extreme anxiety.

Duramorph PF *see Morphine, page 129*

Esgic *See Butalbital, page 90*

ESTAZOLAM

BRAND NAME: ProSom
COMMON STREET NAMES: Candy, downers, sleeping pills, tranks
DEA CLASS: Class IV
PHARMACOLOGIC CLASS: Benzodiazepine, sedative, hypnotic

Description: Estazolam is used for the short-term treatment of sleep disorders such as difficulty falling asleep or staying asleep. Abuse of benzodiazepines is particularly high among heroin and cocaine users.

Method of use: Ingested

Duration of action: Up to 30 hours

Psychological effects of abuse: Confusion, impaired judgment and thinking abilities, irritability, mild euphoria, pressured speech, reduced inhibition, and suicidal ideation. Long-term use may cause psychological dependence.

Physical effects of abuse: Changes in appetite and body weight, constipation, dizziness, impaired muscle coordination, and low blood pressure. Long-term use may cause physical dependence.

Overdose symptoms: The most severe signs of overdose are respiratory depression and coma. Other symptoms may include confusion, diminished reflexes, extreme sleepiness, unrealistic euphoria, and impaired muscle coordination. Death from overdose of a single benzodiazepine is extremely rare. However, there is an increased risk of toxicity when benzodiazepines are combined with alcohol and/or other CNS depressants. Fatalities have been reported in patients who have overdosed with a combination of a single benzodiazepine and alcohol.

Withdrawal symptoms: Abrupt termination following long-term use may precipitate withdrawal symptoms and require hospitalization. Symptoms may include abdominal and muscle cramps, depression, insomnia, sweating, vomiting, tremors, and seizures.

ETHCHLORVYNOL

COMMON STREET NAMES: Not known
DEA CLASS: Class IV
PHARMACOLOGIC CLASS: Sedative, hypnotic

Not commercially available in the U.S.

Description: Ethchlorvynol is used for the short-term treatment of sleep disorders, but it is not superior to the benzodiazepines. For the most part, benzodiazepines have replaced the use of ethchlorvynol because of its high potential for causing addiction and toxic overdose.

Method of use: Ingested

Duration of action: Hypnotic effects last about 5 hours following ingestion of a single therapeutic dose. If given in high doses, the effects may persist for up to 35 hours.

Psychological effects of abuse: Confusion, feelings of intoxication, hallucinations, and depression. Prolonged use of high doses may cause psychological dependence.

Physical effects of abuse: Dizziness, irregular gait, facial numbness, low blood pressure, vomiting, nausea, visual changes, cough, shortness of breath, respiratory distress, and accumulation of fluid in the lungs (with IV injections only). Prolonged use may cause intense physical addiction and withdrawal symptoms.

Overdose symptoms: Tolerance develops rapidly, and the progressively higher doses needed are often in the toxic range. Symptoms include severely low blood pressure, accumulation of fluid in the lungs, and liver damage.

Withdrawal symptoms: Abrupt cessation of use may cause weakness, heightened anxiety, irritability, dizziness, headache, sleeplessness, nausea and vomiting, distortion of visual perception, rapid pulse, and convulsions.

ETHINAMATE
COMMON STREET NAMES: Not known
DEA CLASS: Class IV
PHARMACOLOGIC CLASS: Sedative, hypnotic

Not commercially available in the U.S.

Description: Ethinamate is marketed in other countries for the short-term treatment of insomnia. The drug was withdrawn from the U.S. market in 1990 after safer and more effective agents became available.

Method of use: Ingested

Duration of action: The hypnotic effects start within 20 minutes and last 3 to 5 hours.

Psychological effects of abuse: Behavioral changes, excessive irritability, and paradoxical excitement. Prolonged use may cause psychological dependence.

Physical effects of abuse: Dizziness, drowsiness, confusion, irregular gait, nausea, vomiting, and "hangover" effects. Prolonged use may cause tolerance and physical dependence.

Overdose symptoms: Tolerance develops rapidly, and the progressively higher doses needed are often in the toxic range. Toxicity reactions are similar to barbiturates. Major symptoms of overdose are CNS and respiratory depression, severely low blood pressure, and coma (after high doses). Additional symptoms include severe weakness, confusion, slurred speech, irregular gait, shortness of breath, breathing difficulties, and slowed heartbeat.

Withdrawal symptoms: Abrupt cessation of use may cause confusion, restlessness, nervousness, irritability, trembling, sleeplessness, agitation, dizziness, hyperactive reflexes, hallucinations, and seizures.

ETHYLESTRENOL
COMMON STREET NAMES: Arnolds, gym candy, juice, pumpers, roids, stackers, weight trainers
DEA CLASS: Class III
PHARMACOLOGIC CLASS: Anabolic-androgenic steroid

Not commercially available in the U.S.

Description: Androgens are steroid hormones that develop and maintain male sex characteristics. They are used primarily to replace insufficient levels of testosterone due to poor functioning of the testes. When used in combination with exercise and a high-protein diet, androgens can promote increased muscle size and strength, improve stamina, and decrease recovery time between workouts. Androgens are also used to promote the development of puberty in males with clearly delayed onset. Additionally, androgens are sometimes prescribed for women with advancing, inoperable metastatic breast cancer who are 1 to 5 years postmenopausal.

Method of use: Ingested. Chronic users tend to rotate steroids using various methods known as cycling, stacking, and pyramiding. Sporadic discontinuation of use is believed to allow testosterone levels and sperm counts to return to normal. Taking steroids regularly with periodic "drug-free times" is called cycling. Stacking refers to the concomitant use of two or more steroids at high doses. Pyramiding is when the dose, frequency, or number of steroids taken is gradually increased, followed by progressive tapering of the drug(s).

Duration of action: Depends on the formulation, frequency, and method of use. In general, effects may last up to 6 days.

Psychological effects of abuse: Mood changes, depression, uncontrollable aggressive behavior, euphoria, anxiety, irritability, increased sex drive, and rarely, psychosis. Psychological dependence may also occur.

Physical effects of abuse: Angry or hostile feelings, elevated blood pressure and cholesterol, headache, insomnia, premature balding, psychotic reactions, severe acne, sexual dysfunction, and violent behavior. *In men:* Breast development, impotence, intermittent or painful urination, painful or persistent erections, reduced sperm production, and shrinking of the testicles. *In women:* Decreased body fat and breast size, deepening of the voice, enlarged clitoris, excessive growth of body hair, and menstrual changes. *In adolescents:* Premature termination of growth.

Prolonged use can lead to tolerance. While the long-term effects are not completely known, chronic steroid abuse has been associated with damage to the heart, liver, and brain.

Overdose symptoms: There have been no reports of serious overdose with this drug. Chronic use of high doses may cause excessive sexual stimulation, reduced sperm production, enlarged breasts in males, uncontrolled painful erection, jaundice, and deteriorating liver function. Excessive fluid retention may occur in users who have heart, liver, or kidney disease.

Withdrawal symptoms: Abrupt discontinuation may cause mood changes, tiredness, restlessness, loss of appetite, dissatisfaction with body image, sleeplessness, reduced sex drive, paranoia, and severe depression that can lead to suicide attempts.

FENFLURAMINE
COMMON STREET NAMES: Pep pills, speed, uppers
DEA CLASS: Class IV
PHARMACOLOGIC CLASS: CNS stimulant

Not commercially available in the U.S.

Description: Fenfluramine was previously used as a supplemental agent to help promote weight loss. It was withdrawn from the market worldwide due to its serious adverse effect on heart valves, but can still be found among drug users. Fenfluramine is an indirect-acting sympathomimetic agent related to amphetamines, but at standard doses it usually depresses rather than stimulates the central nervous system.

Method of use: Ingested

Duration of action: Following a single dose, effects may last 4 to 6 hours.

Psychological effects of abuse: Confusion, agitation, depression, restlessness, combative behavior, and hallucinations. Acute paranoia and other psychotic behavior were also reported with the use of this product.

Physical effects of abuse: Constipation, dry mouth, nausea, vomiting, stomach cramps, dizziness, light-headedness, sleeplessness, headache, elevated blood pressure, rapid heartbeat, blurred vision, dilated pupils, and intermittent or painful urination. Valvular heart disease was reported with prolonged use, particularly when ingested with phentermine.

Overdose symptoms: Tolerance may develop after 12 weeks of chronic use, and progressively larger doses are needed to obtain the same effects as before. Toxicity can persist for up to 3 days following a single large dose. Overdose symptoms may include dilated and nonreactive pupils, double vision, rapid and irregular pulse, irregular heart rhythm, respiratory failure, seizures, and coma.

Withdrawal symptoms: Withdrawal symptoms following cessation of fenfluramine are rare, but agitation, irritability, hyperactivity, and interrupted sleep patterns have been reported.

FENTANYL and FENTANYL CITRATE
BRAND NAMES: Actiq, Duragesic, Fentora, Sublimaze
COMMON STREET NAMES: China girl, China white, dance fever, friend, goodfellas, king ivory
DEA CLASS: Class II
PHARMACOLOGIC CLASS: Narcotic analgesic

Description: Fentanyl is used as a sedative prior to surgery, as a supplemental agent to induce general or local anesthesia, and to help manage moderate to severe pain. Transdermal fentanyl is used for chronic pain. Actiq, a raspberry-flavored lozenge, is indicated only for treating breakthrough cancer pain in opiate-tolerant individuals. Actiq is about 80 times more potent than morphine. Although the pharmacologic effects of fentanyl are the same as those of heroin, fentanyl is 50 to 100 times more potent. U.S. authorities have identified at least 12 analogues of fentanyl being produced clandestinely.

Method of use: The most common method is IV injection; other methods include transdermal (absorbed through the skin), transmucosal (buccal, or absorbed through the gums), smoked, and snorted.

Duration of action: Depends on dose and method of use. In general, the effects last for only 1 to 2 hours following administration. However, repeated administration of large doses may result in accumulation and a longer duration of action.

Psychological effects of abuse: Confusion, depression, and hallucinations. Psychological dependence can result after prolonged use, especially with high doses. The psychological dependence associated with narcotic addiction is complex. Long after physical dependence has ended, the addict may continue to think and talk about the drug and feel unable to manage daily activities without it.

Physical effects of abuse: Low blood pressure, drowsiness, dizziness, headache, restlessness, fatigue, muscle rigidity, seizures, paradoxical CNS stimulation, nausea, constipation, vomiting, diminished appetite, dry mouth, stomach cramps, decreased urination, and shortness of breath. Chronic use may cause physical dependence.

Overdose symptoms: The main symptoms are constricted pupils, CNS depression, and slow or labored breathing. Severe overdose may result in interrupted breathing, circulatory depression, severely low blood pressure, muscle rigidity, slow heart rate, seizures, delirium, and shock. Physical activity, such as strenuous exercise or dancing, may cause increased absorption of transdermal fentanyl. Toxicity has been reported with transdermal patches due to heat-induced changes in the delivery system. Risk of overdose increases significantly when the drug is taken with alcohol.

Withdrawal symptoms: Abruptly stopping the drug after chronic use may precipitate withdrawal. The intensity of symptoms is directly related to the total daily dose, frequency and duration of use, and the health of the user. Although withdrawal from narcotics is painful physically and emotionally, it is rarely life-threatening if adequate hydration and nutritional support are maintained. Early symptoms include watery eyes, runny nose, repeated yawning, and excessive sweating. Later-stage symptoms may include restlessness, irritability, loss of appetite, nausea, vomiting, diarrhea, shivering, drug cravings, tremors, and severe depression. Advanced withdrawal symptoms may include chills alternating with flushing, muscle and bone pain in the back and extremities, and elevated heart rate and blood pressure.

Fentora *see Fentanyl and Fentanyl Citrate, page 106*

Fioricet *see Butalbital, page 90*

Fiorinal *see Butalbital, page 90*

FLUNITRAZEPAM

COMMON STREET NAMES: Forget-me pill, Mexican valium, R2, Roche, roofies, roofinol, rope, rophies
DEA CLASS: Class IV
PHARMACOLOGIC CLASS: Benzodiazepine, sedative, hypnotic

Not commercially available in the U.S.

Description: Flunitrazepam is neither approved nor manufactured in the U.S. It is used in other countries for the short-term treatment of insomnia, as a muscle relaxant prior to surgery, and as an aid in the induction of anesthesia. There is widespread abuse of flunitrazepam among drug users, especially those who use opioids or cocaine. Flunitrazepam has also gained a reputation as a "date rape" drug. Victims who are unknowingly given the drug become incapacitated and unable to resist sexual assault.

Method of use: Ingested, snorted, and injected IM or IV

Duration of action: 9 to 30 hours, depending on method of use and dose size.

Psychological effects of abuse: Amnesia, confusion, impaired mental capabilities, mania or hypomania, and suicidal ideation. Long-term use may cause psychological dependence.

Physical effects of abuse: Constipation, decreased blood pressure, dizziness, drowsiness, impaired physical capabilities, loss of muscle tone, sleepiness, slowed psychomotor performance, urinary retention, and visual disturbances. Long-term use may cause physical dependence. Neurological effects can persist for years, particularly in older people.

Overdose symptoms: Overdose with flunitrazepam is particularly dangerous since respiratory arrest can develop rapidly. Other symptoms may include confusion, diminished reflexes, disorientation, impaired coordination, extreme sleepiness, slurred speech, visual disturbances, loss of muscle tone, lowered blood pressure and pulse, and loss of consciousness. Death from overdose of a single benzodiazepine is extremely rare. However, there is an increased risk of toxicity when benzodiazepines are combined with alcohol and/or other CNS depressants. Fatalities have been reported in patients who have overdosed with a combination of a single benzodiazepine and alcohol.

Withdrawal symptoms: Abrupt termination following long-term use may precipitate withdrawal symptoms and require hospitalization. Symptoms may include abdominal and muscle cramps, agitation, delirium, depression, insomnia, rapid pulse, sweating, vomiting, hallucinations, tremors, and seizures.

FLUOXYMESTERONE
BRAND NAME: Halotestin
COMMON STREET NAMES: Arnolds, gym candy, juice, pumpers, roids, stackers, weight trainers
DEA CLASS: Class III
PHARMACOLOGIC CLASS: Anabolic-androgenic steroid

Description: Androgens are steroid hormones that develop and maintain male sex characteristics. They are used primarily to replace insufficient levels of testosterone due to poor functioning of the testes. When used in combination with exercise and a high-protein diet, androgens can promote increased muscle size and strength, improve stamina, and decrease recovery time between workouts. Androgens are also used to promote the development of puberty in males with clearly delayed onset. Additionally, androgens are sometimes prescribed for women with advancing, inoperable metastatic breast cancer who are 1 to 5 years postmenopausal. Fluoxymesterone has also been used in the management of anemias caused by certain cancers or chemotherapy.

Method of use: Ingested. Chronic users tend to rotate steroids using various methods known as cycling, stacking, and pyramiding. Sporadic discontinuation of use is believed to allow testosterone levels and sperm counts to return to normal. Taking steroids regularly with periodic "drug-free times" is called cycling. Stacking refers to the concomitant use of two or more steroids at high doses. Pyramiding is when the dose, frequency, or number of steroids taken is gradually increased, followed by progressive tapering of the drug(s).

Duration of action: Depends on the formulation, frequency, and method of use. In general, effects may last up to 6 days.

Psychological effects of abuse: Anxiety, changes in sex drive, and depression. Psychological dependence may also occur.

Physical effects of abuse: Angry or hostile feelings, elevated blood pressure and cholesterol, headache, insomnia, premature balding, psychotic reactions, severe acne, sexual dysfunction, and violent behavior. *In men:* Breast development, impotence, intermittent or painful urination, painful or persistent erections, reduced sperm production, and shrinking of the testicles. *In women:* Decreased body fat and breast size, deepening of the voice, enlarged clitoris, excessive growth of body hair, and menstrual changes. *In adolescents:* Premature termination of growth.

Prolonged use can lead to tolerance. While the long-term effects are not completely known, chronic steroid abuse has been associated with damage to the heart, liver, and brain.

Overdose symptoms: There have been no reports of serious overdose with this drug. Chronic use of high doses may cause excessive sexual stimulation, reduced sperm production, enlarged breasts in males, uncontrolled painful erection, jaundice, and deteriorating liver function. Excessive fluid retention may occur in users who have heart, liver, or kidney disease.

Withdrawal symptoms: Abrupt discontinuation may cause mood changes, tiredness, restlessness, loss of appetite, dissatisfaction with body image, sleeplessness, reduced sex drive, paranoia, and severe depression that can lead to suicide attempts.

FLURAZEPAM

BRAND NAME: Dalmane
COMMON STREET NAMES: Candy, downers, sleeping pills, tranks
DEA CLASS: Class IV
PHARMACOLOGIC CLASS: Benzodiazepine, sedative, hypnotic

Description: Flurazepam is used for the short-term treatment of sleep disorders such as insomnia. Abuse of benzodiazepines is particularly high among heroin and cocaine users.

Method of use: Ingested

Duration of action: 6 to 8 hours

Psychological effects of abuse: Confusion, impaired judgment and thinking abilities, irritability, mild euphoria, pressured speech, reduced inhibition, and suicidal ideation. Long-term use may cause psychological dependence.

Physical effects of abuse: Changes in appetite and body weight, constipation, dizziness, impaired muscle coordination, and low blood pressure. Long-term use may cause physical dependence.

Overdose symptoms: The most severe signs of overdose are respiratory depression and coma. Other symptoms may include confusion, diminished reflexes, unsteady gait, unrealistic euphoria, extreme sleepiness, and impaired muscle coordination. Death from overdose of a single benzodiazepine is extremely rare. However, there is an increased risk of toxicity when benzodiazepines are combined with alcohol and/or other CNS depressants. Fatalities have been reported in patients who have overdosed with a combination of a single benzodiazepine and alcohol.

Withdrawal symptoms: Abrupt termination following long-term use may precipitate withdrawal symptoms and require hospitalization. Symptoms may include abdominal and muscle cramps, depression, insomnia, sweating, vomiting, tremors, and seizures.

Focalin *see Dexmethylphenidate, page 97*

GHB (GAMMA HYDROXYBUTYRATE or SODIUM OXYBATE)

BRAND NAME: Xyrem
COMMON STREET NAMES: Bodily harm, cherry meth, fantasy, Georgia home boy, grievous bodily harm, liquid ecstasy, liquid E, liquid X, organic quaalude, salty water, scoop, sleep-500, somatomaz, vita-G
DEA CLASS: GHB is Class I; Xyrem is Class III for medical use.
PHARMACOLOGIC CLASS: CNS depressant

Description: GHB is produced naturally in small amounts by the body, but its function is unclear. The drug is used in Europe as a supplemental agent during anesthesia. It is also marketed as a drug that promotes muscle growth. In 2002, the FDA approved GHB to help reduce the number of cataplexy attacks (a condition marked by weak or paralyzed muscles) in patients with narcolepsy, but only under strict distribution control. When produced in clandestine laboratories, its effects are unpredictable. Drug abusers use GHB to reduce the stimulant effects of cocaine, methamphetamine, ephedrine, LSD, and mescaline, as well as to prevent the withdrawal symptoms of these agents. According to government reports, GHB has surpassed Rohypnol as the most common substance used in drug-facilitated sexual assaults. GBL (gamma butyrolactone), an analog of GHB, is also abused.

Method of use: Ingested

Duration of action: GHB is extremely short-acting and quickly leaves the user's system.

Psychological effects of abuse: Agitation, amnesia, confusion, delusion, depression, hallucinations, paranoia, and psychosis.

Physical effects of abuse: GHB is highly addictive, particularly with prolonged use. Early physical effects may include breathing problems, dizziness, excessive sweating, headache, loss of muscle tone, lowered blood pressure, nausea, reduced inhibition, sleepiness, sleepwalking, slowed heart rate and respiration, vertigo, and vomiting. Higher doses may cause complete loss of muscle coordination, decreased level of consciousness, slurred speech, seizures, coma, and death. Mixing GHB with alcohol greatly increases the CNS depressant effects, including respiratory arrest, unconsciousness, and coma.

Overdose symptoms: GHB is frequently combined with alcohol, which increases the risk of severe overdose. Symptoms depend on the amount ingested, whether any other CNS depressants were taken concurrently, and whether the drug was taken with or without food. Signs of overdose may include confusion, agitation, increased combativeness, excessive sweating, headache, impaired coordination, irregular gait, vomiting, blurred vision, memory loss, shortness of breath, respiratory depression, hallucinations, lowered body temperature, slow heart rate, seizures, and death.

Withdrawal symptoms: Abruptly stopping use may cause anxiety, agitation, insomnia, tremors, abnormally fast heart rate, and delirium within 1 to 6 hours after the last dose was taken, and the symptoms can last for months afterward.

GLUTETHIMIDE

COMMON STREET NAMES: Doors; when combined with codeine: doors & fours, loads, pancakes and syrup
DEA CLASS: Class II
PHARMACOLOGIC CLASS: Sedative, hypnotic

Not commercially available in the U.S.

Description: Glutethimide has properties similar to those of barbiturates. It was used previously for the short-term treatment of insomnia, but safer and more effective products have now replaced it. Currently, there is little medical use of the drug in the U.S.

Method of use: Ingested

Duration of action: Sedation occurs 15 to 30 minutes following ingestion, with peak serum levels occurring 1 to 6 hours later.

Psychological effects of abuse: Confusion, false sense of well-being, and impaired perception. Psychological dependence may occur with prolonged use of high doses.

Physical effects of abuse: Anxiety, difficulty swallowing, excessive sleepiness, low blood pressure, loss of coordination, sexual dysfunction, and slowed heart rate and breathing. Excessive use leads to tolerance, physical dependence, and withdrawal symptoms similar to those of the barbiturates.

Overdose symptoms: Tolerance develops rapidly, and progressively higher doses are needed to obtain the same effects as before. Signs of overdose may include extreme tiredness, irregular gait, muscle rigidity, muscular hyperactivity, rapid heart rate, low blood pressure, respiratory failure, heart failure, seizures, and possibly coma.

Withdrawal symptoms: Severity of withdrawal symptoms are similar to those of barbiturates, including weakness, abdominal cramps, nausea, vomiting, disorientation, anxiety, restlessness, elevated body temperature, rapid heart rate, stupor, delirium, visual hallucinations, tremors, seizures, and possibly death.

Halcion *see Triazolam, page 157*

Halotestin *see Fluoxymesterone, page 108*

HYDROCODONE COMBINATION PRODUCTS

GENERIC NAMES: Hydrocodone with acetaminophen (Anexsia, Lorcet, Lortab, Maxidone, Norco, Vicodin, Zydone); hydrocodone with chlorpheniramine (Tussionex); hydrocodone with guaifenesin (Vicodin Tuss); hydrocodone with ibuprofen (Vicoprofen)

COMMON STREET NAMES: Hillbilly heroin, killers, percs, poor man's heroin, schoolboy

DEA CLASS: Class III for combination products; Class II for hydrocodone

PHARMACOLOGIC CLASS: Narcotic analgesic (hydrocodone as a single agent); combination products are classified as cough suppressant, decongestant, expectorant, or antihistamine.

Description: Hydrocodone is used to manage mild to moderate pain and as a cough suppressant.

Method of use: Ingested

Duration of action: Depends on the dose and drug(s) used. In general, when hydrocodone is combined with other analgesics, the painkilling effects may last for up to 8 hours following ingestion.

Psychological effects of abuse: Anxiety, confusion, false sense of well-being, inability to concentrate, mood changes, psychological dependence (after prolonged use). The psychological dependence associated with narcotic addiction is complex. Long after physical dependence has ended, the addict may continue to think and talk about the drug and feel unable to manage daily activities without it.

Physical effects of abuse: Constipation, dizziness, irregular breathing, light-headedness, nausea, respiratory depression, urinary retention, and vomiting. Physical tolerance develops rapidly and is marked by euphoria, sedation, shorter duration of action, and weaker painkilling effects.

Overdose symptoms: Chronic use leads to tolerance, and progressively higher doses are needed to obtain the same effects as before. Signs of overdose may include bluish skin, cold and clammy skin, excessive perspiration, limp muscles, low blood pressure, slow heartbeat, breathing problems, and extreme sleepiness that could progress to a state of nonresponsiveness or coma. Risk of overdose increases significantly when the drug is taken with alcohol.

Withdrawal symptoms: Although the symptoms are similar to those of morphine withdrawal, they are considerably less intense. Abruptly stopping use may cause excessive tearing, yawning, and sweating about 12 to 14 hours after the last dose. Additional symptoms may include diminished appetite, gooseflesh, irritability, confusion, irregular breathing, tremors, seizures and loss of consciousness.

HYDROMORPHONE
BRAND NAMES: Dilaudid, Dilaudid-HP
COMMON STREET NAMES: D, dillies, dust, juice, smack
DEA CLASS: Class II
PHARMACOLOGIC CLASS: Narcotic analgesic, cough suppressant

Description: Hydromorphone is used to help manage moderate to severe pain. In lower doses, it's used as a cough suppressant. Compared with morphine, hydromorphone is two to eight times more potent, has a shorter duration of action, and produces more sedation.

Method of use: Ingested, used rectally, and injected IM, IV, or SC. Narcotic addicts often dissolve the tablets and inject the solution as a substitute for heroin.

Duration of action: About 4 to 5 hours

Psychological effects of abuse: Confusion, depression, hallucination, moodiness, nervousness, psychological dependence (after prolonged use), restlessness, and paradoxical CNS stimulation. The psychological dependence associated with narcotic addiction is complex. Long after physical dependence has ended, the addict may continue to think and talk about the drug and feel unable to manage daily activities without it.

Physical effects of abuse: Constricted pupils, decreased urination, diminished appetite, dry mouth, dizziness, headache, irregular breathing, low blood pressure, light-headedness, nausea, paradoxical CNS stimulation, rash, respiratory depression, seizures, severe constipation, stomach cramps, tiredness, and vomiting. Physical dependence may develop after prolonged use.

Overdose symptoms: Although tolerance develops slowly, the risk of overdose eventually increases as progressively larger doses are needed to obtain the same effects as before. Symptoms of overdose may include severe drowsiness, clammy skin, confusion, constricted pupils, low blood pressure, interrupted breathing, slow pulse, tremors, respiratory depression, convulsions, and coma. Risk of overdose increases significantly when the drug is taken with alcohol.

Withdrawal symptoms: Withdrawal begins slowly, with peak effects occurring 5 days after the last dose; however, sleep disturbances can persist for 13 days afterward. Although withdrawal is painful physically and emotionally, it's rarely life-threatening if adequate hydration and nutritional support are maintained. Early symptoms may include irritability, insomnia, diminished appetite, severe yawning, severe sneezing, tearing, and cold-like symptoms. Later-stage symptoms include nausea, vomiting, diarrhea, abdominal cramps, paradoxical excitability, bone and muscle pain in the back and extremities, fever, chills, excessive sweating, depression, and elevated heart rate and blood pressure.

Infumorph *see Morphine, page 129*

Intensol *see Oxycodone, page 136*

Ionamin *see Phentermine, page 146*

Kadian *see Morphine, page 129*

KETAMINE
BRAND NAME: Ketalar
COMMON STREET NAMES: Cat Valiums, jet, K, K-hole, keets, Lady K, new ecstasy, Special K, super C, vitamin K
DEA CLASS: Class III
PHARMACOLOGIC CLASS: General anesthetic; also identified as a dissociative anesthetic

Description: Ketamine's chemical structure and pharmacologic action are similar to those of phencyclidine (PCP), but it is significantly less potent. The drug's delusional effects are similar to LSD and mescaline. Ketamine produces "dissociative anesthesia," characterized by pain relief and amnesia without causing loss of consciousness. Legally, it is used to induce and maintain general anesthesia, especially when a cardiovascular depression needs to be prevented. Due to its disassociative effects and the fact that it is tasteless and odorless, ketamine is reportedly used as a date-rape drug.

Method of use: Ingested, snorted, used rectally, smoked, and rarely, injected IM or IV

Duration of action: About 2 to 4 hours following the standard dose. Effects of chronic use may take anywhere from several months to 2 years to wear off completely.

Psychological effects of abuse: Visual hallucinations, out-of-body experience, confusion, anxiety, depression, delirium, long-term memory loss, amnesia, aggressive or violent behavior, and vivid dreams. Long-term use may cause tolerance and psychological dependence.

Physical effects of abuse: Ketamine's physical effects are similar to PCP, and it has the same visual effects as LSD. The drug causes impaired motor function, exaggerated sense of strength, elevated blood pressure, rapid heart rate, tremors, slurred speech, nausea, vomiting, loss of appetite, rapid eye movement, and respiratory depression. Rarely, seizures and respiratory arrest may occur.

Overdose symptoms: Disorientation, irrational behavior, hallucinations, rapid heart rate, elevated blood pressure, convulsions, muscle rigidity, respiratory depression, and coma. Death is rare following ketamine abuse or overdose, but 1 gram may cause death.

Withdrawal symptoms: None are reported, since no evidence of physical dependence can be detected when the drug is abruptly withdrawn.

Klonopin *see Clonazepam, page 95*

Levo-Dromoran *see Levorphanol, page 116*

LEVORPHANOL TARTRATE

BRAND NAME: Levo-Dromoran
COMMON STREET NAMES: Dreamer, M, Miss Emma, morph
DEA CLASS: Class II
PHARMACOLOGIC CLASS: Narcotic analgesic

Description: Levorphanol is a potent synthetic opioid that is classified as a morphine derivative. It is used to help manage moderate to severe pain, as a sedative prior to surgery, and as a supplemental agent to nitrous oxide/oxygen anesthesia.

Method of use: Ingested, snorted, and injected IV, IM, or SC

Duration of action: Depends on the dose. Effects generally last 4 to 8 hours but can persist significantly longer in chronic users.

Psychological effects of abuse: Confusion, depression, hallucinations, mood changes, psychological dependence (after prolonged use), and restlessness. The psychological dependence associated with narcotic addiction is complex. Long after physical dependence has ended, the addict may continue to think and talk about the drug and feel unable to manage daily activities without it.

Physical effects of abuse: Blurred vision, constipation, dizziness, excessive sleepiness, low blood pressure, nausea, respiratory depression, slow pulse, and vomiting.

Overdose symptoms: Signs of overdose may include anxiety, cold and clammy skin, confusion, weakness, severe drowsiness and dizziness, constricted pupils, low blood pressure, slow heart rate, CNS and cardiac depression, convulsions, respiratory depression, and unconsciousness.

Withdrawal symptoms: Abruptly stopping the drug after long-term use may precipitate withdrawal symptoms. The intensity and duration of symptoms are directly related to the total daily dose, frequency of use, and health of the user. Although withdrawal from narcotics is painful physically and emotionally, it is rarely life-threatening if adequate hydration and nutritional support are maintained. Early withdrawal symptoms may include watery eyes, runny nose, repeated yawning, and excessive sweating. Later-stage symptoms may include nervousness, muscle twitching, drug cravings, restlessness, irritability, loss of appetite, chills alternating with flushing, nausea, vomiting, bone and muscle pain in the back and extremities, tremors, elevated heart rate and blood pressure, and severe depression.

Librium *see Chlordiazepoxide, page 94*

LORAZEPAM
BRAND NAME: Ativan
COMMON STREET NAMES: Candy, downers, sleeping pills, tranks
DEA CLASS: Class IV
PHARMACOLOGIC CLASS: Benzodiazepine, sedative, antianxiety, antiemetic, anticonvulsant

Description: Lorazepam is used to treat anxiety disorders, including anxiety associated with depression. In addition, it is used intravenously to treat severe epileptic seizures, as a sedative to induce relaxation before anesthesia, and as a supplemental therapy to prevent vomiting. Abuse of benzodiazepines is particularly high among heroin and cocaine users.

Method of use: Ingested and injected IM or IV

Duration of action: 8 to 25 hours

Psychological effects of abuse: Confusion, impaired judgment and thinking abilities, irritability, mild euphoria, pressured speech, reduced inhibition, and suicidal ideation. Long-term use may cause psychological dependence.

Physical effects of abuse: Changes in appetite and body weight, constipation, dizziness, impaired muscle coordination, labored breathing, and low blood pressure. Long-term use may cause physical dependence.

Overdose symptoms: The most severe signs of overdose are respiratory depression and coma. Other symptoms may include confusion, diminished reflexes, unrealistic euphoria, extreme sleepiness, and impaired muscle coordination. Death from overdose of a single benzodiazepine is extremely rare. However, there is an increased risk of toxicity when benzodiazepines are combined with alcohol and/or other CNS depressants. Fatalities have been reported in patients who have overdosed with a combination of a single benzodiazepine and alcohol.

Withdrawal symptoms: Abrupt termination following long-term use may precipitate withdrawal symptoms and require hospitalization. Symptoms may include abdominal and muscle cramps, depression, insomnia, sweating, vomiting, tremors, and seizures.

Lorcet *see Hydrocodone, page 113*

Lortab *see Hydrocodone, page 113*

Luminal *see Phenobarbital, page 145*

Marinol *see Dronabinol and Nabilone, page 101*

Maxidone *see Hydrocodone, page 113*

Mebaral *see Mephobarbital, page 119*

MEPERIDINE HYDROCHLORIDE
BRAND NAMES: Demerol, Meperitab
COMMON STREET NAMES: D, dillies, dust, juice, smack
DEA CLASS: Class II
PHARMACOLOGIC CLASS: Narcotic analgesic

Description: Meperidine is used as a sedative before surgery, as a supplemental agent to induce anesthesia, and to help manage moderate to severe pain. Although it has effects similar to morphine, meperidine has a shorter duration of action and weaker cough suppressing and antidiarrheal activities.

Method of use: Ingested and injected IM, IV, or SC

Duration of action: Depends on the dose and method of use. In general, effects persist 2 to 4 hours following administration.

Psychological effects of abuse: Confusion, depression, and hallucinations. The psychological dependence associated with narcotic addiction is complex. Long after physical dependence has ended, the addict may continue to think and talk about the drug and feel unable to manage daily activities without it. Psychological addiction is a major problem with meperidine, particularly when used in higher doses for prolonged periods.

Physical effects of abuse: Low blood pressure, drowsiness, dizziness, headache, light-headedness, feeling faint, restlessness, fatigue, seizures, nausea, constipation, vomiting, diminished appetite, dry mouth, abdominal cramps, stomach cramps, urine retention, and shortness of breath. Higher doses and long-term use is associated with paradoxical CNS excitement, tremors, and seizures due to the accumulation of the active metabolite normeperidine. Meperidine use has also been associated with symptoms that resemble Parkinson's disease, including jerky movements and tremors. Physical tolerance and addiction can develop, particularly when used in higher doses for prolonged periods.

Overdose symptoms: Chronic use leads to tolerance, and progressively larger doses are needed to obtain the same effects as before. Symptoms of overdose may include severe drowsiness, constricted pupils, clammy skin, confusion, slow pulse, slow or labored breathing, CNS depression, tremors, and seizures. Risk of overdose increases significantly when the drug is taken with alcohol.

Withdrawal symptoms: The intensity of symptoms is directly related to the total daily dose, frequency and duration of use, and the health of the user. Withdrawal symptoms may persist for up to 5 days after the last dose. Although withdrawal from narcotics is painful physically and emotionally, it is rarely life-threatening. Early symptoms appear within 3 hours after the last dose and may include watery eyes, runny nose, yawning, and sweating. Later-stage symptoms may include nervousness, muscle twitching, drug cravings, restlessness, irritability, loss of appetite, chills alternating with flushing, excessive sweating, nausea, vomiting, bone and muscle pain in the back and extremities, tremors, rapid heart rate, elevated blood pressure, and severe depression.

Meperitab *see Meperidine, page 118*

MEPHOBARBITAL
BRAND NAME: Mebaral
COMMON STREET NAME: Downers
DEA CLASS: Class IV
PHARMACOLOGIC CLASS: Barbiturate, sedative, anticonvulsant

Description: Barbiturates depress the sensory cortex, decrease motor activity, alter brain function, and produce drowsiness, sedation, and hypnosis. Mephobarbital is used primarily for daytime sedation and the management of seizure disorders.

Method of use: Ingested

Duration of action: Effects start within an hour and last for about 12 hours.

Psychological effects of abuse: Barbiturates may cause psychological dependence, especially following prolonged use of high doses. Effects may include confusion, alternating euphoria and depression, memory loss, impaired judgment, nervousness, nightmares, and hallucinations.

Physical effects of abuse: The most frequent physical effects are due to CNS depression, including dizziness, headache, excessive sleepiness, drowsiness, and irregular gait. Other symptoms may include headache, stomach pain, and skin rash. Paradoxical excitement and irritability may also occur. In chronic users, blood disorders such as megaloblastic anemia may develop. Short-term therapy has been associated with the development of Stevens-Johnson syndrome and toxic skin eruptions. Rarely, necrotic ulcer of the mouth may occur within 10 days of ingestion. Physical dependence is a significant risk, since it can develop after short-term use.

Overdose symptoms: Unsteady gait, slurred speech, confusion, low body temperature and blood pressure, and dose-dependent respiratory depression. Toxic effects are enhanced when the drug is taken with alcohol and/or other CNS depressants.

Withdrawal symptoms: Symptoms are similar to those of alcohol withdrawal and characterized by severe apprehension, weakness, heightened anxiety, irritability, dizziness, headache, sleeplessness, muscle twitching, nausea and vomiting, distortion of visual perception, and rapid pulse. Severely low blood pressure and convulsions may develop after a day or two, which eventually leads to hallucinations and delirium followed by coma and death.

MEPROBAMATE and CARISOPRODOL

BRAND NAMES: Soma (carisoprodol)
COMMON STREET NAMES: Not known
DEA CLASS: Class IV (meprobamate only)
PHARMACOLOGIC CLASS: Antianxiety agent (meprobamate); muscle relaxant (carisoprodol)

Description: Meprobamate is used to treat anxiety, tension, and muscle spasms associated with tension. Carisoprodol is a muscle relaxant that the body metabolically converts to meprobamate, which probably accounts for some of the drug's pharmacologic properties as well as its tendency to be abused.

Method of use: Ingested

Duration of action: Onset and duration of action of meprobamate are similar to those of the intermediate-acting barbiturates. Its effects peak 2 hours following ingestion and persist for about 10 hours.

Psychological effects of abuse: Confusion, euphoria, and impaired mental abilities. Psychological dependence may develop after prolonged use.

Physical effects of abuse: Chills, diarrhea, drowsiness, elevated heart rate, feeling faint, headache, impaired physical abilities, loss of appetite, nausea, numbness in the extremities, slurred speech, stomach pain, vertigo, and vomiting. Tolerance and physical dependence may develop after excessive use.

Overdose symptoms: Overdose can cause death due to respiratory failure and/or severely low blood pressure. Other signs of overdose may include drowsiness, irregular gait, tiredness, weakness, nausea, vomiting, blurred vision, low blood pressure, shock, and coma.

Withdrawal symptoms: Abruptly stopping use may cause confusion, memory loss, excessive sweating, nervousness, elevated blood pressure, hallucinations, and psychosis.

Metadate *see Methylphenidate, page 124.*

METHADONE

BRAND NAMES: Dolophine, Methadone Intensol, Methadose
COMMON STREET NAMES: D, dillies, dolls, done, dust, frizzies, juice, smack
DEA CLASS: Class II
PHARMACOLOGIC CLASS: Narcotic analgesic

Description: Although methadone's chemical structure is different from morphine and heroin, its pharmacologic effects are the same. It's used for detoxification and maintenance treatment of narcotic addiction and to help manage severe pain. High-dose methadone is useful for treating heroin addicts because it can block the drug's effects.

Method of use: Ingested and injected IM, IV, or SC

Duration of action: About 6 to 8 hours, although effects can last 24 to 48 hours in chronic users.

Psychological effects of abuse: Agitation, change in sexual desires, confusion, depression, disorientation, euphoria, and psychological dependence (after prolonged use). The psychological dependence associated with narcotic addiction is complex. Long after physical dependence has ended, the addict may continue to think and talk about the drug and feel unable to manage daily activities without it.

Physical effects of abuse: Blurred vision, CNS and respiratory depression, constricted pupils, constipation, diminished appetite, dizziness, drowsiness, faintness, headache, insomnia, light-headedness, loss of appetite, low blood pressure, nausea, seizures, slow heartbeat, slow or troubled breathing, stomach cramps, tremors, and vomiting. Chronic use results in tolerance and physical dependence.

Overdose symptoms: Chronic use leads to tolerance, and progressively higher doses are needed to obtain the same effects as before. Signs of overdose include low body temperature, constricted pupils, cold and clammy skin, confusion, severe drowsiness, slow or troubled breathing, CNS and respiratory depression, slow heartbeat, tremors, and seizures.

Withdrawal symptoms: Abruptly stopping the drug after chronic use may precipitate withdrawal symptoms. Although withdrawal from narcotics is painful physically and emotionally, it is rarely life-threatening if adequate hydration and nutritional support are maintained. Methadone withdrawal starts 24 hours after the last dose and can persist for several weeks. The intensity of symptoms is directly related to the total daily dose, frequency and duration of use, and the health of the user.

Early withdrawal symptoms may include watery eyes, runny nose, repeated yawning, and excessive sweating. Later-stage symptoms include restlessness, irritability, loss of appetite, nausea, vomiting, diarrhea, tremors, severe depression, shivering, and drug cravings. Advanced withdrawal symptoms may include elevated heart rate and blood pressure, chills alternating with flushing, and bone and muscle pain in the back and extremities.

Methadone Intensol *see Methadone, page 121*

Methadose *see Methadone, page 121*

METHAMPHETAMINE HYDROCHLORIDE
BRAND NAME: Desoxyn
COMMON STREET NAMES: Chalk, crank, crystal, fire, glass, go fast, ice, meth, speed
DEA CLASS: Class II
PHARMACOLOGIC CLASS: Amphetamine, CNS stimulant

Description: Amphetamine, methamphetamine, and dextroamphetamine are collectively referred to as amphetamines; they have similar chemical properties and pharmacologic actions. Methamphetamine is used as a supplemental agent for treating attention deficit hyperactivity disorder (ADHD). It is also used as a short-term aid for weight loss when combined with caloric restriction, exercise, and behavior modification.

Method of use: Ingested, snorted, smoked (most common use), and injected IV

Duration of action: 8 to 24 hours

Psychological effects of abuse: Anxiety, heightened energy, increased alertness, irritability, restlessness, and talkativeness. Large doses can cause confusion, delusion, rage, violence, visual and auditory hallucinations, delirium, self-destructive behavior, aggressiveness, and panic. Chronic use leads to psychotic behavior, including paranoia, hallucinations, and psychotic rages that may result in violence. Psychological dependence develops rapidly in chronic users.

Physical effects of abuse: Amphetamines are known to increase energy and decrease appetite. Other physical symptoms may include diarrhea, dilated pupils, elevated body temperature, excessive sweating, headache, insomnia, muscle rigidity, rapid heartbeat, rapid breathing, stomach cramps, tremors, and vomiting. Chronic abuse may lead to permanent brain damage. There are characteristic sores on the bodies of chronic users from scratching at "bugs" (the delusional belief that bugs are crawling under the skin). Acute lead poisoning may also develop due to the method of production of methamphetamines that uses lead acetate as a reagent.

Overdose symptoms: Tolerance to the anorectic effect of methamphetamine usually develops within a few weeks. Individuals may need progressively larger doses to obtain the same effects as before. Symptoms of overdose may include nausea, vomiting, diarrhea, restlessness, severe high blood pressure, dangerously high body temperature, tremors, hyperactivity, rapid and irregular heartbeat, rapid breathing, muscle rigidity, severe psychosis, serotonin syndrome, seizures, and coma. High doses may cause stroke. Fatality rates increase significantly if high blood pressure and seizures occur.

Withdrawal symptoms: Methamphetamine is a powerfully addictive drug, and physical and psychological dependence develop rapidly. Abrupt cessation of use may cause anxiety, fatigue, paranoia, aggressive behavior, and strong drug cravings. Severe depression and suicidal ideation have also been reported. Psychotic behavior may persist for months or years after discontinuation of use.

METHENOLONE

COMMON STREET NAMES: Arnolds, gym candy, juice, pumpers, roids, stackers, weight trainers
DEA CLASS: Class III
PHARMACOLOGIC CLASS: Anabolic-androgenic steroid

Not commercially available in the U.S.

Description: Androgens are steroid hormones that develop and maintain male sex characteristics. They are used primarily to replace insufficient levels of testosterone due to poor functioning of the testes. When used in combination with exercise and a high-protein diet, androgens can promote increased muscle size and strength, improve stamina, and decrease recovery time between workouts. Androgens are also used to promote the development of puberty in males with clearly delayed onset. Additionally, androgens are sometimes prescribed for women with advancing, inoperable metastatic breast cancer who are 1 to 5 years postmenopausal. Methenolone has also been effective in the management of aplastic anemia.

Method of use: Ingested and injected IM

Duration of action: Not entirely known but is believed to remain in the body for at least a week.

Psychological effects of abuse: Mood changes, depression, uncontrollable aggressive behavior, euphoria, anxiety, irritability, increased sex drive, and rarely, psychosis. Psychological dependence may also occur.

Physical effects of abuse: Angry or hostile feelings, elevated blood pressure and cholesterol, headache, insomnia, premature balding, psychotic reactions, severe acne, sexual dysfunction, and violent behavior. *In men:* Breast development, impotence, intermittent or painful urination, painful or persistent erections, reduced sperm production, and shrinking of the testicles. *In women:* Decreased body fat and breast size, deepening of the voice, enlarged clitoris, excessive growth of body hair, and menstrual changes. *In adolescents:* Premature termination of growth.

Prolonged use can lead to tolerance. While the long-term effects are not completely known, chronic steroid abuse has been associated with damage to the heart, liver, and brain.

Overdose symptoms: There have been no reports of serious overdose with androgenic steroids. Chronic use of high doses may cause excessive sexual stimulation, reduced sperm production, enlarged breasts in males, uncontrollable painful erection, jaundice, and deteriorating liver function. Excessive fluid retention may occur in users who have heart, liver, or kidney disease.

Withdrawal symptoms: Abrupt discontinuation may cause mood changes, tiredness, restlessness, loss of appetite, dissatisfaction with body image, sleeplessness, reduced sex drive, paranoia, and severe depression that can lead to suicide attempts.

Methitest *see Methyltestosterone, page 125*

Methylin *see Methylphenidate, page 124*

METHYLPHENIDATE HYDROCHLORIDE

BRAND NAMES: Concerta, Daytrana, Metadate, Methylin, Ritalin, Ritalin LA
COMMON STREET NAMES: R-ball, Rit, vitamin R, working man's cocaine
DEA CLASS: Class II
PHARMACOLOGIC CLASS: CNS stimulant, nonamphetamine

Description: Methylphenidate is used to treat attention deficit hyperactivity disorder (ADHD). In addition, it is the preferred drug for treating excessive daytime sleepiness (narcolepsy) due to its rapid action and fewer side effects than other CNS stimulants. Severe complications can occur when methylphenidate tablets are crushed and diluted in water for injection. The tablets contain soluble fibers that can block small blood vessels, causing serious damage to the lungs and eye retina.

Method of use: Ingested; tablets are also crushed and snorted or diluted in water and injected.

Duration of action: 4 to 5 hours following a standard therapeutic dose.

Psychological effects of abuse: Depression, nervousness, and psychotic behavior.

Physical effects of abuse: Anorexia, blurred vision, dizziness, elevated blood pressure, elevated or lowered pulse, headache, high body temperature, insomnia, irregular heart rhythm, nausea, stomach pain, Tourette's syndrome, toxic psychosis, vomiting, and weight loss. Severe blockage in the blood vessels of the lungs and eye retina can occur when the drug is injected.

Overdose symptoms: Signs of overdose include excessive sweating and hyperactivity, vomiting, agitation, tremors, severely elevated body temperature and blood pressure, rapid heart rate, and hallucinations.

Withdrawal symptoms: Withdrawal reactions are less common than with other CNS stimulants. Symptoms may include severe fatigue, depression, nausea, vomiting, stomach cramps, insomnia, and nightmares.

METHYLTESTOSTERONE
BRAND NAMES: Android, Methitest, Testred, Virilon
COMMON STREET NAMES: Arnolds, gym candy, juice, pumpers, roids, stackers, weight trainers
DEA CLASS: Class III
PHARMACOLOGIC CLASS: Anabolic-androgenic steroid

Description: Androgens are steroid hormones that develop and maintain male sex characteristics. They are used primarily to replace insufficient levels of testosterone due to poor functioning of the testes. When used in combination with exercise and a high-protein diet, androgens can promote increased muscle size and strength, improve stamina, and decrease recovery time between workouts. Androgens are also used to promote the development of puberty in males with clearly delayed onset. Additionally, androgens are sometimes prescribed for women with advancing, inoperable metastatic breast cancer who are 1 to 5 years postmenopausal.

Method of use: Ingested and absorbed through the cheek and gum (buccal administration). Chronic users tend to rotate steroids using various methods known as cycling, stacking, and pyramiding. Sporadic discontinuation of use is believed to allow testosterone levels and sperm counts to return to normal. Taking steroids regularly with periodic "drug-free times" is called cycling. Stacking refers to the concomitant use of two or more steroids at high doses. Pyramiding is when the dose, frequency, or number of steroids taken is gradually increased, followed by progressive tapering of the drug(s).

Duration of action: Depends on the dose and method of use. Methyltestosterone remains active for up to 22 hours following use.

Psychological effects of abuse: Mood changes, depression, uncontrollable aggressive behavior, euphoria, anxiety, irritability, increased sex drive, and rarely, psychosis. Psychological dependence may occur.

Physical effects of abuse: Angry or hostile feelings, elevated blood pressure and cholesterol, headache, insomnia, premature balding, psychotic reactions, severe acne, sexual dysfunction, and violent behavior. ***In men:*** Breast development, impotence, intermittent or painful urination, painful or persistent erections, reduced sperm production, and shrinking of the testicles. ***In women:*** Decreased body fat and breast size, deepening of the voice, enlarged clitoris, excessive growth of body hair, and menstrual changes. ***In adolescents:*** Premature termination of growth.

Prolonged use can lead to tolerance. While the long-term effects are not completely known, chronic steroid abuse has been associated with damage to the heart, liver, and brain.

Overdose symptoms: There are no documented reports of overdose with androgens. Chronic use of high doses may cause excessive sexual stimulation, reduced sperm production, enlarged breasts in males, uncontrollable painful erection, jaundice, and deteriorating liver function. Excessive fluid retention may occur in users who have heart, liver, or kidney disease.

Withdrawal symptoms: Abrupt discontinuation may cause mood changes, tiredness, restlessness, loss of appetite, dissatisfaction with body image, sleeplessness, reduced sex drive, paranoia, and severe depression that can lead to suicide attempts.

METHYPRYLON
COMMON STREET NAMES: Not known
DEA CLASS: Class III
PHARMACOLOGIC CLASS: Sedative, hypnotic (nonbarbiturate)

Description: Methyprylon is chemically related to glutethimide and causes CNS depression similar to barbiturates. The drug is marketed in other countries for the short-term treatment of insomnia. Methyprylon was withdrawn from the U.S. market after safer and more effective agents became available.

Method of use: Ingested, used rectally

Duration of action: Usually 5 to 8 hours following a standard therapeutic dose.

Psychological effects of abuse: Confusion, depression, paradoxical excitement, hallucinations, nightmares, and restlessness. Prolonged use may lead to psychological dependence.

Physical effects of abuse: Blurred or double vision, dizziness, drowsiness, fever, headache, insomnia, irregular gait, nausea, vomiting, diarrhea, constipation, stomach cramps, trembling, and weakness. Prolonged use may cause liver damage and/or soft bones or rickets. Respiratory depression, seizures, and coma have also been reported. Prolonged use may lead to tolerance and physical dependence.

Overdose symptoms: Complications with sedative overdose—such as pneumonia, fluid accumulation in the lungs, heart arrhythmias, and heart or kidney failure—may occur in rare cases. Life-threatening signs of overdose include severe confusion, dilated pupils, rapid heartbeat, excessive CNS and respiratory depression, severe drowsiness, loss of reflexes, coma, respiratory arrest, and death. Additional symptoms may include constricted pupils, slurred speech, irregular gait, weakness, and low body temperature.

Withdrawal symptoms: Abrupt cessation of use may cause severe confusion, nightmares, restlessness, paradoxical excitement, sleeplessness, excessive sweating, hallucinations, and seizures. Death has also been reported in individuals not receiving medical treatment during withdrawal.

MIDAZOLAM HYDROCHLORIDE
COMMON STREET NAMES: Candy, downers, sleeping pills, tranks
DEA CLASS: Class IV
PHARMACOLOGIC CLASS: Benzodiazepine, sedative, hypnotic

Description: Midazolam is used to produce drowsiness and relieve anxiety before surgery or diagnostic procedures. It is also used to induce loss of consciousness and amnesia in patients having surgery or those in critical-care settings. It is three to four times more potent than Valium. Abuse of benzodiazepines is particularly high among heroin and cocaine users.

Method of use: Ingested, snorted, and injected IM or IV

Duration of action: Up to 6 hours

Psychological effects of abuse: Amnesia, confusion, depression, impaired judgment and thinking abilities, reduced inhibition, and suicidal ideation. Paradoxical effects include euphoria, hyperactivity, and extreme aggression. Prolonged use may cause psychological dependence.

Physical effects of abuse: Constipation, decreased blood pressure, dizziness, drowsiness, impaired physical capabilities, irregular gait, loss of muscle tone, sleepiness, slowed psychomotor performance, urinary retention, and visual disturbances. Prolonged use may cause physical dependence.

Overdose symptoms: The most severe signs of overdose are respiratory depression, loss of consciousness, and coma. Other symptoms may include confusion, depression, diminished reflexes, slurred speech, impaired coordination, apnea, extreme sleepiness, loss of muscle tone, and severely low blood pressure. Death from overdose of a single benzodiazepine is extremely rare. However, there is an increased risk of toxicity when benzodiazepines are combined with alcohol and/or other CNS depressants. Fatalities have been reported in patients who have overdosed with a combination of a single benzodiazepine and alcohol.

Withdrawal symptoms: Abrupt termination following long-term use may precipitate withdrawal symptoms and require hospitalization. Symptoms may include abdominal and muscle cramps, depression, insomnia, sweating, vomiting, tremors, and seizures.

MODAFINIL
BRAND NAME: Provigil
COMMON STREET NAMES: Not known
DEA CLASS: Class IV
PHARMACOLOGIC CLASS: CNS stimulant, nonamphetamine

Description: Modafinil is used to improve wakefulness in those with excessive daytime sleepiness (narcolepsy). It is also used to treat obstructive sleep apnea/hypopnea syndrome and shift work sleep disorder. The drug is chemically and pharmacologically unrelated to other CNS stimulants such as methylphenidate or amphetamines.

Method of use: Ingested

Duration of action: About 10 to 12 hours

Psychological effects of abuse: Psychoactive and euphoric effects, as well as alterations of mood and perception, are the most common psychological effects of modafinil. Other effects may include anxiety, depression, confusion, paranoid delusions, auditory hallucinations, and amnesia. Eye problems such as floaters and dryness have also been reported.

Physical effects of abuse: High or low blood pressure, irregular heartbeats, headache, nervousness, dizziness, sleeplessness, irregular gait, nausea, diarrhea, vomiting, dry mouth, reduced appetite, ejaculatory difficulties, urinary difficulties, neck pain, tremor, abnormal involuntary movements, tingling sensation, abnormal vision, increased liver enzymes, shortness of breath, and nasal congestion.

Overdose symptoms: Overdose information is limited. The following have been reported with high doses: agitation, irritability, confusion, nervousness, tremor, sleeplessness, and heart palpitations.

Withdrawal symptoms: To date, physical dependence on this drug has not been reported. However, experience with modafinil is limited, and the potential for dependence still exists.

MORPHINE SULFATE
BRAND NAMES: Astramorph PF, Avinza, Duramorph PF, Infumorph, Kadian, MS Contin, MSIR, Oramorph SR, RMS, Roxanol
COMMON STREET NAMES: Dreamer, M, Miss Emma, morph
DEA CLASS: Class II
PHARMACOLOGIC CLASS: Narcotic analgesic

Description: Morphine is the principal constituent of opium. It is used as a sedative prior to surgery, as a supplemental agent to induce anesthesia, and to manage moderate to severe pain. Morphine can also be used to relieve pain associated with heart attack and to relieve anxiety in patients who have shortness of breath due to pulmonary edema or acute heart failure.

Method of use: Ingested, used rectally, and injected IM, IV, or SC

Duration of action: Depends on the dose and method of use. In general, the effects last 3 to 6 hours following administration. However, in chronic users the effects may last significantly longer.

Psychological effects of abuse: Confusion, disorientation, false sense of well-being, hallucinations, and thought disturbances. The psychological dependence associated with narcotic addiction is complex. Long after physical dependence has ended, the addict may continue to think and talk about the drug and feel unable to manage daily activities without it. Psychological dependence on morphine is known to develop slowly.

Physical effects of abuse: Blurred vision, CNS and respiratory depression, constipation, diminished appetite, dizziness, drowsiness, dry mouth, flushing, headache, low blood pressure and pulse, muscle rigidity, nausea, paradoxical CNS stimulation, restlessness, seizures, shortness of breath, stomach cramps, tiredness, urine retention, and vomiting. Physical dependence on morphine develops progressively.

Overdose symptoms: Although tolerance develops slowly, the risk of overdose eventually increases as progressively larger doses are needed to obtain the same effects as before. Signs of overdose may include severe drowsiness, constricted pupils, clammy skin, confusion, low blood pressure, interrupted breathing, slow pulse, tremors, respiratory depression, convulsions, and coma. Risk of overdose increases significantly when the drug is taken with alcohol.

Withdrawal symptoms: Although withdrawal from morphine is painful physically and emotionally, it's rarely life-threatening if adequate hydration and nutritional support are maintained. Symptoms begin slowly, with peak effects observed 5 days after cessation of use; however, sleep disturbances can persist up to 13 days following the last dose. Early withdrawal symptoms may include irritability, sleeplessness, diminished appetite, excessive yawning, severe sneezing, tearing, and head cold. Later-stage symptoms may include nausea, vomiting, severe diarrhea, paradoxical excitability, abdominal cramps, bone and muscle pain in the back and extremities, fever and chills, excessive sweating, and depression. Muscle spasms and kicking movements can also occur, which may explain the expression "kicking the habit."

MS Contin *see Morphine, page 129*

MSIR *see Morphine, page 129*

Mysoline *see Primidone, page 147*

NANDROLONE DECANOATE
COMMON STREET NAMES: Arnolds, gym candy, juice, pumpers, roids, stackers, weight trainers
DEA CLASS: Class III
PHARMACOLOGIC CLASS: Anabolic-androgenic steroid

Description: Androgens are steroid hormones that develop and maintain male sex characteristics. They are used primarily to replace insufficient levels of testosterone due to poor functioning of the testes. When used in combination with exercise and a high-protein diet, androgens can promote increased muscle size and strength, improve stamina, and decrease recovery time between workouts. Androgens are also used to promote the development of puberty in males with clearly delayed onset. Additionally, androgens are sometimes prescribed for women with advancing, inoperable metastatic breast cancer who are 1 to 5 years postmenopausal. Nandrolone has also been shown to positively influence calcium metabolism and increase bone mass in people with osteoporosis.

Method of use: Injected IM. Chronic users tend to rotate steroids using various methods known as cycling, stacking, and pyramiding. Sporadic discontinuation of use is believed to allow testosterone levels and sperm counts to return to normal. Taking steroids regularly with periodic "drug-free times" is called cycling. Stacking refers to the concomitant use of two or more steroids at high doses. Pyramiding is when the dose, frequency, or number of steroids taken is gradually increased, followed by progressive tapering of the drug(s).

Duration of action: Approximately 3 to 4 weeks.

Psychological effects of abuse: Mood changes, depression, and increased sex drive. Psychological dependence may also develop.

Physical effects of abuse: Angry or hostile feelings, elevated blood pressure and cholesterol, headache, insomnia, premature balding, psychotic reactions, severe acne, sexual dysfunction, and violent behavior. *In men:* Breast development, impotence, intermittent or painful urination, painful or persistent erections, reduced sperm production, and shrinking of the testicles. *In women:* Decreased body fat and breast size, deepening of the voice, enlarged clitoris, excessive growth of body hair, and menstrual changes. *In adolescents:* Premature termination of growth.

Prolonged use can lead to tolerance. While the long-term effects are not completely known, chronic steroid abuse has been associated with damage to the heart, liver, and brain.

Overdose symptoms: There have been no reports of serious overdose with this product. Chronic exposure to high doses may cause serious acne, excessive growth of body hair, hoarseness, changes in sex drive, poor sperm production, and menstrual problems in women.

Withdrawal symptoms: Abrupt discontinuation can cause mood changes, tiredness, restlessness, loss of appetite, dissatisfaction with body image, sleeplessness, reduced sex drive, paranoia, and severe depression that can lead to suicide attempts.

Nembutal *see Pentobarbital, page 142*

NITRAZEPAM

COMMON STREET NAMES: Candy, downers, sleeping pills, tranks
DEA CLASS: Class IV
PHARMACOLOGIC CLASS: Benzodiazepine, sedative, hypnotic

Not commercially available in the U.S.

Description: Nitrazepam is neither approved nor manufactured in the U.S. It has similar pharmacologic properties as diazepam (Valium). Nitrazepam is used in other countries for the short-term treatment of insomnia. It has also been used in epilepsy, particularly in infants. Abuse of benzodiazepines is particularly high among heroin and cocaine users.

Method of use: Ingested and injected IM or IV

Duration of action: Up to 30 hours

Psychological effects of abuse: Amnesia, confusion, depression, euphoria, impaired judgment and thinking abilities, mild euphoria, pressured speech, reduced inhibition, and suicidal ideation. Long-term use may cause psychological dependence.

Physical effects of abuse: Constipation, decreased blood pressure, dizziness, drowsiness, impaired physical capabilities, loss of muscle tone, sleepiness, slowed psychomotor performance, urinary retention, and visual disturbances.

Overdose symptoms: The most severe signs of overdose are respiratory depression, loss of consciousness, and coma. Other symptoms may include sensitivity to light, diminished reflexes, slurred speech, impaired coordination, apnea, extreme sleepiness, loss of muscle tone, severely low blood pressure, and tremors. Death from overdose of a single benzodiazepine is extremely rare. However, there is an increased risk of toxicity when benzodiazepines are combined with alcohol and/or other CNS depressants. Fatalities have been reported in patients who have overdosed with a combination of a single benzodiazepine and alcohol.

Withdrawal symptoms: Abrupt termination following long-term use may precipitate withdrawal symptoms and require hospitalization. Symptoms may include abdominal and muscle cramps, depression, insomnia, severe drowsiness, sweating, vomiting, tremors, respiratory depression, seizures, and coma.

NITRITES (amyl nitrite and glyceryl trinitrate)
COMMON STREET NAME: Poppers
DEA CLASS: Not classified
PHARMACOLOGIC CLASS: Coronary vasodilator

Description: Nitrites are volatile liquids that are readily absorbed from the lungs. Amyl nitrite has an action similar to glyceryl trinitrate (also known as nitroglycerin). Nitrites relax and open the blood vessels to the heart and are used therapeutically to relieve acute chest pain (angina) and to help manage heart murmurs. In addition, nitrites are used as supplemental agents to counteract cyanide poisoning, although their effectiveness for this use is still in question. These drugs are often abused because users believe they expand creativity, stimulate music appreciation, promote a sense of abandon in dancing, and intensify sexual experiences.

Method of use: Inhalation

Duration of action: Therapeutic effects of short-acting products usually occur within 30 seconds and last for 3 to 5 minutes.

Psychological effects of abuse: Aggressive behavior, anxiety, restlessness, and rarely, psychosis.

Physical effects of abuse: Anemia and other blood disorders, blurred vision, coma, cough, dizziness, elevated pressure in the eye, face rash, flushing, loss of coordination, low blood pressure or pulse, nausea, paralysis of the face, throbbing headache, rapid heartbeat, shortness of breath, throat irritation, vomiting, weakness, and rarely, death. Cerebrovascular disease can occur due to severely low blood pressure. Tolerance may develop with prolonged use.

Overdose symptoms: Seizures have been reported following severe overdose. Fatalities from nitrite toxicity have occurred due to uncontrolled artery spasm (vasodilation) and/or methemoglobinemia, which causes dangerously low oxygenation of the tissues. Other signs of overdose include bluish skin color, fainting, shortness of breath, increased pressure in the eye, stomach irritation accompanied by nausea and vomiting, severe abdominal pain, muscular weakness, weakness that effects only one side of the body, psychosis, coma, and rarely, death.

Withdrawal symptoms: Sudden withdrawal may cause sharp or persistent contractions of the heart arteries (coronary vasospasm), possibly leading to reduced blood flow and heart damage.

Norco *see Hydrocodone, page 113*

Numorphan *see Oxymorphone, page 139*

OPIUM

BRAND NAMES: Opium Tincture (also known as deodorized tincture of opium), Paregoric
COMMON STREET NAMES: Gee, God's medicine, gondola, great tobacco, gum, gumma
DEA CLASS: Class II for extracts, tinctures, and poppy; Class III for opium combination products such as Paregoric (opium with camphor).
PHARMACOLOGIC CLASS: Narcotic analgesic, antidiarrheal

Description: In the U.S., opium is used in the paregoric form to treat severe diarrhea. Rarely, it's used to relieve pain. Drug traffickers harvest opium from the poppy plant and refine the drug to make morphine or heroin.

Method of use: Ingested

Duration of action: Generally 4 to 5 hours

Psychological effects of abuse: Anxiety, confusion, depression, false sense of well-being, mood changes, psychological dependence (after prolonged use), and restlessness. The psychological dependence associated with narcotic addiction is complex. Long after physical dependence has ended, the addict may continue to think and talk about the drug and feel unable to manage daily activities without it.

Physical effects of abuse: Constipation, dizziness, headache, irregular breathing, light-headedness, loss of appetite, muscle weakness, low blood pressure, nausea, respiratory depression, sleeplessness, slowed heart rate, stomach cramps, urinary retention, and vomiting. Prolonged use may cause physical dependence.

Overdose symptoms: Chronic use leads to tolerance, and progressively higher doses are needed to obtain the same effects as before. Signs of overdose may include constipation, stomach cramps, nausea, vomiting, extreme sleepiness, nonreactive pupils, drowsiness, dizziness, slurred speech, cold and clammy skin, lowered body temperature and blood pressure, CNS and respiratory depression, convulsions, and coma. Death rarely occurs.

Withdrawal symptoms: Opiate withdrawal is considered to be fairly mild. The symptoms begin slowly, with peak effects observed after about 5 days, although sleep disturbances can persist for 13 days following abrupt cessation of use. Symptoms may include excessive yawning, nasal congestion, nausea, vomiting, diarrhea, excessive perspiration, muscle and joint pain, anxiety, fear, mildly elevated blood pressure, and rapid heartbeat. Other signs of withdrawal may include excessive tearing, restlessness, dilated pupils, involuntary twitching, abdominal pain, dehydration, and elevated blood sugar levels.

Oramorph SR *see Morphine, page 129*

Oxandrin *see Oxandrolone, page 134*

OXANDROLONE

BRAND NAMES: Oxandrin
COMMON STREET NAMES: Arnolds, gym candy, juice, pumpers, roids, stackers, weight trainers
DEA CLASS: Class III
PHARMACOLOGIC CLASS: Anabolic-androgenic steroids

Description: Androgens are steroid hormones that develop and maintain male sex characteristics. Oxandrolone is used as a supplemental treatment to promote weight gain following extensive weight loss due to surgery, chronic infections, or severe trauma. It is also used to treat patients who fail to gain or maintain normal weight for unknown medical reasons.

Method of use: Ingested. Chronic users tend to rotate steroids using various methods known as cycling, stacking, and pyramiding. Sporadic discontinuation of use is believed to allow testosterone levels and sperm counts to return to normal. Taking steroids regularly with periodic "drug-free times" is called cycling. Stacking refers to the concomitant use of two or more steroids at high doses. Pyramiding is when the dose, frequency, or number of steroids taken is gradually increased, followed by progressive tapering of the drug(s).

Duration of action: Depends on the formulation, frequency, and method of use. In general, effects last up to 6 days.

Psychological effects of abuse: Altered sex drive, depression, and mood changes. Psychological dependence may also develop.

Physical effects of abuse: Angry or hostile feelings, elevated blood pressure and cholesterol, headache, insomnia, premature balding, psychotic reactions, severe acne, sexual dysfunction, and violent behavior. *In men:* Breast development, impotence, intermittent or painful urination, painful or persistent erections, reduced sperm production, and shrinking of the testicles. *In women:* Decreased body fat and breast size, deepening of the voice, enlarged clitoris, excessive growth of body hair, and menstrual changes. *In adolescents:* Premature termination of growth.

Prolonged use can lead to tolerance. While the long-term effects are not completely known, chronic steroid abuse has been associated with damage to the heart, liver, and brain.

Overdose symptoms: There have been no reports of serious overdose with this drug, but excessive sodium and water retention may occur.

Withdrawal symptoms: Abrupt discontinuation may cause mood changes, tiredness, restlessness, loss of appetite, dissatisfaction with body image, sleeplessness, reduced sex drive, paranoia, and severe depression that can lead to suicide attempts.

OXAZEPAM
COMMON STREET NAMES: Candy, downers, sleeping pills, tranks
DEA CLASS: Class IV
PHARMACOLOGIC CLASS: Benzodiazepine, antianxiety, anticonvulsant

Description: Oxazepam is used to treat anxiety disorders and alcohol withdrawal. Abuse of benzodiazepines is particularly high among heroin and cocaine users.

Method of use: Ingested

Duration of action: 5 to 15 hours

Psychological effects of abuse: Amnesia, confusion, impaired judgment and thinking capabilities, mania or hypomania, pressured speech, reduced inhibition, and suicidal ideation. Long-term use may cause psychological dependence.

Physical effects of abuse: Constipation, dizziness, drowsiness, impaired physical capabilities, low blood pressure, muscle relaxation, sleepiness, slowed psychomotor performance, urinary retention, and visual disturbances. Long-term use may cause physical dependence.

Overdose symptoms: The most severe signs of overdose are respiratory depression and loss of consciousness. Other symptoms may include confusion, diminished reflexes, impaired coordination, slurred speech, extreme sleepiness, and loss of muscle tone. Death from overdose of a single benzodiazepine is extremely rare. However, there is an increased risk of toxicity when benzodiazepines are combined with alcohol and/or other CNS depressants. Fatalities have been reported in patients who have overdosed with a combination of a single benzodiazepine and alcohol.

Withdrawal symptoms: Abrupt termination following long-term use may precipitate withdrawal symptoms and require hospitalization. Symptoms may include abdominal and muscle cramps, depression, insomnia, sweating, vomiting, tremors, and seizures.

OXYCODONE HYDROCHLORIDE

BRAND NAMES: Intensol, OxyContin, OxyDose, OxyIR, Percocet, Percodan, Roxicodone, Tylox
COMMON STREET NAMES: Hillbilly heroin, killers, OC's, Oxycotton, Oxy's, Percs, Poor man's heroin
DEA CLASS: Class II
PHARMACOLOGIC CLASS: Narcotic analgesic

Description: Oxycodone is a semisynthetic opioid derived from the opium alkaloid thebaine. It is used for the management of moderate to severe pain. Oxycodone has pharmacologic actions similar to codeine, heroin, and morphine. It elevates levels of the neurotransmitter dopamine, which is linked to pleasurable experiences. Opiate addicts use oxycodone to control withdrawal symptoms when heroin or morphine is unavailable. The brand OxyContin is especially prone to abuse because it contains higher doses of the medication in a timed-release tablet.

Method of use: Tablets are chewed or crushed into a powder that is snorted or diluted in water for injection. Chewing, crushing, or diluting long-acting tablets disables the timed-release action and allows high doses of the drug to enter the bloodstream quickly. Using oxycodone like this dramatically increases the risk of overdose.

Duration of action: Depends on the dose and method of use. In general, the effects last 4 to 6 hours following administration. The effects of timed-release tablets can persist for 12 hours or more.

Psychological effects of abuse: Abnormal dreams, anxiety, confusion, psychological dependence (after prolonged use), and thought disturbances. The psychological dependence associated with narcotic addiction is complex. Long after physical dependence has ended, the addict may continue to think and talk about the drug and feel unable to manage daily activities without it.

Physical effects of abuse: Abdominal cramps, constipation, decreased urination, diminished appetite, dizziness, dry mouth, euphoria, excessive sweating, gastrointestinal inflammation, headache, hiccups, light-headedness, low blood pressure, nausea, respiratory depression, restlessness, sedation, sleepiness, and vomiting. Chronic use may cause tolerance and physical dependence.

Overdose symptoms: Fatalities have been reported, mostly when the timed-release tablets were crushed and snorted. Signs of overdose include dizziness, constricted pupils, weakness, cold and clammy skin, CNS depression, slowed or interrupted breathing, seizures, loss of consciousness, and coma. Risk of overdose increases significantly when the drug is taken with alcohol.

Withdrawal symptoms: Although withdrawal from oxycodone is painful physically and emotionally, it's rarely life-threatening if adequate hydration and nutritional support are maintained. Although the symptoms are similar to those of morphine withdrawal, they are considerably less intense. Abruptly stopping use may cause excessive tearing, yawning, and sweating about 12 to 14 hours after the last dose. Additional symptoms may include diminished appetite, irritability, restless sleep (sometimes called the "yen"), confusion, irregular breathing, tremors, seizures, and loss of consciousness.

OxyContin *see Oxycodone, page 136*

OxyDose *see Oxycodone, page 136*

OxyIR *see Oxycodone, page 136*

OXYMETHOLONE
BRAND NAME: Anadrol
COMMON STREET NAMES: Arnolds, gym candy, juice, pumpers, roids, stackers, weight trainers
DEA CLASS: Class III
PHARMACOLOGIC CLASS: Anabolic-androgenic steroid

Description: Oxymetholone is a synthetic derivative of testosterone. It is used for the treatment of anemias caused by weak red blood cell production or bone marrow failure.

Method of use: Ingested. Chronic users tend to rotate steroids using various methods known as cycling, stacking, and pyramiding. Sporadic discontinuation of use is believed to allow testosterone levels and sperm counts to return to normal. Taking steroids regularly with periodic "drug-free times" is called cycling. Stacking refers to the concomitant use of two or more steroids at high doses. Pyramiding is when the dose, frequency, or number of steroids taken is gradually increased, followed by progressive tapering of the drug(s).

Duration of action: Depends on the formulation, frequency, and method used. In general, effects may last up to 6 days following use.

Psychological effects of abuse: Mood changes, depression, and reduced sex drive. Psychological dependence may occur.

Physical effects of abuse: Angry or hostile feelings, elevated blood pressure and cholesterol, headache, insomnia, premature balding, psychotic reactions, severe acne, sexual dysfunction, and violent behavior. *In men:* Breast development, impotence, intermittent or painful urination, painful or persistent erections, reduced sperm production, and shrinking of the testicles. *In women:* Decreased body fat and breast size, deepening of the voice, enlarged clitoris, excessive growth of body hair, and menstrual changes. *In adolescents:* Premature termination of growth.
   Prolonged use can lead to tolerance. While the long-term effects are not completely known, chronic steroid abuse has been associated with damage to the heart, liver, and brain.

Overdose symptoms: There have been no reports of severe overdose with this drug, and toxicity is unlikely following acute overdose. Chronic exposure to high doses may result in severe acne, excessive growth of body hair, hoarseness, change in sex drive, poor sperm production, and menstrual problems in women.

Withdrawal symptoms: Abrupt discontinuation may cause mood changes, tiredness, restlessness, loss of appetite, dissatisfaction with body image, sleeplessness, reduced sex drive, paranoia, and severe depression that can lead to suicide attempts.

OXYMORPHONE HYDROCHLORIDE

BRAND NAME: Numorphan
COMMON STREET NAMES: Dreamer, M, Miss Emma
DEA CLASS: Class II
PHARMACOLOGIC CLASS: Narcotic analgesic

Description: Oxymorphone is used to help manage moderate to severe pain, as a sedative prior to surgery, and as a supplemental agent during anesthesia. It's also used to relieve anxiety in patients who have difficulty breathing due to pulmonary edema caused by heart dysfunction.

Method of use: Rectal and injected IV, IM, or SC

Duration of action: Generally 3 to 6 hours (rectal and IV administration)

Psychological effects of abuse: Confusion, depression, hallucinations, and paradoxical CNS stimulation. The psychological dependence associated with narcotic addiction is complex. Long after physical dependence has ended, the addict may continue to think and talk about the drug and feel unable to manage daily activities without it.

Physical effects of abuse: Blurred vision, CNS and respiratory depression, constipation, diminished appetite, dizziness, drowsiness, dry mouth, flushing, headache, low blood pressure, lowered pulse, muscle rigidity, nausea, paradoxical CNS stimulation, restlessness, seizures, shortness of breath, stomach cramps, tiredness, urinary retention, and vomiting. Physical dependence develops progressively.

Overdose symptoms: Although tolerance develops slowly, the user eventually needs progressively larger doses to obtain the same effects as before. Symptoms of overdose may include severe drowsiness, clammy skin, confusion, constricted pupils, low blood pressure, interrupted breathing, slow pulse, tremors, respiratory depression, convulsions, and coma. Risk of overdose increases significantly when the drug is taken with alcohol.

Withdrawal symptoms: Although withdrawal from narcotics is painful physically and emotionally, it's rarely life-threatening if adequate hydration and nutritional support are maintained. Symptoms begin slowly, with peak effects observed 5 days after cessation of use; however, sleep disturbances can persist up to 13 days following the last dose. Early withdrawal symptoms may include irritability, sleeplessness, diminished appetite, excessive yawning, severe sneezing, tearing, and head cold. Later-stage symptoms may include nausea, vomiting, severe diarrhea, paradoxical excitability, abdominal cramps, bone and muscle pain in the back and extremities, fever and chills, excessive sweating, and depression. Elevated heart rate and blood pressure may also develop.

PARALDEHYDE

COMMON STREET NAMES: Blue angels, blue devils, downers, goofers, nebbies, Peter, pink ladies, rainbows, softballs, yellow bullets
DEA CLASS: Class IV
PHARMACOLOGIC CLASS: Sedative, hypnotic

Description: Paraldehyde is marketed in other countries for the short-term treatment of insomnia. It is also used for treating symptoms of alcohol, barbiturate, and opiate withdrawal. High doses have sometimes been used to treat delirium and seizures. Paraldehyde was withdrawn from the U.S. market after safer and more effective agents became available.

Method of use: Ingested, used rectally, and injected IM or IV. Intravenous administration is extremely hazardous and could cause internal bleeding, accumulation of fluid in the lungs, heart damage, and circulatory collapse. Intramuscular injections are painful and could cause severe tissue damage, skin infection, and nerve damage at the injection site. Oral use can cause mouth and stomach irritation; rectal use can also cause irritation.

Duration of action: Depends on method of use. Hypnotic effects generally last 8 to 12 hours following a standard therapeutic dose.

Psychological effects of abuse: Nervousness, restlessness, irritability, and severe anxiety. Prolonged use may cause psychological dependence.

Physical effects of abuse: Coughing, low blood pressure, rapid heartbeat, fluid in the lungs, increased blood clotting, infection at the injection site, drowsiness, dizziness, "hangover" effects, stomach pain, nausea, and seizures. Paraldehyde decomposes during long-term storage, and deaths from corrosive poisoning have occurred after use of the decomposed drug. Prolonged use can lead to tolerance and physical dependence, especially in alcoholics.

Overdose symptoms: Death due to heart failure has been reported. Signs of overdose include weakness, depression, nausea, vomiting, rapid or labored breathing, slowed heartbeat, severely low blood pressure, and kidney or liver damage. Severe overdose could lead to respiratory depression and stupor followed by coma.

Withdrawal symptoms: Abrupt discontinuation can cause muscle and stomach cramps, excessive sweating, nausea, vomiting, tremors, hallucinations, and convulsions.

PEMOLINE

COMMON STREET NAMES: Not known
DEA CLASS: Class IV
PHARMACOLOGIC CLASS: CNS stimulant, nonamphetamine

Not commercially available in the U.S.

Description: Pemoline works much like dextroamphetamine and is used to treat attention deficit hyperactivity disorder (ADHD). However, pemoline is not recommended as first-line therapy due to its possible connection with liver failure.

Method of use: Ingested

Duration of action: For children, 7 hours; in other patients effects may last up to 13 hours.

Psychological effects of abuse: Depression, irritability, mild euphoria, and paranoid psychosis.

Physical effects of abuse: Dizziness, drowsiness, seizures, sleeplessness, headache, hallucinations, liver problems, loss of appetite, movement disorders, nausea, stuttering, stomach discomfort, severe muscle weakness, Tourette's syndrome, and weight loss. Prolonged use can lead to physical dependence.

Overdose symptoms: Prolonged use can lead to tolerance, and the progressively higher doses needed are often in the toxic range. Signs of overdose include agitation, confusion, restlessness, excessive sweating, severe muscle weakness, vomiting, rapid heartbeat, high blood pressure or body temperature, and hallucinations.

Withdrawal symptoms: Abrupt cessation of use may cause severe fatigue, sleepiness, headache, nausea, vomiting, abdominal pain, depression, paranoid psychosis, and seizures.

PENTAZOCINE HYDROCHLORIDE

BRAND NAME: Talwin
COMMON STREET NAMES: Poor man's heroin, Ts and Bs, Ts and Blues
DEA CLASS: Class IV
PHARMACOLOGIC CLASS: Narcotic analgesic, sedative

Description: Pentazocine is an opioid-type pain medication. It is used to treat moderate to severe pain, as a sedative prior to surgery, and as a supplemental agent during anesthesia. Combined preparations with aspirin may also be used in the treatment of moderate pain.

Method of use: Ingested and injected IM, IV, or SC

Duration of action: After ingestion: 4 to 5 hours; after injection: 2 to 3 hours.

Psychological effects of abuse: Confusion, disorientation, hallucinations, nightmares, and thought disturbances. The psychological dependence associated with narcotic addiction is complex. Long after physical dependence has ended, the addict may continue to think and talk about the drug and feel unable to manage daily activities without it.

Physical effects of abuse: Abdominal pain, blurred vision, chills, constipation, diminished appetite, dry mouth, feeling faint, flushing, headache, light-headedness, low blood pressure, nausea, sleeplessness, and vomiting. High doses can lead to rapid heart rate and respiratory depression. Chronic use may cause physical dependence.

Overdose symptoms: Although tolerance develops slowly, the user eventually needs progressively larger doses to obtain the same effects as before. Signs of overdose may include severe drowsiness, constricted pupils, severe high blood pressure, interrupted breathing, slow pulse, tremors, respiratory depression, convulsions, and coma. Risk of overdose increases significantly when the drug is taken with alcohol.

Withdrawal symptoms: Although pentazocine may cause physical dependence, withdrawal symptoms are much less severe than those of morphine. Early withdrawal symptoms may include irritability, sleeplessness, diminished appetite, excessive yawning, severe sneezing, tearing, and head cold. Later-stage symptoms may include nausea, vomiting, severe diarrhea, abdominal cramps, bone and muscle pain in the back and extremities, fever and chills, excessive sweating, depression, and elevated heart rate and blood pressure.

Pentothal *see Thiopental, page 155*

PENTOBARBITAL SODIUM
BRAND NAME: Nembutal
COMMON STREET NAMES: Downers, jackets, yellows
DEA CLASS: Class II
PHARMACOLOGIC CLASS: Barbiturate, sedative, anticonvulsant

Description: Barbiturates depress the sensory cortex, decrease motor activity, alter cerebral function, and produce drowsiness, sedation, and hypnosis. Pentobarbital is used as a sedative prior to surgery and to help induce anesthesia and alleviate anxiety. In addition, it is used for the emergency treatment of acute convulsive episodes such as status epilepticus.

Method of use: Used rectally and injected IM or IV

Duration of action: 3 to 4 hours following administration of a standard therapeutic dose.

Psychological effects of abuse: Barbiturates may cause psychological dependence, especially following prolonged use of high doses. Principal side effects include confusion, alternating euphoria and depression, and memory loss.

Physical effects of abuse: The most frequent physical side effects are due to CNS depression, including dizziness, headache, excessive sleepiness, drowsiness, and irregular gait. Other symptoms may include headache, stomach pain, and skin rash. Paradoxical excitement and irritability may also occur. In chronic users, blood disorders such as megaloblastic anemia may develop. Physical dependence is a significant risk, since it can develop after short-term use.

Overdose symptoms: Pentobarbital overdose may be complicated by the development of kidney necrosis, muscle necrosis, skin lesions, pneumonia, and low blood sugar. Seizures are not expected, except upon abrupt withdrawal from the drug.

Withdrawal symptoms: Pentobarbital is one of the most commonly abused barbiturates. Severe and life-threatening symptoms may occur within 48 hours of abrupt withdrawal, including continuous seizures, acute delirium syndromes with toxic psychosis, and coma, eventually resulting in death.

Percocet *see Oxycodone, page 136*

Percodan *see Oxycodone, page 136*

PHENDIMETRAZINE TARTRATE

BRAND NAMES: Bontril
COMMON STREET NAMES: Not known
DEA CLASS: Class III
PHARMACOLOGIC CLASS: CNS stimulant, anorexiant

Description: Phendimetrazine is related to amphetamines both chemically and pharmacologically. It is a CNS stimulant and an indirect-acting sympathomimetic with actions similar to those of dextroamphetamine. Phendimetrazine is used as a short-term aid to help promote weight loss in conjunction with caloric restriction, exercise, and behavior modification.

Method of use: Ingested

Duration of action: 9 to 12 hours

Psychological effects of abuse: Agitation, paranoia, delusions, and hyperactivity. Rarely, psychotic episodes may occur following a single dose.

Physical effects of abuse: Elevated blood pressure, rapid heart rate, sleep disturbances, headache, dizziness, dry mouth, thirst, constipation, nausea, diarrhea, and increased urinary frequency. Effects of chronic abuse include hyperactivity, severe sleeplessness, severe irritability, personality changes, and psychosis. Pulmonary hypertension and valvular heart defects have been reported in patients receiving phendimetrazine in combination with other weight-loss-promoting drugs.

Overdose symptoms: Although overdose with phendimetrazine is rare, the following symptoms have been reported: agitation, hyperactivity, significantly elevated blood pressure and body temperature, and seizures.

Withdrawal symptoms: Although there are no reports of withdrawal reactions, the potential still exists for long-term users.

PHENMETRAZINE
BRAND NAME: Preludin
COMMON STREET NAMES: Black Cadillacs, beans, blue devils, bolt, cartwheels, fives, hearts, jellybeans, pep pills, snap
DEA CLASS: Class II
PHARMACOLOGIC CLASS: CNS stimulant, appetite suppressant

Not commercially available in the U.S.

Description: Phenmetrazine is related to amphetamines both chemically and pharmacologically. It is a CNS stimulant and indirect-acting sympathomimetic with actions similar to those of dextroamphetamine. It is used as a short-term aid to help promote weight loss in conjunction with caloric restriction, exercise, and behavior modification. Phenmetrazine is not recommended as first-line therapy due to the potential for serious CNS side effects.

Method of use: Ingested, used rectally, and injected IV

Duration of action: Depends on the formulation. The effects of shorter-acting agents can last 4 to 6 hours, while the sustained-release version can last for 24 hours or more.

Psychological effects of abuse: Mild euphoria, nervousness, irritability, altered sexual desire, depression, mania, and rarely, psychotic behavior. Prolonged use may cause psychological dependence.

Physical effects of abuse: Rapid heartbeat, high blood pressure, heart palpitations, sleeplessness, headache, tremor, dizziness, dry mouth, excessive thirst, constipation, stomach discomfort, diarrhea, frequent urination, impotence, and blurred vision. Severe physical effects may include pulmonary hypertension, heart murmurs, and valvular heart disease. Prolonged use may cause physical dependence.

Overdose symptoms: Tolerance develops rapidly, and the progressively higher doses needed are often in the toxic range. Overdose symptoms include sleeplessness, hyperactivity, personality changes, psychosis, hallucinations, irregular heart rhythm, aggressive behavior, panic state, elevated body temperature, hyperactive reflexes, convulsions, and coma. Fatalities due to heart failure have been reported with high doses.

Withdrawal symptoms: Abrupt cessation of high doses may cause extreme fatigue, depression, and sleeping problems. Additional symptoms include hyperactivity, irritability, nausea, vomiting, nightmares, and tremors.

PHENOBARBITAL SODIUM
BRAND NAME: Luminal sodium
COMMON STREET NAMES: Barbs, downers, goofballs
DEA CLASS: Class IV
PHARMACOLOGIC CLASS: Barbiturate, sedative, hypnotic, anticonvulsant

Description: Barbiturates depress the sensory cortex, decrease motor activity, alter brain function, and produce drowsiness, sedation, and hypnosis. Phenobarbital is used to treat grand-mal and partial seizures. In addition, the injected form is effective for inducing sedation prior to surgery and facilitating the induction of anesthesia.

Method of use: Ingested and injected IM, IV, or SC

Duration of action: Effects begin in 20 to 60 minutes and can last for days, depending on the dose.

Psychological effects of abuse: Barbiturates may cause psychological dependence, especially following prolonged use of high doses. Psychological side effects may include confusion, alternating euphoria and depression, memory loss, impaired judgment, nervousness, nightmares, and hallucinations.

Physical effects of abuse: The most frequent physical effects are due to CNS depression, including dizziness, headache, excessive sleepiness, drowsiness, and irregular gait. Other symptoms may include headache, stomach pain, and skin rash. Paradoxical excitement and irritability may also occur. Short-term therapy with phenobarbital has been associated with the development of Stevens-Johnson syndrome and toxic skin eruptions. Physical dependence is a significant risk, since it can develop after short-term use.

Overdose symptoms: Phenobarbital overdose is associated with unusual reactions, including red, blistering skin lesions and neurological problems, that can appear 1 to 2 hours after ingestion. Other symptoms of overdose may include unsteady gait, slurred speech, confusion, low body temperature and blood pressure, and dose-dependent respiratory depression. Toxic effects may be enhanced when the drug is taken with alcohol and/or other CNS depressant drugs.

Withdrawal symptoms: Phenobarbital is abused less frequently because it is a long-acting barbiturate. Nevertheless, abrupt withdrawal may cause continuous seizures. Withdrawal symptoms can occur following discontinuation of chronic phenobarbital use, but are rare following an acute overdose. Symptoms are similar to those of alcohol withdrawal and may include generalized weakness, heightened anxiety, irritability, dizziness, headache, sleeplessness, muscle twitching, nausea and vomiting, and rapid pulse. Severely low blood pressure and convulsions may develop after a day or two, which eventually leads to hallucinations and delirium followed by coma and death.

PHENTERMINE HYDROCHLORIDE
BRAND NAMES: Adipex-P, Ionamin
COMMON STREET NAMES: Pep pills, speed, uppers
DEA CLASS: Class IV
PHARMACOLOGIC CLASS: CNS stimulant, anorexiant

Description: Phentermine is related to amphetamines both chemically and pharmacologically. It is used as a short-term aid to help promote weight loss in conjunction with caloric restriction, exercise, and behavior modification.

Method of use: Ingested

Duration of action: Up to 20 hours

Psychological effects of abuse: Confusion, agitation, reduced sexual desire, and restlessness. Acute paranoia and other psychotic behavior have also been reported. Psychological dependence can occur after chronic abuse.

Physical effects of abuse: Elevated blood pressure, rapid heart rate, constipation, diarrhea, nausea, dry mouth, sleeplessness, headache, and dizziness. Pulmonary hypertension and valvular heart defects have been reported, particularly when given concomitantly with fenfluramine or dexfenfluramine. Ischemic cerebrovascular disease, severe headache, and numbness have been associated with the use of phentermine.

Overdose symptoms: Overdose with phentermine is rare, but symptoms may include agitation, hyperactivity, significantly elevated blood pressure and body temperature, and seizures.

Withdrawal symptoms: Abrupt withdrawal may cause extreme fatigue and depression.

PRIMIDONE
BRAND NAME: Mysoline
COMMON STREET NAMES: Barb, downers, goofers
DEA CLASS: Not classified
PHARMACOLOGIC CLASS: Barbiturate, anticonvulsant

Description: Primidone is used in the management of grand-mal, psychomotor, and focal seizures. One of its active metabolites is phenobarbital.

Method of use: Ingested

Duration of action: Effects are age- and dose-dependent, but usually persist for up to 5 days due to the drug's active metabolites.

Psychological effects of abuse: Barbiturates may cause psychological dependence, especially following prolonged use of high doses. Psychological side effects may include behavioral changes and excessive irritability.

Physical effects of abuse: Drowsiness, vertigo, tiredness, irregular gait, loss of appetite, nausea, vomiting, sexual dysfunction, double vision, and rapid eye movements.

Overdose symptoms: Unsteady gait, confusion, slurred speech, low blood pressure, lowered or elevated body temperature, dose-dependent respiratory depression, and coma. The drug's toxic effects are enhanced when taken with alcohol and/or other CNS depressants.

Withdrawal symptoms: Symptoms are similar to those of alcohol withdrawal and characterized by severe apprehension, weakness, heightened anxiety, irritability, dizziness, headache, sleeplessness, muscle twitching, nausea and vomiting, distortion of visual perception, and rapid pulse. Severely low blood pressure and convulsions may develop after a day or two, which eventually leads to hallucinations, delirium, and continuous seizures, followed by coma and death.

PROPOXYPHENE HYDROCHLORIDE and PROPOXYPHENE NAPSYLATE
BRAND NAME: Darvon
COMMON STREET NAMES: D, dillies, dust, juice, smack
DEA CLASS: Class IV
PHARMACOLOGIC CLASS: Narcotic analgesic

Description: Propoxyphene is an opioid analgesic that is structurally related to methadone. It is used to alleviate mild to moderate pain.

Method of use: Ingested

Duration of action: Generally, effects persist 6 to 12 hours following use, but can last 30 to 36 hours in chronic users.

Psychological effects of abuse: Confusion, depression, hallucinations, nervousness, and paradoxical excitement. The psychological dependence associated with narcotic addiction is complex. Long after physical dependence has ended, the addict may continue to think and talk about the drug and feel unable to manage daily activities without it.

Physical effects of abuse: Blurred vision, CNS and respiratory depression, constricted pupils, constipation, diminished appetite, dizziness, drowsiness, faintness, headache, insomnia, light-headedness, loss of appetite, low blood pressure, nausea, seizures, slow heartbeat, slow or troubled breathing, stomach cramps, tremors, and vomiting. Chronic use results in tolerance and physical dependence.

Overdose symptoms: Chronic use can lead to tolerance, and progressively higher doses are needed to obtain the same effects as before. Toxic accumulations of propoxyphene and its metabolites can occur quickly with repeated doses, and the effects are often complicated by the addition of alcohol or other drugs. A disturbing number of fatalities have occurred from accidental or intentional overdose with propoxyphene; death within an hour of overdosing is not uncommon. Psychotic reactions and possibly fatal CNS depression—including decreased or labored breathing, temporary stoppage of breathing, and decreased heart function—can develop rapidly. Other symptoms of propoxyphene overdose may include bluish skin, extreme sleepiness, pupil constriction later followed by dilation, irregular heartbeat, low blood pressure, stupor, seizures, and coma.

Withdrawal symptoms: Severe withdrawal syndromes have been reported, particularly in older individuals. Symptoms may include restlessness, muscle and bone pain, severe diarrhea, sleeplessness, involuntary leg movements, chills alternating with hot flashes, depression, nausea, vomiting, elevated heart rate and blood pressure, convulsions, and coma.

ProSom *see Estazolam, page 102*

Provigil *see Modafinil, page 128*

QUAZEPAM
BRAND NAME: Doral
COMMON STREET NAMES: Candy, downers, sleeping pills, tranks
DEA CLASS: Class IV
PHARMACOLOGIC CLASS: Benzodiazepine, sedative, hypnotic

Description: Quazepam is used for the short-term treatment of sleep disorders such as insomnia. Abuse of benzodiazepines is particularly high among heroin and cocaine users.

Method of use: Ingested

Duration of action: 25 to 41 hours

Psychological effects of abuse: Confusion, impaired judgment and thinking abilities, irritability, mild euphoria, pressured speech, reduced inhibition, and suicidal ideation. Long-term use may cause psychological dependence.

Physical effects of abuse: Changes in appetite and body weight, constipation, dizziness, impaired muscle coordination, and low blood pressure. Long-term use may cause physical dependence.

Overdose symptoms: The most severe signs of overdose are respiratory depression and coma. Other symptoms may include confusion, diminished reflexes, manic behavior, unrealistic euphoria, extreme sleepiness, and impaired muscle coordination. Death from overdose of a single benzodiazepine is extremely rare. However, there is an increased risk of toxicity when benzodiazepines are combined with alcohol and/or other CNS depressants. Fatalities have been reported in patients who have overdosed with a combination of a single benzodiazepine and alcohol.

Withdrawal symptoms: Abrupt termination may lead to withdrawal symptoms and require hospitalization. Symptoms may include abdominal and muscle cramps, depression, insomnia, sweating, vomiting, tremors, and seizures.

Repan *see Butalbital, page 90*

Restoril *see Temazepam, page 153*

Ritalin *see Methylphenidate, page 124*

RMS *see Morphine, page 129*

Roxanol *see Morphine, page 129*

Roxicodone *see Oxycodone, page 136*

SECOBARBITAL
BRAND NAME: Seconal
COMMON STREET NAMES: Downers, reds, red devils
DEA CLASS: Class II
PHARMACOLOGIC CLASS: Barbiturate (short-acting), sedative, hypnotic, anticonvulsant

Description: Barbiturates depress the sensory cortex, decrease motor activity, alter brain function, and produce drowsiness, sedation, and hypnosis. Secobarbital is used as an emergency aid in the management of acute convulsive episodes. In addition, it is used for the short-term treatment of insomnia and as a sedative before surgery to help induce anesthesia and alleviate anxiety.

Method of use: Ingested and injected IV or IM

Duration of action: 3 to 4 hours

Psychological effects of abuse: Barbiturates may cause psychological dependence, especially following prolonged use of high doses. Psychological effects may include confusion, alternating euphoria and depression, and memory loss.

Physical effects of abuse: The most frequent physical effects are due to CNS depression, including dizziness, headache, excessive sleepiness, drowsiness, and irregular gait. Other symptoms may include headache, stomach pain, and skin rash. Paradoxical excitement and irritability may also occur. In chronic users, blood disorders such as megaloblastic anemia may develop. Physical dependence is a significant risk, since it can develop after short-term use.

Overdose symptoms: Symptoms may include unsteady gait, slurred speech, confusion, low body temperature and blood pressure, and dose-dependent respiratory depression. Toxic effects are enhanced when secobarbital is taken with alcohol and/or other CNS depressant drugs.

Withdrawal symptoms: Addiction may result following chronic use. Withdrawal symptoms may include anorexia, nausea, vomiting, muscle weakness, tremors, and low blood pressure, followed by seizures within 16 to 24 hours after the last dose. Acute delirium with toxic psychosis may occur within 48 hours following termination of use.

Seconal *see this page*

Soma *see Meprobamate and Carisoprodol, page 120*

Somnote *see Chloral hydrate, page 92*

Sonata *see Zaleplon, page 158*

Stadol *see Butorphanol, page 91*

Sufenta *see Sufentanil, page 151*

SUFENTANIL CITRATE
BRAND NAME: Sufenta
COMMON STREET NAMES: China white, China girl, dance fever, friend, good-fellas, king ivory
DEA CLASS: Class II
PHARMACOLOGIC CLASS: Narcotic analgesic/agonist, general anesthetic

Description: Sufentanil has three main uses: 1) as a primary agent for induction and maintenance of anesthesia administered with oxygen; 2) as a supplemental agent during maintenance of general anesthesia; and 3) as a combined agent used with low-dose bupivacaine during labor.

Method of use: Injected IV

Duration of action: Depends on dose size and the user's weight (duration is longer in obese individuals). Effects generally last 2 to 3 hours, but repeated use of large doses may result in accumulation and a longer duration of action.

Psychological effects of abuse: Confusion, depression, hallucinations, and restlessness. Prolonged use causes psychological dependence, particularly when high doses are used.

Physical effects of abuse: Blurred vision, CNS depression, constipation, decreased urination, diminished appetite, dizziness, drowsiness, dry mouth, excessive sleepiness, headache, high blood pressure (depending on dose), muscle rigidity, nausea, respiratory depression (depending on dose), slow heart rate or pulse, stomach cramps, and vomiting. Chronic use may cause physical dependence.

Overdose symptoms: The primary signs of overdose include CNS and respiratory depression and constricted pupils. Serious overdose may result in interrupted breathing, circulatory depression, severely low blood pressure, muscle rigidity, slow heart rate, delirium, seizures, and shock.

Withdrawal symptoms: Abruptly stopping the drug after long-term use may precipitate withdrawal symptoms. The intensity of symptoms is directly related to the total daily dose, frequency and duration of use, and the health of the user. Although painful physically and emotionally, withdrawal from narcotics is rarely life-threatening. Early symptoms may include watery eyes, runny nose, yawning, and sweating. Later-stage symptoms may include nervousness, muscle twitching, drug cravings, restlessness, irritability, loss of appetite, chills alternating with flushing, nausea, vomiting, bone and muscle pain in the back and extremities, tremors, elevated heart rate and blood pressure, and severe depression.

STANOZOLOL

COMMON STREET NAMES: Arnolds, gym candy, juice, pumpers, roids, stackers, weight trainers
DEA CLASS: Class III
PHARMACOLOGIC CLASS: Anabolic-androgenic steroid

Description: Androgens are steroid hormones that develop and maintain male sex characteristics. They are used primarily to replace insufficient levels of testosterone due to poor functioning of the testes. When used in combination with exercise and a high-protein diet, androgens can promote increased muscle size and strength, improve stamina, and decrease recovery time between workouts. Androgens are also used to promote the development of puberty in males with clearly delayed onset. Additionally, androgens are sometimes prescribed for women with advancing, inoperable metastatic breast cancer who are 1 to 5 years postmenopausal. This product is also effective for treating excessive swelling and welts below the skin (angioedema).

Method of use: Ingested. Chronic users tend to rotate steroids using various methods known as cycling, stacking, and pyramiding. Sporadic discontinuation of use is believed to allow testosterone levels and sperm counts to return to normal. Taking steroids regularly with periodic "drug-free times" is called cycling. Stacking refers to the concomitant use of two or more steroids at high doses. Pyramiding is when the dose, frequency, or number of steroids taken is gradually increased, followed by progressive tapering of the drug(s).

Duration of action: Depends on the formulation, frequency, and method used. In general, effects can last up to 6 days following use.

Psychological effects of abuse: Mood changes, decreased or increased sexual drive, anxiety, and depression. Psychological dependence may occur.

Physical effects of abuse: Angry or hostile feelings, elevated blood pressure and cholesterol, headache, insomnia, premature balding, psychotic reactions, severe acne, sexual dysfunction, and violent behavior. *In men:* Breast development, impotence, intermittent or painful urination, painful or persistent erections, reduced sperm production, and shrinking of the testicles. *In women:* Decreased body fat and breast size, deepening of the voice, enlarged clitoris, excessive growth of body hair, and menstrual changes. *In adolescents:* Premature termination of growth.

Prolonged use can lead to tolerance. While the long-term effects are not completely known, chronic steroid abuse has been associated with damage to the heart, liver, and brain.

Overdose symptoms: There have been no reports of severe overdose with this product. Chronic abuse of high doses may result in acne, excessive body hair, changes in hormonal and lipid metabolism, nausea, vomiting, jaundice, behavioral changes, stroke, heart function deterioration, psychosis, and sudden death.

Withdrawal symptoms: Abrupt discontinuation may cause mood changes, tiredness, restlessness, loss of appetite, dissatisfaction with body image, sleeplessness, reduced sex drive, paranoia, and severe depression that can lead to suicide attempts.

Talwin *see Pentazocine, page 141*

TEMAZEPAM
BRAND NAME: Restoril
COMMON STREET NAMES: Candy, downers, sleeping pills, tranks
DEA CLASS: Class IV
PHARMACOLOGIC CLASS: Benzodiazepine, sedative, hypnotic

Description: Temazepam is used for the short-term treatment of sleep disorders such as insomnia. Abuse of benzodiazepines is particularly high among heroin and cocaine users.

Method of use: Ingested

Duration of action: 5 to 17 hours

Psychological effects of abuse: Confusion, impaired judgment and thinking abilities, irritability, mild euphoria, pressured speech, reduced inhibition, and suicidal ideation. Long-term use may cause psychological dependence.

Physical effects of abuse: Changes in appetite and body weight, constipation, dizziness, impaired muscle coordination, impaired physical capabilities, and low blood pressure. Long-term use may cause physical dependence.

Overdose symptoms: The most severe signs of overdose are respiratory depression and coma. Other symptoms may include confusion, diminished reflexes, manic behavior, unrealistic euphoria, extreme sleepiness, and impaired coordination. Death from overdose of a single benzodiazepine is extremely rare. However, there is an increased risk of toxicity when benzodiazepines are combined with alcohol and/or other CNS depressants. Fatalities have been reported in patients who have overdosed with a combination of a single benzodiazepine and alcohol.

Withdrawal symptoms: Abrupt termination following long-term use may precipitate withdrawal symptoms and require hospitalization. Symptoms may include abdominal and muscle cramps, agitation, delirium, depression, insomnia, rapid pulse, sweating, vomiting, hallucinations, tremors, and seizures.

Tenuate *see Diethylpropion, page 99*

TESTOSTERONE ENANTHATE

BRAND NAME: Delatestryl
COMMON STREET NAMES: Arnolds, gym candy, juice, pumpers, roids, stackers, weight trainers
DEA CLASS: Class III
PHARMACOLOGIC CLASS: Anabolic-androgenic steroid

Description: Androgens are steroid hormones that develop and maintain male sex characteristics. Testosterone enanthate is a derivative of the male hormone testosterone. Androgens are used primarily to replace insufficient levels of testosterone due to poor functioning of the testes. When used in combination with exercise and a high-protein diet, androgens can promote increased muscle size and strength, improve stamina, and decrease recovery time between workouts. Androgens are also used to promote the development of puberty in males with clearly delayed onset. Additionally, androgens are sometimes prescribed for women with advancing, inoperable metastatic breast cancer who are 1 to 5 years postmenopausal. This product has also been used in premenopausal women with breast cancer who have benefited from removal of one or both ovaries and are considered to have a hormone-responsive tumor.

Method of use: Injected IM. Chronic users tend to rotate steroids using various methods known as cycling, stacking, and pyramiding. Sporadic discontinuation of use is believed to allow testosterone levels and sperm counts to return to normal. Taking steroids regularly with periodic "drug-free times" is called cycling. Stacking refers to the concomitant use of two or more steroids at high doses. Pyramiding is when the dose, frequency, or number of steroids taken is gradually increased, followed by progressive tapering of the drug(s).

Duration of action: Up to 24 hours following IM administration.

Psychological effects of abuse: Mood changes, depression, and reduced sex drive. Psychological dependence may occur.

Physical effects of abuse: Angry or hostile feelings, elevated blood pressure and cholesterol, headache, insomnia, premature balding, psychotic reactions, severe acne, sexual dysfunction, and violent behavior. *In men:* Breast development, impotence, intermittent or painful urination, painful or persistent erections, reduced sperm production, and shrinking of the testicles. *In women:* Decreased body fat and breast size, deepening of the voice, enlarged clitoris, excessive growth of body hair, and menstrual changes. *In adolescents:* Premature termination of growth.

Prolonged use can lead to tolerance. While the long-term effects are not completely known, chronic steroid abuse has been associated with damage to the heart, liver, and brain.

Overdose symptoms: There have been no reports of severe overdose with this product. Chronic abuse of high doses may result in blurred vision, headache, sudden and severe inability to speak, seizures, slurred speech, temporary blindness, and sudden, severe weakness in the arm and/or leg on one side of the body.

Withdrawal symptoms: Abrupt discontinuation may cause mood changes, tiredness, restlessness, loss of appetite, dissatisfaction with body image, sleeplessness, reduced sex drive, paranoia, and severe depression that can lead to suicide attempts.

Testred *see Methyltestosterone, page 125*

THIOPENTAL SODIUM
BRAND NAME: Pentothal
COMMON STREET NAMES:
DEA CLASS: Class III
PHARMACOLOGIC CLASS: Barbiturate, anticonvulsant, general anesthetic, sedative

Description: Barbiturates depress the sensory cortex, decrease motor activity, alter brain function, and produce drowsiness, sedation, and hypnosis. Thiopental is used to control convulsions by inducing anesthesia. It is also used to treat grand-mal, psychomotor, and focal seizures. One of the drug's active metabolites is phenobarbital.

Method of use: Ingested

Duration of action: Effects are age- and dose-dependent but are usually brief.

Psychological effects of abuse: Barbiturates may cause psychological dependence, especially following prolonged use of high doses. Effects may include behavioral changes, excessive irritability, nightmares, hallucinations, nervousness, anxiety, and impaired judgment.

Physical effects of abuse: Low heart rate and blood pressure, feeling faint, drowsiness, tiredness, dizziness, headache, chills, coughing, irregular gait, loss of appetite, excessive sleeplessness, nausea, vomiting, sexual dysfunction, double vision, rapid eye movements, respiratory depression, and interrupted breathing.

Overdose symptoms: Unsteady gait, confusion, slurred speech, low blood pressure, high or low body temperature, sleepiness, dose-dependent respiratory depression, shock, and coma. The drug's toxic effects are enhanced when taken with alcohol and/or other CNS depressants.

Withdrawal symptoms: Symptoms are similar to those of alcohol withdrawal and characterized by severe apprehension, weakness, heightened anxiety, irritability, dizziness, headache, sleeplessness, muscle twitching, nausea and vomiting, distortion of visual perception, and rapid pulse. Severely low blood pressure and convulsions may develop after a day or two, which eventually lead to hallucinations, delirium, and continuous seizures, followed by coma and death.

Tranxene *see Clorazepate, page 93*

TRENBOLONE ACETATE

COMMON STREET NAMES: Arnolds, gym candy, juice, pumpers, roids, stackers, weight trainers
DEA CLASS: Class III
PHARMACOLOGIC CLASS: Anabolic-androgenic steroid

Not commercially available in the U.S.

Description: Androgens are steroid hormones that develop and maintain male sex characteristics. They are used primarily to replace insufficient levels of testosterone due to poor functioning of the testes. When used in combination with exercise and a high-protein diet, androgens can promote increased muscle size and strength, improve stamina, and decrease recovery time between workouts. Androgens are also used to promote the development of puberty in males with clearly delayed onset. Additionally, androgens are sometimes precribed for women with advancing, inoperable metastatic breast cancer who are 1 to 5 years postmenopausal.

Method of use: Ingested. Chronic users tend to rotate steroids using various methods known as cycling, stacking, and pyramiding. Sporadic discontinuation of use is believed to allow testosterone levels and sperm counts to return to normal. Taking steroids regularly with periodic "drug-free times" is called cycling. Stacking refers to the concomitant use of two or more steroids at high doses. Pyramiding is when the dose, frequency, or number of steroids taken is gradually increased, followed by progressive tapering of the drug(s).

Duration of action: Depends on the formulation, frequency, and method of use. In general, effects may last up to 6 days.

Psychological effects of abuse: Mood changes, depression, uncontrollable aggressive behavior, euphoria, anxiety, irritability, increased sex drive, and rarely, psychosis. Psychological dependence may also occur.

Physical effects of abuse: Angry or hostile feelings, elevated blood pressure and cholesterol, headache, insomnia, premature balding, psychotic reactions, severe acne, sexual dysfunction, and violent behavior. *In men:* Breast development, impotence, intermittent or painful urination, painful or persistent erections, reduced sperm production, and shrinking of the testicles. *In women:* Decreased body fat and breast size, deepening of the voice, enlarged clitoris, excessive growth of body hair, and menstrual changes. *In adolescents:* Premature termination of growth.

Prolonged use can lead to tolerance. While the long-term effects are not completely known, chronic steroid abuse has been associated with damage to the heart, liver, and brain.

Overdose symptoms: There have been no reports of serious overdose with this drug. Chronic use of high doses may cause excessive sexual stimulation, reduced sperm production, enlarged breasts in males, uncontrolled painful erection, jaundice, and deteriorating liver function. Excessive fluid retention may occur in users who have heart, liver, or kidney disease.

Withdrawal symptoms: Abrupt discontinuation may cause mood changes, tiredness, restlessness, loss of appetite, dissatisfaction with body image, sleeplessness, reduced sex drive, paranoia, and severe depression that can lead to suicide attempts.

TRIAZOLAM

BRAND NAME: Halcion
COMMON STREET NAMES: Candy, downers, sleeping pills, tranks
DEA CLASS: Class IV
PHARMACOLOGIC CLASS: Benzodiazepine, sedative, hypnotic

Description: Triazolam is used for the short-term treatment of sleep disorders such as insomnia. Abuse of benzodiazepines is particularly high among heroin and cocaine users.

Method of use: Ingested

Duration of action: 6 to 7 hours

Psychological effects of abuse: Confusion, impaired judgment and thinking abilities, irritability, mild euphoria, pressured speech, reduced inhibition, and suicidal ideation. Long-term use may cause psychological dependence.

Physical effects of abuse: Changes in appetite and body weight, constipation, dizziness, impaired muscle coordination, and low blood pressure. Long-term use may cause physical dependence.

Overdose symptoms: The most severe signs of overdose are respiratory depression and coma. Other symptoms may include confusion, diminished reflexes, manic behavior, unrealistic euphoria, extreme sleepiness, and impaired coordination. Death from overdose of a single benzodiazepine is extremely rare. However, there is an increased risk of toxicity when benzodiazepines are combined with alcohol and/or other CNS depressants. Fatalities have been reported in patients who have overdosed with a combination of a single benzodiazepine and alcohol.

Withdrawal symptoms: Abrupt termination following long-term use may precipitate withdrawal symptoms and require hospitalization. Symptoms may include abdominal and muscle cramps, depression, insomnia, sweating, vomiting, tremors, and seizures.

Tylox *see Oxycodone, page 136*

Valium *see Diazepam, page 98*

Vicodin *see Hydrocodone, page 113*

Virilon *see Methyltestosterone, page 125*

Xanax *see Alprazolam, page 84*

Xyrem *see GHB, page 110*

ZALEPLON
BRAND NAME: Sonata
COMMON STREET NAMES: Candy, downers, sleeping pills, tranks
DEA CLASS: Class IV
PHARMACOLOGIC CLASS: Hypnotic (not a benzodiazepine, but interacts with the same receptors in the brain)

Description: Zaleplon is used for the short-term treatment of insomnia. Abuse of benzodiazepine-type hypnotics is particularly high among heroin and cocaine users.

Method of use: Ingested

Duration of action: 6 to 8 hours

Psychological effects of abuse: Abnormal dreams, amnesia, changes in sexual desire, confusion, depersonalization, depression, hallucinations, impaired judgment and thinking abilities, reduced inhibition, and suicidal ideation. Paradoxical effects include euphoria, hyperactivity, and extreme aggression. Prolonged use may cause psychological dependence.

Physical effects of abuse: Abdominal pain, constipation, decreased blood pressure, dizziness, drowsiness, fatigue, impaired physical capabilities, irregular gait, light-headedness, loss of appetite, menstrual irregularities, migraine, nausea, sleepiness, slowed psychomotor performance, urinary retention, vertigo, and visual disturbances. Prolonged use may cause physical dependence.

Overdose symptoms: The most severe signs of overdose with benzodiazepine-type hypnotics are respiratory depression, loss of consciousness, and coma. Other symptoms may include sensitivity to light, confusion, diminished reflexes, slurred speech, impaired coordination, apnea, extreme sleepiness, loss of muscle tone, and severely low blood pressure. Death from overdose of a single benzodiazepine-type hypnotic is extremely rare. However, there is an increased risk of toxicity when benzodiazepine-type drugs are combined with alcohol and/or other CNS depressants. Fatalities have been reported in patients who have overdosed with a combination of a single benzodiazepine-type hypnotic and alcohol.

Withdrawal symptoms: Abrupt termination following long-term use may precipitate withdrawal symptoms and require hospitalization. Symptoms may include abdominal and muscle cramps, depression, insomnia, severe drowsiness, sweating, vomiting, tremors, respiratory depression, seizures, and coma.

Zebutal *see Butalbital, page 90*

ZOLPIDEM

BRAND NAME: Ambien, Ambien CR
COMMON STREET NAMES: Candy, downers, sleeping pills, tranks
DEA CLASS: Class IV
PHARMACOLOGIC CLASS: Hypnotic, sedative (not a benzodiazepine, but interacts with the same receptors in the brain)

Description: Zolpidem is used for the short-term treatment of insomnia. Abuse of benzodiazepine-type hypnotics is particularly high among heroin and cocaine users.

Method of use: Ingested

Duration of action: 6 to 8 hours

Psychological effects of abuse: Abnormal dreams, amnesia, confusion, depression, impaired judgment and thinking abilities, reduced inhibition, and suicidal ideation. Paradoxical effects include euphoria, hyperactivity, and extreme aggression. Prolonged use may cause psychological dependence.

Physical effects of abuse: Changes in sexual desire, constipation, decreased blood pressure, dizziness, drowsiness, fatigue, impaired physical capabilities, irregular gait, light-headedness, sleepiness, slowed psychomotor performance, urinary retention, and visual disturbances. Prolonged use may cause physical dependence.

Overdose symptoms: The most severe signs of overdose with benzodiazepine-type hypnotics are respiratory depression, loss of consciousness, and coma. Other symptoms may include confusion, diminished reflexes, slurred speech, impaired coordination, apnea, extreme sleepiness, loss of muscle tone, and severely low blood pressure. Death from overdose of a single benzodiazepine-type hypnotic is extremely rare. However, there is an increased risk of toxicity when benzodiazepine-type drugs are combined with alcohol and/or other CNS depressants. Fatalities have been reported in patients who have overdosed with a combination of a single benzodiazepine-type hypnotic and alcohol.

Withdrawal symptoms: Abrupt termination following long-term use may precipitate withdrawal symptoms and require hospitalization. Symptoms may include abdominal and muscle cramps, depression, insomnia, sweating, vomiting, tremors, and seizures.

Part 4.
Illegal Drugs

AMT (ALPHA-METHYLTRYPTAMINE)
COMMON STREET NAMES: Amthrax, Amtrak, spirals
DEA CLASS: Class I
PHARMACOLOGIC CLASS: Hallucinogen

Description: AMT is a chemical found in a variety of South American plants. The drug has a similar structure and pharmacologic characteristics as other tryptamine-based Class I hallucinogens.

Method of use: Ingested (often as a tea), smoked or used as snuff, and rarely, injected.

Duration of action: 1 to 6 hours, but in chronic users the effects can last 18 to 24 hours.

Psychological effects: AMT can produce similar psychological effects as other hallucinogens, including changes in perception, visual distortions, agitation, hyperactivity, confusion, euphoria, anxiety, mood alterations, slowed thinking, delirium, and unpredictable behavior. Long-term use may cause tolerance and psychological dependence.

Physical effects: AMT can produce similar physical effects as other hallucinogens, including CNS depression or stimulation, nausea, vomiting, diarrhea, elevated blood pressure and body temperature, abnormally fast heart rate, blurred vision, excessive salivation, irregular gait, loss of appetite, irregular breathing, numbness in the extremities, dizziness, drowsiness, decreased REM sleep, enhanced color awareness, and time distortion.

Overdose symptoms: AMT is not considered addictive; it does not produce compulsive drug-seeking behavior as do cocaine, amphetamines, heroin, and alcohol. However, it does produce tolerance, and chronic users must take progressively higher doses to achieve the same effects as before. This is particularly dangerous due to the unpredictability of the drug's effects. Symptoms of overdose may include irregular gait, rapid heart rate, tremors, and elevated blood pressure and body temperature.

Withdrawal symptoms: None are reported, since no evidence of physical dependence can be detected when the drug is abruptly withdrawn.

4-BROMO-2,5-DIMETHOXYPHENETHYLAMINE

COMMON STREET NAMES: 2C-B, B-DMPEA, bromo, MFT, Nexus, two's
DEA CLASS: Class I
PHARMACOLOGIC CLASS: CNS stimulant

Description: This drug is an illegally manufactured variation of mescaline and amphetamine and has the same pharmacologic actions as amphetamine. Because the drug is manufactured in clandestine laboratories, it's rarely pure, and the amount of active drug in an oral dose can vary considerably.

Method of use: Ingested and snorted

Duration of action: Up to 8 hours; effects begin 20 to 30 minutes after use and reach their peak within 1 to 2 hours.

Psychological effects: Aggressive and impulsive behavior, agitation, anxiety, confusion, delusions, depression, drug cravings, hallucinations, and paranoia. Psychological dependence can develop rapidly.

Physical effects: Dilated pupils, elevated heart rate, and increased blood pressure. Long-term effects may include psychiatric disturbances, impaired cognitive functions, and memory loss.

Overdose symptoms: In general, toxicity results in mild symptoms that may include agitation, dilated pupils, fatigue, poor concentration, excessive sweating, elevated blood pressure, and rapid heart rate. Occasionally, severe depression, anxiety, and delirium can occur. Severe overdose may cause dangerously high body temperature, blood-clotting problems, severe muscle weakness and pain, seizures, and acute kidney failure.

Withdrawal symptoms: Abruptly stopping the drug after long-term use may cause extreme fatigue, overeating, depression, and stupor.

COCAINE and CRACK COCAINE

COMMON STREET NAMES: Big C, blow, coke, crack, crank, flake, lady, nose candy, rocks, snow, snowbirds, white, zip
DEA CLASS: Class II
PHARMACOLOGIC CLASS: CNS stimulant

Description: Cocaine is prepared from an extract of the coca plant. It is one of the most potent CNS stimulants and is widely abused. Crack cocaine is processed with baking soda or ammonia to produce a form that can be smoked. Currently, controlled doses of cocaine can be administered by a doctor for legitimate medical use, primarily as a local anesthetic for certain eye, ear, and throat surgeries.

Method of use: Ingested, snorted, smoked (also called "freebasing"), and injected IV. Each method has significant health risks for the user.

Duration of action: Depends on the method of use. Snorting produces a slow onset that lasts 15 to 30 minutes. The effects of smoking or IV injection last 5 to 10 minutes and produce a more intense high.

Psychological effects: Cocaine use causes psychological dependence. *Moderate doses:* Agitation, argumentative behavior, irritability, nervousness, and talkativeness. *High doses:* Anxiety, delusions, extreme irritability, paranoia, and restlessness.

Physical effects: Cocaine is highly addictive due to its rapid onset of action. Compulsive use appears to develop more quickly in smokers than in users who snort. *Moderate doses:* Abdominal pain, constricted blood vessels, decreased appetite, dilated pupils, disturbances in heart rhythm, elevated blood pressure, headaches, increased body temperature, nausea, and rapid heart and respiratory rates. *High doses:* Abdominal pain, blurred vision, chest pain, coma, convulsions, dizziness, excessive sweating, headaches, heart attacks, muscle spasms, nausea, respiratory failure, shortness of breath, and stroke. *Warning:* Cocaine use can cause sudden death, even after the first time the drug is taken.

Overdose symptoms: An overdose can be fatal. Tolerance develops rapidly, and chronic users must take progressively higher doses to obtain the same effects as before. Cocaine-related deaths are usually caused by cardiac arrest or seizures followed by respiratory arrest. Other symptoms of overdose include high body temperature, hallucinations, and convulsions. Smoking or injecting cocaine is more dangerous than snorting it. Risk of harmful effects also increases when the drug is combined with alcohol.

Withdrawal symptoms: Abruptly stopping chronic use of high doses may produce relatively mild withdrawal symptoms, including depression, anxiety, sleep disturbances, and increased appetite. These usually occur within 24 to 48 hours following the last dose and can last 7 to 10 days. Long-term users may develop acute tolerance and can suffer from depression, headache, fatigue, and irritability after they stop using the drug. Crack cocaine users appear to develop a greater dependence on the drug and therefore have more severe withdrawal symptoms, including major psychiatric complications and severe depression.

(4-METHYL-2,5-DIMETHOXYAMPHETAMINE) and DOB (4-BROMO-2,5-ᴅMETHOXYAMPHETAMINE)

COMMON STREET NAME: STP, an acronym for Serenity, Tranquility, and Peace
DEA CLASS: Class I
PHARMACOLOGIC CLASS: CNS stimulant

Description: These drugs are an illegally manufactured variation of mescaline and amphetamine. They are sold as drug-laced pieces of paper. Because these drugs are manufactured in clandestine laboratories, they are rarely pure, and the amount of active drug in an oral dose can vary considerably.

Method of use: Ingested, snorted, and rarely, injected IV

Duration of action: Depends on method of use. Effects can last 12 to 36 hours. Symptoms start about an hour after use and reach their peak after 4 to 10 hours.

Psychological effects: The main effects are perceptual distortions that can vary with dose, setting, and the user's mood. Tolerance and psychological dependence can develop rapidly following chronic use.

Physical effects: The most common effects are elevated heart rate, increased blood pressure, and dilated pupils. Because DOB and DOM are hallucinogens, their effects are unpredictable and could be substantially different each time they are used.

Overdose symptoms: In general, toxicity with these drugs results in mild symptoms that may include agitation, elevated blood pressure, rapid heart rate, dilated pupils, and excessive sweating. Fatigue and poor concentration are also common. Occasionally, severe depression, anxiety, and delirium can occur. Severe overdose may cause dangerously high body temperature, blood-clotting problems, muscle weakness, seizures, and acute kidney failure.

Withdrawal symptoms: These drugs are highly addictive, and physical and psychological dependence develops rapidly. Abrupt cessation of use may cause anxiety, paranoia, aggressive behavior, and strong drug cravings. Suicidal ideation has been reported. Psychotic behavior may persist for months or years after discontinuation of use.

HASHISH

COMMON STREET NAMES: Boom, chronic, gangster, hash, hash oil, hemp
DEA CLASS: Class I
PHARMACOLOGIC CLASS: Cannabinoid

Description: Hashish contains the psychoactive chemical delta-9-tetrahydrocannabinol (THC). It is made from the THC-rich resinous material of the cannabis plant, which is collected, dried, and then compressed into ι variety of forms, such as balls, cakes, or cookie-like sheets. Pieces are then broken off, placed in pipes, and smoked. The Middle East, North Africa, Pakistan, and Afghanistan are the main sources of hashish.

Hashish (and hash oil) are stronger forms of marijuana. The drug's effects depend on the potency of the THC content. Hashish averages 2 to 8 percent THC, but it can contain as much as 20 percent. The drug has no legitimate medical use, but THC and a synthetic cannabinol (nabilone) are used to prevent vomiting in patients receiving cancer chemotherapy. In some studies, cannabis was found to have effects similar to analgesics, muscle relaxants, and appetite stimulants.

Hash oil is a tar-like solution distilled from hashish; it can contain anywhere from 15 to 70 percent THC. Cannabis growers usually try to maximize the plant's THC content.

Method of use: Hashish is usually smoked as a cigarette (called a joint or nail) or in a pipe (bong).

Duration of action: Hashish produces an effect almost immediately and reaches its peak in about 30 minutes. The effects usually wear off after 3 to 4 hours. Chronic users may not experience anything until 30 to 90 minutes after the first inhalation, but the effects can last for up to 8 hours.

Psychological effects: Distortion of time and space, loss of memory, impaired judgment, panic and anxiety attacks, and a false sense of well-being. Users taking cannabis in large doses have had psychotic episodes with paranoid or schizophrenic characteristics. Prolonged use of cannabis may lead to tolerance and psychological dependence.

Physical effects: Early physical effects may include nausea and vomiting. Later-stage effects may include memory loss, poor coordination, impaired learning skills, elevated heart rate and blood pressure, dry mouth, dry eyes, and blurred vision. Experts continue to debate whether physical dependence can occur.

Overdose symptoms: Heavy users rapidly develop tolerance and need progressively higher doses to obtain the same effects as before. Symptoms of overdose may include increased appetite, red and swollen eyes, dry mouth, poor motor coordination, and elevated heart rate and blood pressure.

Withdrawal symptoms: Withdrawal symptoms may include loss of appetite, anxiety, sleeplessness, irritability, restlessness, visual abnormalities, excessive sweating, headache, and stomach upset.

...ION STREET NAMES: Brown sugar, cheese (black tar heroin), dope, H, ...rse, junk, skag, skunk, smack, white horse

DEA CLASS: Class I

PHARMACOLOGIC CLASS: Narcotic analgesic

Description: Heroin is derived from the resin of the poppy plant. Pure heroin is a white powder with a bitter taste but is rarely sold on the street. Most heroin is distributed as powder that varies in color due to additives and manufacturing impurities. Another form of heroin, "black tar," has become increasingly available in the United States. The color and consistency of black tar heroin results from the crude processing methods used to manufacture the substance in Mexico. When mixed with Tylenol PM and crushed into powder form, black tar heroin is sold very inexpensively to minors, who then snort it. Heroin, which is illegal in the United States, is used in very limited treatment applications in other countries.

Method of use: Ingested, snorted, smoked, and injected IV (also called mainlining), IM, or SC (also called skin popping). Injection is the most efficient way to administer low-purity heroin, and until recently was the preferred method of use. The availability of higher-purity heroin now allows users to snort or smoke the narcotic.

Duration of action: The euphoric effects usually occur 7 to 8 seconds after injection. IM injection produces a relatively slow onset, typically 5 to 8 minutes. When heroin is sniffed or smoked, the peak effects usually occur within 10 to 15 minutes.

Psychological effects: Enhanced sexual pleasure, euphoria, psychological dependence, and significantly impaired mental function. The psychological dependence associated with narcotic addiction is complex. Long after physical dependence has ended, the addict may continue to think and talk about the drug and feel unable to manage daily activities without it.

Physical effects: Short-term physical effects include drowsiness, dry mouth, flushing, and a heavy feeling in the extremities. Long-term effects may include alternating wakefulness and drowsiness, slowed breathing, and reduced mental functioning. The development of infectious diseases—such as HIV/AIDS, infection of the heart lining, various abscesses, pneumonia, and hepatitis—is a major problem in heroin users. In addition, the impurities in the drug—especially talc—may clog blood vessels and damage the lungs, liver, kidneys, and brain.

Overdose symptoms: Tolerance and physical dependence may develop after only 2 to 3 days of continued heroin use. This greatly increases the risk of overdose as progressively higher doses are needed to obtain the same effects as before. Overdose may cause shallow breathing, convulsions, coma, and possibly death. In addition, heroin suppresses breathing and can cause the lungs to fill with fluid, which may also lead to death. Since heroin is manufactured in clandestine laboratories and drug impurities are unknown, abusers are at great risk of overdose or death.

Withdrawal symptoms: Withdrawal from heroin is extremely painful and dangerous. Symptoms are worse in people who have used large doses for prolonged periods. Abrupt withdrawal of heroin in a chronic user may be fatal. Symptoms may begin to appear within 6 hours after the last dose and continue to manifest within 24 hours. Withdrawal symptoms reach their peak at 48 to 72 hours following the last dose but may continue for weeks. Early symptoms include irritability, insomnia, diminished appetite, gooseflesh, hot and cold flashes, dilated pupils, runny nose, severe yawning, severe sneezing, excessive tearing, and cold-like symptoms. Later-stage symptoms include abdominal cramps, bone and muscle pain in the back and extremities, pronounced depression, nausea, vomiting, diarrhea, alternating fever and chills, excessive sweating, and elevated heart rate and blood pressure. Muscle spasms and kicking movements can also occur, which may explain the expression "kicking the habit."

KHAT

COMMON STREET NAMES: Khat has more than 40 street names, including Cadillac express, cat, chat, ephedrine, gat, go fast, kat, qat, slick, sniff, superspeed, tohai, tschat, wonderstar

DEA CLASS: Class I (cathine, one of the ingredients in khat, is Class IV)

PHARMACOLOGIC CLASS: CNS stimulant

Description: Khat is a naturally occurring stimulant derived from the *Catha edulis* shrub. This shrub is cultivated mainly in East Africa and the Arabian Peninsula, where the use of khat is an established cultural tradition for many social occasions. Khat is illegal in the U.S. but is used in some countries to aid weight loss.

The stimulating effects of khat are due to cathinone (a phenylpropylamine agent) and, to a much lesser extent, cathine (a norpseudoephedrine agent). Cathinone is about 10 times more potent than cathine and is only present in fresh leaves. As the leaves mature or dry, cathinone is converted to cathine. The effects of these alkaloids resemble those of amphetamines, particularly cathinone.

Methcathinone is an illegal synthetic drug that is sold as an alternative to methamphetamine. It has a chemical structure similar to cathinone but has stronger addictive properties and side effects.

Method of use: Usually ingested but can be snorted. The leaves are often chewed like tobacco and the juice swallowed; occasionally the chewed are also swallowed. In addition, khat can be brewed as a tea or ...shed and mixed with honey to make a paste.

Duration of action: Several hours

Psychological effects: Aggressive verbal outbursts, behavioral changes, euphoria, pressured speech, and psychotic reactions. Rarely, schizophrenic behavior or manic-like psychosis may occur. Psychological dependence develops rapidly.

Physical effects: Anorexia, constipation, dilated pupils, dry mouth, elevated blood pressure and body temperature, headache, increased heart rate with palpitations, insomnia, mouth inflammation or infection, severe nausea, swollen cornea, and tremors. Rarely, abnormal heart rhythm and severe chest pain may occur. Cathinone is very addictive, and physical dependence develops rapidly with chronic use.

Overdose symptoms: The main symptoms are hyperactivity, severely elevated blood pressure and body temperature, and seizures. Serious overdose symptoms from chewing khat are due to the phenylpropylamine content of the leaves.

Withdrawal symptoms: Cathinone is highly addictive, and physical and psychological dependence develop rapidly. Abruptly stopping the drug may precipitate withdrawal symptoms such as anxiety, paranoia, aggressive behavior, and strong drug cravings. Suicidal ideation has also been reported. Psychotic behavior may persist for months or years after discontinuation of use.

LSD (LYSERGIC ACID DIETHYLAMIDE)

COMMON STREET NAMES: Acid, blotter, boomers, cubes, dots, L, mellow yello, microdots, tabs, trips, window pane, yellow sunshines

DEA CLASS: Class I

PHARMACOLOGIC CLASS: Hallucinogen

Description: LSD is a potent hallucinogenic substance. It has no legitimate medical use. LSD, commonly referred to as acid, is usually sold as "dots" on blotter paper, but it can also be found as tablets, square gel caps, and rarely, in liquid form. Rogue chemists manufacturer the drug as a crystalline powder that can be reduced to a clear liquid for dosing purposes.

Method of use: Ingested

Duration of action: Up to 12 hours

Psychological effects: Psychological effects depend on the individual. The user may feel various emotions at once or swing rapidly from one mood to another. Depending on the dose, the drug may produce delusions, visual hallucinations, flashbacks, severe depression, and panic attacks. The user often refers to this experience as a "bad trip." Some LSD users experience severe, terrifying thoughts, and become fearful of losing control, going insane, or dying. Long-term use may cause tolerance and psychological dependence.

Physical effects: The effects of LSD are unpredictable, but the drug is not physically addictive. Physical reactions to LSD depend on the dose; the user's personality, mood, and expectations; and the surroundings in which the drug is used. Initial effects may include dilated pupils, elevated body temperature, increased heart rate and blood pressure, excessive sweating, loss of appetite, sleeplessness, dry mouth, and tremors.

Overdose symptoms: LSD is not considered addictive; it does not produce compulsive drug-seeking behavior as do cocaine, amphetamines, heroin, and alcohol. However, it does produce tolerance, and chronic users must take progressively higher doses to achieve the same effects as before. This is particularly dangerous due to the unpredictability of LSD. Symptoms of overdose may include excessive tearing, irregular gait, dilated pupils, rapid heart rate, tremors, and elevated blood pressure and body temperature. Overdose with LSD can be frightening and cause panic. Injuries and fatal accidents have been reported during states of LSD intoxication.

Withdrawal symptoms: None are reported, since no evidence of physical dependence can be detected when the drug is abruptly withdrawn.

MARIJUANA

COMMON STREET NAMES: Blunt, budah, chronic, dope, ganja, grass, herb, homegrown, indo, joints, Mary Jane, pot, reefer, schwag, sinsemilla, skunk, weed
DEA CLASS: Class I
PHARMACOLOGIC CLASS: Cannabinoid

Description: Marijuana is a green, brown, or gray mixture of dried, shredded leaves, stems, seeds, and flowers of the hemp plant (*Cannabis sativa*). Cannabis is a term that refers to marijuana and other drugs made from the same plant. The active ingredient in marijuana is delta-9-tetrahydrocannabinol (THC), which is responsible for its psychoactive effects.

Method of use: Smoked as a cigarette (joint) or in a pipe (bong). Users also smoke blunts, the street name for cigars that have had their tobacco contents replaced with marijuana and other illicit drugs such as crack. Marijuana can also be mixed into foods or used to brew a tea.

Duration of action: Effects begin as soon as the drug enters the brain and can last from 1 to 3 hours.

Psychological effects: All cannabis products are mind-altering drugs. Users initially feel euphoric but then become extremely sleepy and depressed. Other effects include distorted perception, mood changes, anxiety or panic attacks, and difficulty with thinking and problem solving.

Physical effects: Short-term effects may include memory loss, poor coordination, impaired learning skills, elevated heart rate and blood pressure, dry mouth, dry eyes, and blurred vision. The potential for heart attack increases within the first hour of use due to the drug's effects on heart rate and blood pressure. Marijuana may also impair the immune system, which greatly increases the risk of bacterial infections. Tolerance and physical dependence may develop with long-term use.

In addition, smoking marijuana causes similar effects on the lungs as smoking tobacco, including daily cough and phlegm production, frequent chest illnesses, heightened risk of lung infections, and greater tendency toward obstructed airways. Marijuana contains 50 to 70 percent more carcinogenic hydrocarbons than tobacco, and cancer of the respiratory tract and lungs can result from marijuana smoking.

Overdose symptoms: Heavy users rapidly develop tolerance and need progressively higher doses to obtain the same effects as before. Serious health effects are more likely to be secondary to impaired judgment and behavioral problems rather than direct overdose effects. Early symptoms of overdose may include excessive sleepiness, mild euphoria, short-term memory loss, difficulty in accomplishing tasks, and lapses of attention. Serious overdose effects may include extreme tiredness, severe weakness and drowsiness, dizziness, slurred speech, irregular gait, decreased motor coordination and muscle strength, and rarely, psychosis.

Withdrawal symptoms: Abrupt discontinuation of use may cause drug cravings, irritability, agitation, apprehension, aggressiveness, tremulousness, sleeplessness, excessive sweating, and elevated anxiety. Additional symptoms may include increased aggression that reaches its peak effects about a week after the last smoked dose.

MDMA (3,4-METHYLENEDIOXYMETHAMPHETAMINE)

COMMON STREET NAMES: Adam, clarity, ecstasy, Eve, lover's speed, peace, STP, X, XTC
DEA CLASS: Class I
PHARMACOLOGIC CLASS: Amphetamine, CNS stimulant

Description: MDMA is an illegally manufactured variation of mescaline and amphetamine. It has both psychedelic and stimulant effects. It is a so-called "club drug" used at all-night dance parties known as "raves." Because MDMA is manufactured in clandestine laboratories, it is rarely pure, and the amount of active drug in an oral dose can vary considerably.

Method of use: Ingested and snorted

Duration of action: Psychedelic effects last 4 to 6 hours.

Psychological effects: Anxiety, confusion, depression, paranoia, drug craving, and aggressive and impulsive behavior. Tolerance and psychological dependence may develop with chronic use.

Physical effects: High blood pressure, increased heart rate, elevated body temperature, jaw and teeth clenching, muscle tension, chills and/or sweating, nausea, blurred vision, faintness, dizziness, and drug craving. MDMA can increase heart rate significantly during strenuous physical activity, but the heart does not respond normally. Since MDMA use is associated with such strenuous activities as dancing for hours, the drug's effects on the heart could increase the risk of heart damage and cardiovascular collapse.

Overdose symptoms: Large doses may cause extremely high fever, severely high blood pressure, rapid heart rate, and kidney and heart failure. *Warning:* Drinking too much water after taking MDMA can be lethal. MDMA significantly increases the blood levels of vasopressin (an antidiuretic hormone). Vasopressin causes the body to retain more water, which dilutes the amount of sodium and other salts in the blood. This can swell the brain, causing damage to the brain and nerve tissue.

Withdrawal symptoms: MDMA is a powerfully addictive drug, and physical and psychological dependence develops rapidly. Abrupt cessation may precipitate withdrawal symptoms such as anxiety, paranoia, aggressive behavior, and strong drug cravings. Suicidal ideation has been reported. Psychotic behavior may persist for months or years after discontinuation of use.

MESCALINE (PEYOTE CACTUS)
COMMON STREET NAMES: Buttons, cactus, mesc
DEA CLASS: Class I
PHARMACOLOGIC CLASS: Hallucinogen

Description: Peyote is a small cactus whose principal active ingredient is mescaline (3, 4, 5-trimethoxyphenethylamine), a compound that is structurally similar to amphetamines. It can be either extracted from the plant or produced synthetically.

Method of use: Ingested (sometimes brewed as a tea) and smoked

Duration of action: 6 to 12 hours

Psychological effects: Common effects include visual and auditory hallucinations, abnormal sensory perception, amnesia, and anxiety. The following may also occur: suicidal thoughts, emotional instability, fear, anxiety, paranoia, and flashbacks.

Physical effects: Dizziness, drowsiness, headache, light-headedness, excessive salivation, tremors, weakness, increased muscle tone, blurred vision, dilated pupils, irregular gait, elevated blood pressure, stomach cramps, nausea, vomiting, abnormal reflexes, shivering, feelings of hot or cold, and respiratory depression. The drug can also cause numbness of the tongue and mouth. Tolerance has been documented but decreases rapidly within a few days following cessation of use. Although physiological drug addiction generally does not occur, cross-tolerance with other hallucinogens can develop.

Overdose symptoms: Overdose can cause death due to homicidal, psychotic, or suicidal behavior. Signs of mescaline overdose resemble those of LSD. A wide range of symptoms can be present, since users often take other drugs simultaneously with mescaline. Concomitant administration of alcohol with mescaline may produce prolonged seizures and coma.

Withdrawal symptoms: None are reported, since no evidence of physical dependence can be detected when the drug is abruptly withdrawn.

METHAQUALONE
COMMON STREET NAMES: Ludes, mandrex, Quaalude, quad, quay
DEA CLASS: Class I
PHARMACOLOGIC CLASS: Sedative, hypnotic

Description: Methaqualone has properties similar to those of barbiturates. It was used previously for the short-term treatment of insomnia but was withdrawn from the market in the U.S. and other countries due to a high risk of abuse.

Method of use: Ingested

Duration of action: Methaqualone absorbs rapidly following ingestion. The drug reaches peak serum levels within 2 hours, with the effects lasting 5 to 8 hours.

Psychological effects: Anxiety, confusion, false sense of well-being, and impaired perception. Psychological dependence may occur with prolonged use of high doses.

Physical effects: Excessive sleepiness, loss of coordination, low blood pressure, sexual dysfunction, and slowed heart rate and breathing. Excessive use leads to tolerance, physical dependence, and withdrawal symptoms similar to those of barbiturates.

Overdose symptoms: Tolerance develops rapidly, and progressively higher doses are needed to obtain the same effects as before. Signs of overdose may include extreme tiredness, irregular gait, muscle rigidity, muscular hyperactivity, rapid heart rate, low blood pressure, respiratory failure, heart failure, seizures, and coma.

Withdrawal symptoms: Methaqualone withdrawal may lead to death if left untreated. Symptoms include weakness, abdominal cramps, nausea, vomiting, disorientation, anxiety, restlessness, rapid heart rate, visual hallucinations, stupor, delirium, tremors, and seizures.

5-MeO-DIPT (5-METHOXY-N, N-DIISOPROPYLTRYPTAMINE)
COMMON STREET NAMES: Foxy, foxy methoxy
DEA CLASS: Class I
PHARMACOLOGIC CLASS: Hallucinogen

Description: This drug has the same chemical properties and effects as other tryptamine-based Class I hallucinogens.

Method of use: Ingested, snorted, and smoked

Duration of action: 3 to 6 hours

Psychological effects: This drug can cause the same psychological effects as other hallucinogens, including changes in perception, visual distortions, agitation, hyperactivity, confusion, euphoria, anxiety, mood alterations, slowed thinking, delirium, and unpredictable behavior. Long-term use may cause tolerance and psychological dependence.

Physical effects: This drug can produce the same physical effects as other hallucinogens, including CNS depression or stimulation, nausea, vomiting, diarrhea, elevated blood pressure and body temperature, abnormally fast heart rate, blurred vision, excessive salivation, irregular gait, loss of appetite, irregular breathing, numbness in the extremities, dizziness, drowsiness, decreased REM sleep, enhanced color awareness, and time distortion.

Overdose symptoms: This drug is not considered addictive; it does not produce compulsive drug-seeking behavior as do cocaine, amphetamine, heroin, and alcohol. However, it does produce tolerance, and chronic users must take progressively higher doses to achieve the same effects as before. This is particularly dangerous due to the unpredictability of the drug's effects. Symptoms of overdose may include irregular gait, rapid heart rate, tremors, and elevated blood pressure and body temperature.

Withdrawal symptoms: None are reported, since no evidence of physical dependence can be detected when the drug is abruptly withdrawn.

PCP (PHENCYCLIDINE)
COMMON STREET NAMES: Angel dust, boat, hog, love boat, peace pill
DEA CLASS: Class I and II
PHARMACOLOGIC CLASS: Hallucinogen

Description: PCP is a dissociative anesthetic with sympathomimetic and hallucinogenic properties. It is a bitter-tasting, white crystalline powder that can dissolve in water and be mixed with dyes. PCP is manufactured illegally by rogue chemists in places known as "bucket labs." It is related chemically to ketamine and is a potent analgesic and anesthetic. The drug was originally developed as a tranquilizer for animals. PCP was formerly used in humans as an intravenous anesthetic, but severe adverse effects—especially postoperative psychosis—precluded its use. However, the drug still has some veterinary applications.

Method of use: Ingested, smoked, snorted, and injected IV. The most popular method is to apply the drug to a marijuana joint or menthol cigarette and smoke it, known as a "kool-dip."

Duration of action: If smoked, the effects start in 2 to 5 minutes and last about 15 to 30 minutes. In chronic users the effects can last 4 to 6 hours but may also linger for 1 to 2 days.

Psychological effects: PCP is a highly addictive drug that can cause psychological dependence. Frequent use can result in tolerance and drug craving. Effects may include mood and perception alteration, paranoia, panic attacks, anxiety, decreased awareness, compulsive drug-seeking behavior, and suicidal ideation. It can induce psychosis that is indistinguishable from schizophrenia. The following have also been reported: hallucinations, euphoria, agitation, hyperactivity, disorientation, and violent delusional behavior.

Physical effects: The physical effects of PCP are unpredictable, but the following have been reported: elevated pulse and heart rate, increased blood pressure and body temperature, muscle relaxation, dilated pupils, rapid eye movement, nausea, vomiting, blurred vision, dizziness, tremors, shallow breathing, loss of coordination, excessive salivation, excessive perspiration, convulsions, numbness and tingling in the extremities, and occasionally, excessively high fever. Constricted pupils and seizures are more common in children. Substantially increased blood pressure is the hallmark sign that usually resolves within 4 hours but can persist for more than 24 hours. Respiratory effects are uncommon without concurrent use of sedatives, narcotics, or alcohol.

Overdose symptoms: An overdose can cause death due to respiratory depression and coma. Other symptoms include unpredictable behavior, depression, convulsions, flashbacks, psychosis, delusions, and dangerously high fever.

Withdrawal symptoms: None are reported, since no evidence of physical dependence can be detected when the drug is abruptly withdrawn.

PMA (PARAMETHOXYAMPHETAMINE)
COMMON STREET NAMES: Death, Mitsubishi, double-stack
DEA CLASS: Class I
PHARMACOLOGIC CLASS: Amphetamine, hallucinogen, CNS stimulant

Description: PMA is a synthetic hallucinogen that is structurally related to MDMA but is significantly more lethal, even in smaller doses. It is produced legally in the U.S. for limited commercial applications and scientific research.

Method of use: Ingested, but the powder form may be injected or snorted.

Duration of action: Up to 8 hours; effects begin 30 to 60 minutes after use and reach their peak after approximately 90 minutes.

Psychological effects: Initial feelings include a rush of euphoria followed by a general sense of happiness and well-being. These effects are followed by a "coming down" phase 3 to 6 hours later, resulting in depression, anxiety, and general negativity that can persist for several days. Prolonged use may cause tolerance and psychological dependence.

Physical effects: Depends on the dose. A single small dose can cause labored breathing, erratic eye movement, elevated pulse rate and body temperature, high blood pressure, muscle spasms, nausea, and heightened visual stimulation. Larger doses may cause irregular heart rhythm, serious breathing difficulties, severely elevated body temperature, vomiting, kidney failure, and cardiac arrest.

Overdose symptoms: Illicit drug makers sometimes stamp MDMA logos on their PMA "products" in order to pass them off as MDMA. This could increase the risk of fatal overdose because users may unknownly mix PMA with MDMA. Signs of overdose can include vomiting, severely elevated body temperature, convulsions, coma, and death.

Withdrawal symptoms: None are reported, since no evidence of physical dependence can be detected when the drug is abruptly withdrawn.

PSILOCYBIN
COMMON STREET NAMES: Magic mushroom, musk, purple passion, shrooms
DEA CLASS: Class I
PHARMACOLOGIC CLASS: Hallucinogen

Description: Psilocybin, or psilocyn, is obtained from certain mushrooms indigenous to tropical and subtropical regions of South America, Mexico, and the United States. These mushrooms are available fresh or dried. The effects produced by dried or brewed mushrooms are far less predictable and largely depend on the particular mushrooms used and the age and preservation of the extract. Psilocybin has properties similar to LSD but is less potent. It has no legitimate medical use.

Method of use: Ingested; the mushrooms are sometimes brewed as a tea or added to food to mask the bitter flavor.

Duration of action: 4 to 6 hours

Psychological effects: Vivid visual and auditory hallucinations, panic attacks, and emotional disturbances. Long-term use may cause tolerance and psychological dependence.

Physical effects: There are many species of mushrooms that contain varying amounts of psilocybin as well as uncertain amounts of other chemicals. It is nearly impossible to predict the physical effects of this compound. The most commonly reported effects include drowsiness, vomiting, muscle weakness, and panic attacks. The exact mechanism of action and extent of toxicity are unknown.

Overdose symptoms: Symptoms of overdose may occur 30 to 60 minutes (and sometimes as late as 3 hours) following ingestion. Signs include a pleasant yet apprehensive mood, impaired judgment, compulsive movements, vertigo, dilated pupils, irregular gait, tingling sensations, muscle weakness, loss of muscle tone, and drowsiness that almost progresses to sleep. Children may develop high temperatures with seizures.

Withdrawal symptoms: None are reported, since no evidence of physical dependence can be detected when the drug is abruptly withdrawn.

SALVIA DIVINORUM
COMMON STREET NAMES: Diviner's sage, herbal ecstasy, Mexican mint, ska Maria Pastora
DEA CLASS: Not classified
PHARMACOLOGIC CLASS: Hallucinogen

Description: S. divinorum is a perennial herb in the mint family. It's one of several vision-inducing plants used by the Mazatec Indians of Mexico.

The herb's active ingredient is Salvinorin A, a psychoactive chemical that can cause intense hallucinations.

Method of use: Ingested (usually as a tea), smoked, and chewed. The herb is most effective when it's vaporized and inhaled.

Duration of action: Hallucinogenic effects can last up to 1 hour.

Psychological effects: S. *divinorum* may cause similar psychological effects as ketamine, mescaline, and psilocybin, including changes in perception, hallucinations, and delirium. Long-term use may cause tolerance and psychological dependence.

Physical effects: S. *divinorum* may induce similar physical effects as ketamine, mescaline, and psilocybin, including CNS depression or stimulation, nausea, vomiting, diarrhea, elevated blood pressure, and abnormally fast heart rate.

Overdose symptoms: This drug is not considered addictive; it does not produce compulsive drug-seeking behavior as do cocaine, amphetamines, heroin, and alcohol. However, it does produce tolerance, and chronic users must take progressively higher doses to achieve the same effects as before. This is particularly dangerous due to the unpredictability of the drug's effects. Signs of overdose may include irregular gait, rapid heart rate, tremors, and elevated blood pressure and body temperature.

Withdrawal symptoms: None are reported, since no evidence of physical dependence can be detected when the drug is abruptly withdrawn.

Psychotropic Drug Profiles

ABILIFY/ABILIFY DISCMELT

Generic name: Aripiprazole

What is this medication?

Abilify is an antipsychotic drug used for the treatment of schizophrenia in adults and adolescents 13 to 17 years of age. It is also used to treat manic and mixed episodes associated with bipolar disorder. Abilify may also be used with antidepressants to treat major depressive disorder in adults.

What is the most important information I should know about this medication?

Abilify is not approved for elderly patients with dementia-related psychosis due to the risk of death.

If you or a family member notices new signs of nervousness, agitation, panic attacks, sleeplessness, irritability, aggressiveness, and other mood changes on a day-to-day basis, notify your doctor right away. These signs may be associated with an increased risk of suicidal thinking.

Hyperglycemia, or elevated blood sugar, may occur when taking Abilify. If you have diabetes mellitus, monitor your blood sugar levels carefully.

Report any sudden changes in temperature, heart rate (arrhythmia), or heart palpitations to your doctor, as these may be symptoms of a serious side effect. Also report any involuntary movements, seizures, or the inability to swallow while taking Abilify.

An extreme drop in blood pressure when standing rapidly from a lying or sitting position may cause extreme dizziness and/or fainting. Sitting up slowly, then standing up slowly may help prevent this.

Who should not take this medication?

Elderly patients with dementia-related psychosis should not receive Abilify.

If you have kidney and/or liver disease, you should be monitored closely.

If you are taking antidepressants, you should be monitored closely for changes in mood and/or behavior.

What should I tell my doctor before I take the first dose of this medication?

Tell your doctor about all prescription, over-the-counter, and herbal medications you are taking before beginning treatment with Abilify. Also, talk to your doctor about your complete medical history, especially if you have diabetes mellitus, high blood pressure, heart disease, or are recovering from a heart attack.

What is the usual dosage?

The information below is based on the dosage guidelines your doctor uses. Depending on your condition and medical history, your doctor may prescribe a different regimen. Do not change the dosage or stop taking your medication without your doctor's approval.

Bipolar Disorder

Adults: Initial dose is 15 milligrams (mg) daily, which can be increased to 30 mg daily if needed. Treatment may be as long as 6 weeks.

Children: The recommended dose of Abilify is 10 mg daily, as monotherapy or adjuvant therapy with lithium or valproate. Start with 2 mg daily, then titrate to 10 mg daily over a period of 4 days.

Major Depressive Disorder

Adults: The recommended starting dose for Abilify as adjuvant treatment for patients already taking an antidepressant is 2 to 5 mg daily. The dose may be increased up to 15 mg daily if necessary.

Schizophrenia

Adults: The recommended starting dose for Abilify is 10 to 15 mg daily. Dosage increases, if necessary, should not be made before 2 weeks of initiation of therapy. Adolescents aged 13-17 should be started at 10 mg daily, and increased to 15 mg daily if needed.

How should I take this medication?

Abilify tablets should be taken as one dose, with or without food, as directed.

For the Abilify Discmelt orally disintegrating tablets, use dry hands to remove the tablet, and place the entire tablet on your tongue. Tablet disintegration occurs rapidly in saliva. Although it is recommended to take the disintegrating tablet without liquid, you may do so if needed. Do not attempt to split the tablets.

What should I avoid while taking this medication?

Because Abilify has the potential to impair judgment, thinking, or motor skills, use caution when operating machinery, including automobiles, until you learn how Abilify affects you.

Avoid alcohol intake while taking Abilify.

Avoid rapid movements, such as quickly rising from a seated or lying position, as this can cause severe dizziness and/or fainting.

Avoid strenuous exercise, or prolonged exposure to heat, since this could contribute to a rise in core body temperature, and dehydration.

Avoid excessive sugar intake if you have diabetes, since Abilify may elevate blood sugar levels.

What are possible food and drug interactions associated with this medication?

If Abilify is used with certain other drugs, the effects of either could be increased, decreased, or altered. It is especially important to check with your doctor before combining Abilify with the following: alcohol, antihypertensive drugs (drugs used to treat blood pressure), carbamazepine, fluoxetine, ketoconazole, paroxetine, and quinidine.

What are the possible side effects of this medication?

Side effects cannot be anticipated. If any develop or change in intensity, tell your doctor as soon as possible. Only your doctor can determine if it is safe for you to continue taking this drug.

Side effects may include: nausea, vomiting, constipation, headache, dizziness, nervousness, sleeplessness, restlessness, tremors

Can I receive this medication if I am pregnant or breastfeeding?

The effects of Abilify during pregnancy and breastfeeding are unknown. Tell your doctor immediately if you are pregnant, plan to become pregnant, or are breastfeeding.

What should I do if I miss a dose of this medication?

Since Abilify is taken once daily, take the missed dose as soon as you remember. If the next dose is within 12 hours, skip the missed dose and continue with your normal dosing schedule. Never double the dose.

How should I store this medication?

Store at room temperature.

ADDERALL

Generic name: Amphetamine salts

What is this medication?

Adderall is indicated for the treatment of attention-deficit/hyperactivity disorder (ADHD) and narcolepsy.

What is the most important information I should know about this medication?

The following have been reported with use of Adderall and other stimulant medications.

Heart-related problems such as sudden death in patients who have heart problems or heart defects; stroke and heart attack in adults; and increased blood pressure and heart rate. Call your doctor right away if you or your child show any signs of heart problems such as chest pain, shortness of breath, or fainting while taking Adderall XR.

Mental problems such as new or worsening behavior and thought problems; new or worsening bipolar disorder; or new or worsening aggressive behavior or hostility.

Monitor children and teenagers for any new psychotic or manic symptoms.

Who should not take this medication?

Adderall should not be taken if you or your child: have heart disease or hardening of the arteries; have moderate to severe high blood pressure; have an overactive thyroid; have an eye disease called glaucoma; are very anxious, tense, or agitated; have a history of drug abuse; are taking or have taken within the past 14 days a type of antidepressive medication called a monoamine oxidase inhibitor or MAOI; are sensitive to, allergic to, or had a reaction to other stimulant medicines.

Adderall is not recommended for use in children under 3 years old.

What should I tell my doctor before I take the first dose of this medication?

Tell your doctor about all prescription, over-the-counter, and herbal medications you are taking before beginning treatment with Adderall. Also, talk to your doctor about you or your child's complete medical history, including: heart problems, heart defects, high blood pressure, or a family history of these problems; a history of mental problems or a family history of suicide, bipolar disorder, or depression; tics or Tourette's syndrome; liver or kidney problems; thyroid problems; or seizures or have had an abnormal brain wave test (EEG).

Tell your doctor if you or your child are pregnant, planning to become pregnant, or breastfeeding.

What is the usual dosage?

The information below is based on the dosage guidelines your doctor uses. Depending on your condition and medical history, your doctor may prescribe a different regimen. Do not change the dosage or stop taking your medication without your doctor's approval.

Attention-Deficit/Hyperactivity Disorder

Not recommended for children under 3 years of age. In children from 3 to 5 years of age, start with 2.5 milligrams (mg) daily; daily dosage may be raised in increments of 2.5 mg at weekly intervals until optimal response in obtained. In children 6 years and older, start with 5 mg once or twice daily; daily dosage may be raised in increments of 5 mg at weekly intervals until optimal response is obtained. Only in rare cases will it be necessary to exceed a total of 40 mg per day.

Narcolepsy

Usual dose 5 to 60 mg per day in divided doses, depending on the individual patient response.

How should I take this medication?

Adderall tablets are usually taken two or three times a day. The first dose is usually taken when you first wake in the morning. One or two more doses may be taken during the day, 4 to 6 hours apart. Adderall can be taken with or without food.

What should I avoid while taking this medication?

Amphetamines may impair your ability to engage in potentially hazardous activities such as operating machinery or vehicles; use caution while taking Adderall.

What are possible food and drug interactions associated with this medication?

If Adderall is taken with certain other drugs, the effects of either could be increased, decreased, or altered. It is especially important to check with your doctor before combining Adderall with the following: antidepressant medications, including MAOIs, blood pressure medications, blood thinner medications, cold or allergy medications that contain decongestants, seizure medications, stomach acid medications.

What are the possible side effects of this medication?

Side effects cannot be anticipated. If any develop or change in intensity, tell your doctor as soon as possible. Only your doctor can determine if it is safe for you to continue taking this drug.

Serious side effects may include: slowing of growth (height and weight) in children; seizures, mainly in patients with a history of seizures; eyesight changes or blurred vision

Common side effects may include: headache, stomachache, trouble sleeping, decreased appetite, nervousness, dizziness

Can I receive this medication if I am pregnant or breastfeeding?

The effects of Adderall during pregnancy and breastfeeding are unknown. Tell your doctor immediately if you are pregnant, plan to become pregnant, or are breastfeeding.

What should I do if I miss a dose of this medication?

Take it as soon as you remember. If it is almost time for your next dose, skip the missed dose and return to your regular schedule. Never take 2 doses at the same time.

How should I store this medication?

Store in a cool, dry place in a tightly closed, light-resistant container.

ADDERALL XR
Generic name: Amphetamine salts

What is this medication?

Adderall XR is a once-daily central nervous system stimulant medicine used for the treatment of attention-deficit/hyperactivity disorder (ADHD). Adderall XR may help increase attention and decrease impulsiveness and hyperactivity in patients with ADHD.

What is the most important information I should know about this medication?

The following have been reported with use of Adderall XR and other stimulant medications.

Heart-related problems such as sudden death in patients who have heart problems or heart defects; stroke and heart attack in adults; and increased blood pressure and heart rate. Call your doctor right away if you or your child show any signs of heart problems such as chest pain, shortness of breath, or fainting while taking Adderall XR.

Mental problems such as new or worsening behavior and thought problems; new or worsening bipolar disorder; or new or worsening aggressive behavior or hostility.

Monitor children and teenagers for any new psychotic or manic symptoms.

Who should not take this medication?

Adderall XR should not be taken if you or your child have heart disease or hardening of the arteries; have moderate to severe high blood pressure; have an overactive thyroid; have an eye disease called glaucoma; are very anxious, tense, or agitated; have a history of drug abuse; are taking or have taken within the past 14 days a type of antidepressive medication called a monoamine oxidase inhibitor or MAOI; are sensitive to, allergic to, or had a reaction to other stimulant medicines.

Adderall XR is not recommended for use in children under 3 years old.

What should I tell my doctor before I take the first dose of this medication?

Tell your doctor about all prescription, over-the-counter, and herbal medications you are taking before beginning treatment with Adderall XR. Also, talk to your doctor about you or your child's complete medical history, including heart problems, heart defects, high blood pressure, or a family history of these problems; a history of mental problems or a family history of suicide, bipolar disorder, or depression; tics or Tourette's syndrome; liver or kidney problems; thyroid problems; or seizures or have had an abnormal brain wave test (EEG).

Tell your doctor if you or your child are pregnant, planning to become pregnant, or breastfeeding.

What is the usual dosage?
The information below is based on the dosage guidelines your doctor uses. Depending on your condition and medical history, your doctor may prescribe a different regimen. Do not change the dosage or stop taking your medication without your doctor's approval.

Adults: In adults with ADHD who are either starting treatment for the first time or switching from another medication, the recommended dose is 20 milligrams (mg) a day. Patients taking divided doses of immediate-release Adderall, for example twice a day, may be switched to Adderall XR at the same total daily dose taken once a day.

Adolescents: The recommended starting dose for adolescents who are 13 to 17 years of age with ADHD is 10 mg/day. The dose may be increased to 20 mg/day after one week if ADHD symptoms are not adequately controlled.

Children: Children with ADHD who are 6 years of age and older and are either starting treatment for the first time or switching from another medication should start with 10 mg once daily in the morning; daily dosage may be adjusted in increments of 5 mg or 10 mg at weekly intervals. The maximum recommended dose for children is 30 mg/day.

How should I take this medication?
Take Adderall XR once a day in the morning when you first wake up. Adderall XR is an extended-release capsule that releases medicine into your body throughout the day. Swallow Adderall XR capsules whole with water or other liquids. If you or your child cannot swallow the capsule, open it and sprinkle the medicine over a spoonful of applesauce. Swallow the applesauce and medicine mixture without chewing. Follow with a drink of water or other liquid. Adderall XR may be taken with or without food.

What should I avoid while taking this medication?
Amphetamines may impair your ability to engage in potentially hazardous activities such as operating machinery or vehicles; use caution while taking Adderall XR.

What are possible food and drug interactions associated with this medication?
If Adderall XR is taken with certain other drugs, the effects of either could be increased, decreased, or altered. It is especially important to check with your doctor before combining Adderall XR with the following: antidepressive medicines (including MAOIs), antipsychotic medicines, blood pressure medicines, blood thinner medicines, cold or allergy medicines that contain decongestants, lithium, narcotic pain medications, seizure medicines, and stomach acid medicines.

What are the possible side effects of this medication?

Side effects cannot be anticipated. If any develop or change in intensity, tell your doctor as soon as possible. Only your doctor can determine if it is safe for you to continue taking this drug.

Serious side effects may include: slowing of growth (height and weight) in children; seizures, mainly in patients with a history of seizures; eyesight changes or blurred vision

Common side effects may include: headache, stomachache, trouble sleeping, decreased appetite, nervousness, mood swings, dizziness

Can I receive this medication if I am pregnant or breastfeeding?

The effects of Adderall XR during pregnancy and breastfeeding are unknown. Amphetamines are secreted in human milk. Mothers taking amphetamines such as Adderall XR should refrain from nursing. Tell your doctor immediately if you are pregnant, plan to become pregnant, or are breastfeeding.

What should I do if I miss a dose of this medication?

Take it as soon as you remember. If it is almost time for your next dose, skip the missed dose and return to your regular schedule. Never take 2 doses at the same time.

How should I store this medication?

Store in a cool, dry place in a tightly closed, light-resistant container.

AMBIEN

Generic name: Zolpidem tartrate

What is this medication?

Ambien is used for the short-term treatment of insomnia, which includes trouble falling asleep, waking up too early in the morning, or waking up often during the night.

What is the most important information I should know about this medication?

Do not take Ambien if you are allergic to any of its ingredients.

Do not drive or engage in hazardous activities that require mental alertness or coordination after taking Ambien until you feel fully awake.

After you stop taking Ambien, you may experience lightheadedness, trouble sleeping, nausea, and nervousness for 1 to 2 days.

When sleep medicines are used every night for more than a few weeks, they may lose their effectiveness or cause dependence.

Call your doctor if your insomnia worsens or does not improve within 7 to 10 days of beginning treatment. This may mean that there is another condition causing your sleeping problems.

Tell your doctor if you experience abnormal thinking, mood problems, behavior changes, anxiety, or memory loss while taking this medication.

Who should not take this medication?
Do not take Ambien if you are allergic to any of its ingredients.

What should I tell my doctor before I take the first dose of this medication?
Tell your doctor about all prescription, over-the-counter, and herbal medications you are taking before beginning treatment with Ambien. Also, talk to your doctor about your complete medical history, especially if you have ever abused or have been dependent on alcohol, or prescription or street drugs. In addition, tell your doctor if you have a history of suicidal thoughts, depression, or mental illness.

What is the usual dosage?
The information below is based on the dosage guidelines your doctor uses. Depending on your condition and medical history, your doctor may prescribe a different regimen. Do not change the dosage or stop taking your medication without your doctor's approval.

Adults: The recommended adult dose of Ambien is 10 milligrams (mg) immediately before bedtime.
Elderly or liver problems: Your doctor may prescribe a lower dose.

How should I take this medication?
Take Ambien immediately before going to bed. Do not take Ambien with or immediately after a meal.

Do not take Ambien unless you are able to stay in bed for a full night (7-8 hours) before you must be active again.

What should I avoid while taking this medication?
Do not drink alcohol while taking Ambien because it can increase the drug's side effects.

When you first start taking Ambien, you may be drowsy the next day. Use extreme care while doing anything that requires complete alertness, such as driving or operating machinery.

Do not take Ambien with other medications that can make you sleepy.

What are possible food and drug interactions associated with this medication?
If Ambien is taken with certain other drugs, the effects of either could be increased, decreased, or altered. It is especially important to check with your doctor before combining Ambien with the following: alcohol, chlorpromazine, imipramine, ketoconazole, and rifampin.

What are the possible side effects of this medication?
Side effects cannot be anticipated. If any develop or change in intensity, tell your doctor as soon as possible. Only your doctor can determine if it is safe for you to continue taking this drug.

Side effects may include: diarrhea, dizziness, drowsiness, "drugged feeling"

Can I receive this medication if I am pregnant or breastfeeding?
The effects of Ambien during pregnancy are unknown. Sleep medicines may cause sedation of your unborn baby when used during the last weeks of pregnancy. Ambien should not be used if you are breastfeeding. Tell your doctor immediately if you are pregnant, planning to become pregnant, or are breastfeeding.

What should I do if I miss a dose of this medication?
Skip the missed dose and go back to your regular dosing schedule. Do not take two doses at once. Do not take more than your total daily dose in any 24-hour period.

How should I store this medication?
Store at room temperature.

AMBIEN CR
Generic name: Zolpidem tartrate, extended-release

What is this medication?
Ambien CR belongs to a group of medicines known as sedative/hypnotics, or sleep medicines. Ambien CR is used for the short-term treatment of insomnia, which includes trouble falling asleep, waking up too early in the morning, or waking up often during the night.

What is the most important information I should know about this medication?
Do not take Ambien CR if you are allergic to any of its ingredients.

Do not take Ambien CR unless you are able to stay in bed for a full night (7-8 hours) before you must be active again.

Do not drive or engage in hazardous activities that require mental alertness or coordination after taking Ambien CR until you are fully awake.

After you stop taking Ambien CR you may experience lightheadedness, trouble sleeping, nausea, or nervousness for 1 to 2 days.

When sleep medicines are used every night for more than a few weeks, they may lose their effectiveness or cause dependence.

Call your doctor if your insomnia worsens or does not improve within 7 to 10 days of beginning treatment. This may mean that there is another condition causing your sleep problems.

Tell your doctor if you experience abnormal thinking, mood problems, behavior changes, anxiety, or memory loss while taking this medication.

Who should not take this medication?

Do not take Ambien CR if you are allergic to any of its ingredients.

What should I tell my doctor before I take the first dose of this medication?

Tell your doctor about all prescription, over-the-counter, and herbal medications you are taking before beginning treatment with Ambien CR. Also, talk to your doctor about your complete medical history, especially if you have ever abused or have been dependent on alcohol, or prescription or street drugs. In addition, tell your doctor if you have a history of suicidal thoughts, depression, or mental illness.

What is the usual dosage?

The information below is based on the dosage guidelines your doctor uses. Depending on your condition and medical history, your doctor may prescribe a different regimen. Do not change the dosage or stop taking your medication without your doctor's approval.

Adults: The recommended dose of Ambien CR is 12.5 milligrams (mg) taken immediately before bedtime.

Elderly or liver problems: Your doctor may prescribe a lower dose of Ambien CR. The recommended dose is 6.25 mg.

The safety and efficacy of Ambien CR have not been established in children.

How should I take this medication?

Take Ambien CR immediately before going to bed. Swallow Ambien CR tablets whole. Do not divide, crush, or chew the tablets. Taking Ambien CR with or immediately after a meal may slow the medication's effects. Do not take Ambien CR unless you are able to stay in bed for a full night (7-8 hours) before you must be active again.

What should I avoid while taking this medication?

Do not drink alcohol while taking Ambien CR because it can increase the drug's side effects.

Take Ambien CR exactly as prescribed. Do not take a larger dose of Ambien CR than you need.

When you first start taking Ambien CR, you may be drowsy the next day. Use extreme care while doing anything that requires complete alertness, such as driving, operating machinery, or piloting an aircraft.

Do not take Ambien CR with other medications that can make you sleepy.

What are possible food and drug interactions associated with this medication?

If Ambien CR is taken with certain other drugs, the effects of either could be increased, decreased, or altered. It is especially important to check with your doctor before combining Ambien CR with the following: alcohol, chlorpromazine, imipramine, ketoconazole, rifampin, and other sedative/hypnotic drugs that slow the central nervous system, which may prolong the sedative effects of Ambien CR.

What are the possible side effects of this medication?
Side effects cannot be anticipated. If any develop or change in intensity, tell your doctor as soon as possible. Only your doctor can determine if it is safe for you to continue taking this drug.

Side effects may include: daytime drowsiness, dizziness, headache, sleepiness

Can I receive this medication if I am pregnant or breastfeeding?
The effects of Ambien CR during pregnancy are unknown. Sleep medicines may cause sedation of your unborn baby when used during the last weeks of pregnancy. The use of Ambien CR in nursing mothers is not recommended. Tell your doctor immediately if you are pregnant, planning to become pregnant, or are nursing.

What should I do if I miss a dose this medication?
This drug should be taken only if needed, at bedtime. If you miss a dose, skip it. Do not take an extra dose to make up for missed doses.

How should I store this medication?
Store Ambien CR at room temperature.

AMITRIPTYLINE HYDROCHLORIDE

What is this medication?
Amitriptyline is used to treat depression. It is a member of the group of drugs called tricyclic antidepressants.

What is the most important information I should know about this medication?
Amitriptyline is not approved for use in children less than 12 years old.

Antidepressant medicines may increase suicidal thoughts or actions in some children, teenagers, and young adults when the medicine is first started. Depression and other serious mental illnesses are the most important causes of suicidal thoughts and actions. Some people may have a particularly high risk of having suicidal thoughts or actions. These include people who have (or have a family history of) bipolar disorder (also called manic-depressive illness) or suicidal thoughts or actions.

Pay close attention to any changes, especially sudden ones, in mood, behaviors, thoughts, or feelings. This is very important when an antidepressant medicine is first started or when the dose is changed.

Call the doctor right away to report new or sudden changes in mood, behavior, thoughts, or feelings. Signs to watch for include new or worsening depression, new or worsening anxiety, agitation, insomnia, hostility, panic attacks, restlessness, extreme hyperactivity, and suicidal thinking or behavior.

Keep all follow-up visits as scheduled, and call the doctor between visits as needed, especially if you have concerns about symptoms.

Do not stop taking antidepressant therapy without first consulting with your physician, as this can cause a variety of side effects.

Who should not take this medication?

If you are sensitive to or have ever had an allergic reaction to amitriptyline or similar drugs such as desipramine and imipramine, you should not take this medication. Make sure your doctor is aware of any drug reactions you have experienced.

Do not take amitriptyline while taking other drugs known as monoamine oxidase inhibitors (MAOIs). Drugs in this category include the antidepressants phenelzine and tranylcypromine.

Unless you are directed to do so by your doctor, do not take this medication if you are recovering from a heart attack.

Do not take this medication if you are currently taking Cisapride. Concurrent use of the two medications increases the risk for arrhythmia, and irregular heart rhythm.

Consult with your doctor if you are breastfeeding as to whether amitriptyline should be used.

What should I tell my doctor before I take the first dose of this medication?

Tell your doctor about all prescription, over-the-counter, and herbal medications you are taking before beginning treatment with amitriptyline. Also, talk to your doctor about your complete medical history, especially if you have ever had any of the following: seizures, urinary retention, glaucoma or other chronic eye conditions, a heart or circulatory system disorder, liver problems, bipolar disorder (manic-depression), schizophrenia, or other mental illnesses. Also, let your doctor know if you are receiving thyroid medication or have diabetes, since amitriptyline may raise or lower blood sugar levels.

Before having surgery, dental treatment, or any diagnostic procedure, tell the doctor that you are taking amitriptyline. Certain drugs used during surgery, such as anesthetics and muscle relaxants, and drugs used in certain diagnostic procedures, may react badly with amitriptyline.

What is the usual dosage?

The information below is based on the dosage guidelines your doctor uses. Depending on your condition and medical history, your doctor may prescribe a different regimen. Do not change the dosage or stop taking your medication without your doctor's approval.

Adults: The usual starting dosage is 75 milligrams (mg) per day divided into 2 or more smaller doses. Your doctor may gradually increase this dose to 150 mg per day. The total daily dose is generally never higher than 200 mg.

Alternatively, your doctor may want you to start with 50 to 100 mg at bedtime and may increase this bedtime dose by 25 or 50 mg, up to a total of 150 mg a day.

For long-term use, the usual dose ranges from 40 to 100 mg taken once daily, usually at bedtime.

Children ≥12 years: The usual dose is 10 mg, 3 times a day, with 20 mg taken at bedtime.

How should I take this medication?

Take this drug exactly as prescribed. Amitriptyline may cause dry mouth. Sucking a hard candy, chewing gum, or melting bits of ice in your mouth can provide relief.

What should I avoid while taking this medication?

Do not stop taking amitriptyline abruptly, especially if you have been taking large doses for a long time. Your doctor will probably want to decrease your dosage gradually. This will help prevent a possible relapse and will reduce the possibility of withdrawal symptoms.

Amitriptyline may make your skin more sensitive to sunlight. Try to stay out of the sun, wear protective clothing, and apply a sun block.

Amitriptyline may cause you to become drowsy or less alert; therefore, you should not drive or operate dangerous machinery or participate in any hazardous activity that requires full mental alertness until you know how this drug affects you.

Amitriptyline may intensify the effects of alcohol. Do not drink alcohol while taking this medication.

What are possible food and drug interactions associated with this medication?

If amitriptyline is taken with certain other drugs, the effects of either could be increased, decreased, or altered. It is especially important that you consult with your doctor before taking amitriptyline in combination with the following: airway-opening drugs such as albuterol and pseudoephedrine; antiarrhythmic drugs, such as flecainide and propafenone; antidepressants that raise serotonin levels, such as fluoxetine, paroxetine, and sertraline; other antidepressants; antihistamines such as diphenhydramine and clemastine fumarate; antispasmodic drugs, such as dicyclomine; barbiturates such as phenobarbital; blood pressure medicines such as clonidine; cimetidine; disulfiram; estrogen-containing drugs and oral contraceptives; ethchlorvynol; MAOIs, such as phenelzine and tranylcypromine; painkillers; Parkinson's disease drugs such as benztropine and levodopa; quinidine; seizure medications such as carbamazepine and phenytoin; sleep medicines such as flurazepam and triazolam; thyroid hormones; tranquilizers such as chlorpromazine, thioridazine, alprazolam and chlordiazepoxide; warfarin (a blood thinner).

What are the possible side effects of this medication?
Side effects cannot be anticipated. If any develop or change in intensity, inform your doctor as soon as possible. Only your doctor can determine if it is safe for you to continue taking amitriptyline.

Older adults are especially liable to experience certain side effects of amitriptyline, including rapid heartbeat, constipation, dry mouth, blurred vision, sedation, and confusion, and are in greater danger of sustaining a fall.

Side effects may include: blurred vision, bone marrow depression, bowel problems, breast enlargement (in males and females), constipation, dizziness upon standing, dry mouth, hair loss, heart attack, high body temperature, problems urinating, rash, seizure, stroke, swelling of the testicles, water retention

Side effects due to a rapid decrease in dose or abrupt withdrawal include: headache, nausea, vague feeling of bodily discomfort

Side effects due to gradual dosage reduction may include: dream and sleep disturbances, irritability, restlessness

Can I receive this medication if I am pregnant or breastfeeding?
The effects of amitriptyline during pregnancy have not been adequately studied. If you are pregnant or planning to become pregnant, tell your doctor immediately. This medication appears in breast milk; consult your doctor before breastfeeding.

What should I do if I miss a dose of this medication?
If you miss a dose of this drug, skip it. Do not take an extra dose to make up for missed doses.

How should I store this medication?
Store at room temperature. Protect from light and excessive heat.

AMITRIPTYLINE HYDROCHLORIDE WITH PERPHENAZINE
What is this medication?
Amitriptyline HCl with perphenazine is used to treat patients with nervousness and/or agitation and depressed mood, or patients with depression and any of the above in association with a long-term physical disease.

What is the most important information I should know about this medication?
Amitriptyline HCl with perphenazine is not recommended for use in children.

Antidepressant medications may increase suicidal thoughts or actions in some children, teenagers, and young adults when first started. Depression and other serious mental illnesses are the most important causes of suicidal thoughts and actions. Some people may have a particularly high risk of having suicidal thoughts or actions. These include people who have (or have a family history of) bipolar disorder (also called manic-depressive illness) or suicidal thoughts or actions.

Pay close attention to any changes, especially sudden changes, in mood, behaviors, thoughts, or feelings. This is very important when an antidepressant medicine is first started or when the dose is changed.

Call the doctor right away to report new or sudden changes in mood, behavior, thoughts, or feelings. Signs to watch for include new or worsening depression, new or worsening nervousness, agitation, sleeplessness, hostility, panic attacks, restlessness, extreme hyperactivity, and suicidal thinking or behavior.

Keep all follow-up visits as scheduled, and call the doctor between visits as needed, especially if you have concerns about symptoms.

Do not stop taking antidepressant medications without consulting with your doctor first.

Who should not take this medication?
Do not take amitriptyline HCl with perphenazine if you are sensitive to or have ever had an allergic reaction to amitriptyline or phenothiazines, or if you are taking other drugs known as monoamine oxidase inhibitors (MAOIs). This medication should also be avoided if you have a certain blood disorder known as bone marrow suppression or if you are recovering from a heart attack.

What should I tell my doctor before I take the first dose of this medication?
Tell your doctor about all prescription, over-the-counter, and herbal medications you are taking before beginning treatment with amitriptyline HCl with perphenazine. Also, talk to your doctor about your complete medical history, especially if you have had trouble urinating, or have a history of seizure disorders, heart problems, certain conditions of the eyes, or thyroid problems. If you have any of the above problems, your doctor may change your dose.

What is the usual dosage?
The information below is based on the dosage guidelines your doctor uses. Depending on your condition and medical history, your doctor may prescribe a different regimen. Do not change the dosage or stop taking your medication without your doctor's approval.

Adults: The usual recommended dose of amitriptyline HCl with perphenazine is one tablet of 25 milligrams (mg)/2 mg or 25 mg/4 mg three to four times daily or one tablet of 50 mg/4 mg twice daily.

The total daily dose of amitriptyline HCl with perphenazine tablets should not exceed 200 mg of amitriptyline HCl or 16 mg of perphenazine.

How should I take this medication?
Take this drug exactly as indicated by your doctor.

What should I avoid while taking this medication?
You should never stop taking this medication without consulting your doctor first. Driving or operating dangerous machinery or participating in any hazardous activity that requires full mental alertness should be avoided until you know how this drug affects you. Avoid the consumption of alcohol.

What are possible food and drug interactions associated with this medication?
If amitriptyline HCl with perphenazine is taken with certain other drugs, the effects of either could be increased, decreased, or altered. It is especially important to check with your doctor before combining this medication with any the following: allergy medications, antidepressants, cimetidine, ethchlorvynol, flecainide, pain medications, propafenone, quinidine.

What are the possible side effects of this medication?
Side effects cannot be anticipated. If any develop or change in intensity, inform your doctor as soon as possible. Only your doctor can determine if it is safe for you to continue taking this drug.

Side effects may include: drowsiness, mental impairments, high blood pressure, and dry mouth

Can I receive this medication if I am pregnant or breastfeeding?
The effects of amitriptyline HCl with perphenazine during pregnancy or nursing mothers are unknown; therefore, its use is not recommended. If you are pregnant or planning to become pregnant, tell your doctor immediately.

What should I do if I miss a dose of this medication?
If you miss a dose of this drug, skip it. Never take an extra dose to make up for a missed dose.

How should I store this medication?
Store at room temperature and protect from light.

AMOXAPINE

What is this medication?

Amoxapine is an antidepressant used for the relief of symptoms of depression in patients with neurotic or reactive depressive disorders as well as endogenous and psychotic depression. It is also used to treat depression accompanied by anxiety or agitation.

What is the most important information I should know about this medication?

Amoxapine, along with other antidepressants, may increase the risk of suicidal thinking and behavior in children, adolescents, and young adults. Patients, their families, and their caregivers are encouraged to be alert to the emergence of anxiety, agitation, irritability, hostility, aggressiveness, and suicidal ideation, especially early during antidepressant treatment, and when the dose is adjusted up or down.

Amoxapine may cause drowsiness, and impair your ability to drive or operate machinery.

Amoxapine should not be administered with a class of drugs known as monoamine oxidase inhibitors (MAOIs), as this could cause severe convulsions or death. Allow a minimum of 14 days after stopping an MAOI before starting amoxapine therapy.

You should not use amoxapine of you are recovering from a heart attack.

Patients in whom chronic or long-term use of amoxapine is contemplated are at higher risk of developing tardive dyskinesia, a syndrome consisting of potentially irreversible, involuntary movements.

Who should not take this medication?

Patients currently taking MAOIs, pediatric patients, and patients with known allergies to dubenzoxazepine compounds should not take this medication.

What should I tell my doctor before I take the first dose of this medication?

Tell your doctor about all prescription, over-the-counter, and herbal medications you are taking before beginning treatment with amoxapine. Also, talk to your doctor about your complete medical history, especially if you have been diagnosed with bipolar (manic-depressive) disorder in the past. Also, tell your doctor if you are taking any other neuroleptic drugs.

What is the usual dosage?

The information below is based on the dosage guidelines your doctor uses. Depending on your condition and medical history, your doctor may prescribe a different regimen. Do not change the dosage or stop taking your medication without your doctor's approval.

Adults: The usual starting dose is 50 milligrams (mg) two or three times daily. Depending upon tolerance, dosage may be increased to 100 mg 2 or 3 times daily by the end of the first week. Increases above 300 mg daily should be made only if 300 mg daily has been ineffective during a trial period of at least 2 weeks. When effective dosage is established, the drug may be given in a single dose at bedtime.

Elderly patients should start with 25 mg 2 to 3 times daily and gradually increase the dose until effective dose is established.

How should I take this medication?
Take this medication at bedtime exactly as directed by your physician.

What should I avoid while taking this medication?
Avoid other antidepressants and MAOIs. Avoid alcohol and central nervous system depressants.

Since this drug may cause drowsiness, avoid performing activities that require alertness until you learn how this medication affects you.

What are possible food and drug interactions associated with this medication?
If amoxapine is used with certain other drugs, the effects of either could be increased, decreased, or altered. It is especially important to check with your doctor before combining amoxapine with the following: alcohol, antidepressants, central nervous system depressants, cimetidine, flecainide, MAOIs, propafenone, quinidine.

What are the possible side effects of this medication?
Side effects cannot be anticipated. If any develop or change in intensity, tell your doctor as soon as possible. Only your doctor can determine if it is safe for you to continue taking this drug.

Side effects may include: drowsiness, dry mouth, constipation, blurred vision, insomnia, anxiety, restlessness, headache, fatigue

Can I receive this medication if I am pregnant or breastfeeding?
The effects of amoxapine during pregnancy and breastfeeding are unknown. Tell your doctor immediately if you are pregnant, plan to become pregnant, or are breastfeeding.

What should I do if I miss a dose of this medication?
Skip the dose and continue with your normal dosing regimen. Never double the dose.

How should I store this medication?
Store at room temperature.

ANAFRANIL
Generic name: Clomipramine hydrochloride

What is this medication?
Anafranil is used to treat obsessions and compulsions in patients with obsessive-compulsive disorder (OCD).

What is the most important information I should know about this medication?
Patients with major depressive disorder (MDD) may experience worsening of their depression and/or the emergence of suicidal ideation and behavior or unusual changes in behavior. Suicide is a known risk of depression and certain other psychiatric disorders.

During studies, seizures were the most significant risk of Anafranil use.

Who should not take this medication?
Anafranil should be used with caution in patients with the following: overactive thyroid or who are on thyroid medication; a history of glaucoma or urinary retention; certain brain tumors; impaired kidney function; those on MAOIs currently or within the past 14 days.

Anafranil should not be taken in patients with a history of hypersensitivity to Anafranil or other tricyclic antidepressants.

What should I tell my doctor before I take the first dose of this medication?
Tell your doctor about all prescription, over-the-counter, and herbal medications you are taking before beginning treatment with Anafranil. Also, talk to your doctor about your complete medical history, including: thoughts of suicide, history of seizures, if you are pregnant or plan on becoming pregnant, if you are breastfeeding, a family history of bipolar disorder, depression, or suicide.

What is the usual dosage?
The information below is based on the dosage guidelines your doctor uses. Depending on your condition and medical history, your doctor may prescribe a different regimen. Do not change the dosage or stop taking your medication without your doctor's approval.

Adults: Treatment should be initiated at a dosage of 25 milligrams (mg) daily and is gradually increased, as tolerated, to approximately 100 mg during the first two weeks up to a maximum of 250 mg daily.

Children/Adolescents: The starting dose is 25 mg daily and is gradually increased during the first two weeks, as tolerated, up to a daily maximum of 3 mg/kg or 100 mg, whichever is smaller. The daily maximum after the titration period is 200 mg.

How should I take this medication?
During initial titration, Anafranil should be given in divided doses with meals in order to reduce stomach upset. After the titration period, it is best taken at bedtime to minimize daytime sedation.

What should I avoid while taking this medication?
Never stop an antidepressant medicine without first talking to a health-care provider.

Avoid activities requiring mental alertness or coordination until drug effects are realized, as drug may cause dizziness and somnolence.

Do not drink alcohol while taking this drug.

Do not take MAOIs during or within 14 days before or after Anafranil therapy.

What are possible food and drug interactions associated with this medication?
If Anafranil is taken with certain other drugs, the effects of either could be increased, decreased, or altered. It is especially important to check with your doctor before combining Anafranil with the following: central nervous system medications, cimetidine, clonidine, digoxin, fluoxetine, guanethidine, phenobarbital, phenytoin, quinidine, warfarin.

What are the possible side effects of this medication?
Side effects cannot be anticipated. If any develop or change in intensity, tell your doctor as soon as possible. Only your doctor can determine if it is safe for you to continue taking this drug.

Side effects may include: stomach upset, dry mouth, constipation, nausea, loss of appetite, dizziness, nervousness, sexual dysfunction, fatigue, sweating, vision changes

Can I receive this medication if I am pregnant or breastfeeding?
The effects of Anafranil during pregnancy are unknown. Tell your doctor immediately if you are pregnant or plan to become pregnant. Anafranil has been found to pass through breast milk; because of this potential for fetal harm, consult with your physician before breastfeeding.

What should I do if I miss a dose of this medication?
Take it as soon as you remember. If it is almost time for your next dose, skip the missed dose and return to your regular schedule. Never take 2 doses at the same time.

How should I store this medication?
Store in a cool, dry place and in a light-resistant container.

ANTABUSE

Generic name: Disulfiram

What is this medication?

Antabuse is an alcohol-abuse deterrent used for the treatment of alcohol dependence. It works by blocking the breakdown of alcohol, causing unpleasant side effects such as vomiting and upset stomach when even a small amount of alcohol is consumed.

What is the most important information I should know about this medication?

Avoid all alcohol including that found in sauces, vinegars, mouthwash, liquid medicines, lotions, after shave, or backrub products. A reaction to alcohol may cause flushing, nausea, thirst, abdominal pain, chest pain, dizziness, vomiting, rapid breathing, fast heartbeat, fainting, difficulty breathing, or confusion.

Use caution when using topical products containing alcohol, such as cologne or perfume. Before using alcohol-containing products on the skin, test the product by applying some to a small area of the skin. If no redness, itching, headache, or nausea occurs after 1 or 2 hours, you should be able to use the product.

You may have a reaction if you drink alcohol or use a product that contains alcohol for 2 weeks after your last dose of Antabuse.

Do not take the first dose of Antabuse for at least 12 hours after your last consumption of alcohol.

Antabuse may cause drowsiness. Do not drive, operate machinery, or do anything else that could be dangerous until you know how you react to Antabuse. Using Antabuse alone, with certain other medicines, or with alcohol may lessen your ability to drive or perform other potentially dangerous tasks.

Notify your doctor immediately if you experience yellowing of the skin or eyes, dark urine, weakness, tiredness, loss of appetite, or nausea and vomiting. These may be signs of a liver problem.

Before you have any medical or dental treatments, emergency care, or surgery, tell the doctor or dentist that you are using Antabuse.

Carry an identification card at all times that says you are taking Antabuse.

Because of the possibility of an accidental disulfiram-alcohol reaction, Antabuse should be used with extreme caution in patients with any of the following conditions: diabetes mellitus, hypothyroidism, epilepsy, cerebral damage, chronic and acute nephritis (kidney inflammation), liver cirrhosis or insufficiency.

Who should not take this medication?

Patients who are receiving or have recently received metronidazole, paraldehyde, alcohol, or alcohol-containing preparations such as cough syrups, tonics and the like, should not be given Antabuse.

Antabuse should not be administered to those who have severe heart disease, psychoses, or hypersensitivity to disulfiram or to thiuram derivatives used in pesticides and rubber vulcanization.

What should I tell my doctor before I take the first dose of this medication?

Tell your doctor about all prescription, over-the-counter, and herbal medications you are taking before beginning treatment with Antabuse. Also, talk to your doctor about your complete medical history, especially if you have a history of brain damage, diabetes, heart or lung disease, mental or mood problems such as depression, an underactive thyroid, seizures, liver or kidney problems. In addition, tell your doctor if you are pregnant, planning to become pregnant, or are nursing.

What is the usual dosage?

The information below is based on the dosage guidelines your doctor uses. Depending on your condition and medical history, your doctor may prescribe a different regimen. Do not change the dosage or stop taking your medication without your doctor's approval.

Adults: Antabuse should not be taken for at least 12 hours following your last consumption of alcohol.

When beginning treatment with Antabuse, a maximum of 500 milligrams (mg) daily is taken in a single dose for 1 to 2 weeks. Although usually taken in the morning, Antabuse may be taken at night by those who experience sedative effects. Alternatively, to minimize or eliminate the sedative effects, dosage may be adjusted downward.

The average maintenance dose is 250 mg daily but can range from 125 to 500 mg. The dose may be increased but should not exceed 500 mg daily.

Safety and effectiveness in pediatric patients have not been established.

How should I take this medication?

Antabuse should be taken exactly as prescribed by your doctor. Antabuse should not be used for at least 12 hours following your last consumption of alcohol. Antabuse may be taken with or without food. Antabuse may be swallowed whole, chewed, or crushed and mixed with food.

What should I avoid while taking this medication?

Avoid all alcohol and alcohol-containing products. See **"What is the most important information I should know about this medication?"** above.

Do not drive, operate machinery, or do anything else that could be dangerous until you know how you react to Antabuse.

What are possible food and drug interactions associated with this medication?

If Antabuse is taken with certain other drugs, the effects of either could be increased, decreased, or altered. It is especially important to check with your doctor before combining Antabuse with the following: alcohol-containing medicine such as amprenavir, cough syrup or metronidazole; anticoagulants such as warfarin; benzodiazepines such as diazepam; isoniazid; phenytoin.

What are the possible side effects of this medication?

Side effects cannot be anticipated. If any develop or change in intensity, tell your doctor as soon as possible. Only your doctor can determine if it is safe for you to continue taking this drug.

Side effects may include: drowsiness, headache, metallic or garlic taste in the mouth, blurred vision, changes in color vision, dark urine, loss of appetite, mental or mood problems, or severe allergic reactions (such as rash, hives, swelling in the mouth, face, lips, or tongue)

Can I receive this medication if I am pregnant or breastfeeding?

The effects of Antabuse during pregnancy and breastfeeding are unknown. Tell your doctor immediately if you are pregnant, plan to become pregnant, or are breastfeeding.

This drug should only be used during pregnancy if the benefits clearly outweigh the risks in the judgment of your doctor.

Women receiving Antabuse should not breastfeed due to the possible excretion of the drug into breast milk.

What should I do if I miss a dose of this medication?

If you missed a dose of Antabuse, take the dose as soon as possible unless it is almost time for the next dose. If a dose is skipped, you should not double the next dose.

How should I store this medication?

Store Antabuse at room temperature.

APLENZIN

Generic name: Bupropion hydrobromide

What is this medication?

Aplenzin is used to treat adults with major depressive disorder.

What is the most important information I should know about this medication?

Antidepressant medicines may increase suicidal thoughts or actions in some children, teenagers, and young adults when the medicine is first started. Depression and other serious mental illnesses are the most important causes of suicidal thoughts and actions. Some people may have a particularly high risk of having suicidal thoughts or actions. These include people who have (or have a family history of) bipolar disorder (also called manic-depressive illness) or suicidal thoughts or actions.

Pay close attention to any changes, especially sudden changes, in mood, behaviors, thoughts, or feelings. This is very important when an antidepressant medicine is first started or when the dose is changed.

Call the doctor right away to report new or sudden changes in mood, behavior, thoughts, or feelings. Signs to watch for include new or worsening depression, new or worsening anxiety, agitation, insomnia, hostility, panic attacks, restlessness, extreme hyperactivity, and suicidal thinking or behavior.

Keep all follow-up visits as scheduled, and call the doctor between visits as needed, especially if you have concerns about symptoms.

There is a chance of having a seizure in some people with certain medical conditions and people on some medications.

Who should not take this medication?

Do not take Aplenzin if you have a seizure disorder or epilepsy.

Do not take simultaneously with Zyban (a drug that helps people to overcome smoking) or any medication containing bupropion, such as Wellbutrin.

Do not take if you have taken antidepressants called monoamine oxidase inhibitors (MAOIs) within 14 days.

Do not take if you have an eating disorder called anorexia nervosa or bulimia or if you are allergic to the active ingredient in Aplenzin.

What should I tell my doctor before I take the first dose of this medication?

Tell your doctor about all prescription, over-the-counter, and herbal medications you are taking before beginning treatment with Aplenzin. Also, talk to your doctor about your complete medical history, especially if you have a history of kidney or liver problems, eating disorders, head injury, seizures, tumors of the spine or nervous system, had a heart attack, heart problems, high blood pressure, are a diabetic taking insulin or other medicines to control blood sugar, drink alcohol in excess, or if you abuse prescription medicines or street drugs.

What is the usual dosage?

The information below is based on the dosage guidelines your doctor uses. Depending on your condition and medical history, your doctor may prescribe a different regimen. Do not change the dosage or stop taking your medication without your doctor's approval.

Adults: The usual adult dose is 348 milligrams (mg) a day given once daily in the morning.

How should I take this medication?

Take Aplenzin as prescribed by your doctor. Do not chew or crush the tablet. You must swallow the tablet whole.

Take Aplenzin at the same time each day and at least 24 hours apart.

Aplenzin can be taken with or without food. If you have nausea, take your medicine with food.

If you have trouble sleeping, do not take your medicine too close to bedtime.

What should I avoid while taking this medication?

Avoid alcohol while taking Aplenzin. If you usually drink a lot of alcohol, talk with your doctor before suddenly stopping.

Avoid driving or operating machinery until you know how Aplenzin affects you, as it may impair your ability to perform these tasks.

What are possible food and drug interactions associated with this medication?

If Aplenzin is taken with certain other drugs, the effects of either could be increased, decreased, or altered. It is especially important to check with your doctor before combining Aplenzin with the following: amantadine, antipsychotics, antidepressants, levodopa, MAOIs, phenelzine, systemic steroids, theophylline.

What are the possible side effects of this medication?

Side effects cannot be anticipated. If any develop or change in intensity, tell your doctor as soon as possible. Only your doctor can determine if it is safe for you to continue taking this drug.

Side effects may include: weight loss, skin rash, ringing in the ears, stomach pain, agitation, muscle pain, sore throat, fast heartbeat, frequent urination, sweating, high blood pressure, unusual thoughts and behavior (including delusions, hallucinations, and paranoia), seizures, allergic reactions (signs of severe allergic reactions may include hives, difficulty breathing, and swelling of the throat); if any of these events occur, seek immediate medical attention

Can I receive this medication if I am pregnant or breastfeeding?

Aplenzin should be avoided during pregnancy and breastfeeding. Talk with your doctor before taking this drug if you are pregnant, plan to become pregnant, or are breastfeeding.

What should I do if I miss a dose of this medication?

Wait and take your next tablet at the regular time if you miss a dose. Never take an extra tablet to make up for a missed dose.

How should I store this medication?

Store at room temperature and away from direct light.

ATIVAN
Generic name: Lorazepam

What is this medication?
Ativan is an antianxiety agent, belonging to the drug class of benzodiazepines. Ativan is used for the management of anxiety disorders or for the short-term relief of the symptoms of anxiety or anxiety associated with depressive symptoms.

What is the most important information I should know about this medication?
Patients with acute narrow-angle glaucoma should not take Ativan.

Patients with a primary depressive disorder or psychosis should not take Ativan, since pre-existing depression may emerge or worsen during use of benzodiazepines.

Use of benzodiazepines, including Ativan, whether used alone or in combination with other central nervous system depressants, may lead to potentially fatal respiratory depression.

Prolonged or excessive use of Ativan or other benzodiazepines may lead to physical and psychological dependence.

Patients taking Ativan may have a decreased tolerance for alcohol and other central nervous system depressants. Use caution when operating a vehicle or other machinery.

Who should not take this medication?
Patients with acute narrow-angle glaucoma should not take Ativan, nor should patients with a primary depressive disorder unless they are being treated with antidepressants.

Elderly patients, as well as patients with liver or kidney diseases, should start on a low dose to minimize side effects, and should be monitored closely.

What should I tell my doctor before I take the first dose of this medication?
Tell your doctor about all prescription, over-the-counter, and herbal medications you are taking before beginning treatment with Ativan. Also, talk to your doctor about your complete medical history, especially if you have been diagnosed with depression, acute narrow-angle glaucoma, liver or kidney disease, respiratory disorders, or cardiovascular disorders.

What is the usual dosage?
The information below is based on the dosage guidelines your doctor uses. Depending on your condition and medical history, your doctor may prescribe a different regimen. Do not change the dosage or stop taking your medication without your doctor's approval.

Adults: For anxiety, most patients require an initial dose of 2 to 3 milligrams (mg) daily, divided in 2 to 3 doses.

For insomnia due to anxiety, a single daily dose of 2 to 4 mg may be given at bedtime.

For elderly patients, an initial dose of 1 to 2 mg per day in divided doses is recommended to reduce side effects.

The dose of Ativan may be increased gradually as needed, with the higher portion of the daily dose taken at bedtime.

How should I take this medication?

Take Ativan exactly as directed, with the larger portion of the daily dose taken at bedtime. Do not take more than the prescribed dose, as serious side effects may occur.

What should I avoid while taking this medication?

Avoid operating dangerous machinery, including motor vehicles, as Ativan may cause drowsiness.

Avoid alcohol and other central nervous system depressants, as this can cause serious respiratory disorders.

Do not stop taking this medication without first consulting your doctor.

What are possible food and drug interactions associated with this medication?

If Ativan is used with certain other drugs, the effects of either could be increased, decreased, or altered. It is especially important to check with your doctor before combining Ativan with the following: alcohol, anticonvulsants, antidepressants, antihistamines, clozapine, probenecid.

What are the possible side effects of this medication?

Side effects cannot be anticipated. If any develop or change in intensity, tell your doctor as soon as possible. Only your doctor can determine if it is safe for you to continue taking this drug.

Side effects may include: sedation, dizziness, weakness, unsteadiness, dose-dependant respiratory depression, fatigue, amnesia

Can I receive this medication if I am pregnant or breastfeeding?

Because the use of these drugs is rarely a matter of urgency, the use of Ativan during pregnancy should be avoided. Ativan has been detected in human breast milk, therefore, it should not be administered to breastfeeding women, unless the expected benefit to the woman outweighs the potential risk to the infant.

What should I do if I miss a dose of this medication?

Skip the dose and continue with your normal dosing schedule; never double a dose.

How should I store this medication?
Store at room temperature.

BUSPAR
Generic name: Buspirone hydrochloride

What is this medication?
BuSpar is used to treat anxiety disorders or to relieve symptoms of anxiety.

What is the most important information I should know about this medication?
BuSpar should not be used with antidepressant drugs known as monoamine oxidase inhibitors (MAOIs) such as phenelzine or tranyl-cypromine.

Until you know how this medication affects you, do not drive a car or operate potentially dangerous machinery.

During your treatment with BuSpar, avoid drinking large amounts of grapefruit juice.

Who should not take this medication?
Do not take BuSpar if you are sensitive or allergic to it.

Anxiety or tension related to everyday stress usually does not require treatment with BuSpar. Discuss your symptoms thoroughly with your doctor.

BuSpar is not recommended if you have severe kidney or liver damage.

The safety and effectiveness of BuSpar have not been established in children younger than 18 years of age.

What should I tell my doctor before I take the first dose of this medication?
Tell your doctor about all prescription, over-the-counter, and herbal medications you are taking before beginning treatment with BuSpar. Also, talk to your doctor about your complete medical history, especially if you use alcohol, take MAOIs, or if you have kidney or liver damage. Inform your doctor of any other anti-anxiety medications you may be taking or if you are pregnant, planning to become pregnant, or are breastfeeding.

What is the usual dosage?
The information below is based on the dosage guidelines your doctor uses. Depending on your condition and medical history, your doctor may prescribe a different regimen. Do not change the dosage or stop taking your medication without your doctor's approval.

Adults: The recommended initial dose is 15 milligrams (mg) daily divided into 2 doses. Your doctor may increase the dosage by 5 mg per day every 2-3 days. The maximum daily dose is 60 mg.

How should I take this medication?
Take BuSpar consistently at the same time. Always either take with food or always take without food.

What should I avoid while taking this medication?
Avoid drinking large amounts of grapefruit juice.

Avoid driving or operating machinery until you know how this medication affects you.

What are possible food and drug interactions associated with this medication?
If BuSpar is taken with certain other drugs, the effects of either drug could be increased, decreased, or altered. It is especially important to check with your doctor before combining BuSpar with the following: alcohol, blood thinners such as warfarin, haloperidol, MAOIs such as phenelzine or tranylcypromine, trazodone.

What are the possible side effects of this medication?
Side effects cannot be anticipated. If any develop or change in intensity, tell your doctor as soon as possible. Only your doctor can determine if it is safe for you to continue taking this drug.

Side effects may include: dizziness, excitement, headache, lightheadedness, nausea, nervousness

Can I receive this medication if I am pregnant or breastfeeding?
The effects of BuSpar during pregnancy and breastfeeding are unknown. Talk with your doctor before taking this drug if you are pregnant, plan to become pregnant, or are breastfeeding.

What should I do if I miss a dose of this medication?
Take the missed dose as soon as you remember. If it is almost time for your next dose, skip the one you missed and go back to your regular schedule. Never take 2 doses at the same time.

How should I store this medication?
Store at room temperature in a tightly closed container away from light.

CAMPRAL
Generic name: Acamprosate

What is this medication?
Campral is used for treating alcohol dependence. It is thought to work by restoring the balance of certain chemicals in the brain of patients who have used large amounts of alcohol and is most effective when used in combination with a treatment program that includes social support.

What is the most important information I should know about this medication?

Campral may cause dizziness. Do not drive, operate machinery, or do anything else that could be dangerous until you know how you react to Campral. Using Campral alone, with certain other medicines, or with alcohol may lessen your ability to drive or perform other potentially dangerous tasks.

Do not drink alcohol while you are using Campral. Continue taking Campral even if you begin drinking alcohol again.

Alcohol-dependent patients should be monitored for the development of depression or suicidal thinking. Patients and their families or caregivers should pay close attention to changes in moods or actions, especially if changes occur suddenly. Contact your health care provider right away if any of the following effects occur or worsen: depression, anxiety, restlessness or irritability, panic attacks, thoughts or attempts of suicide, or other unusual changes in behavior or mood.

Campral will not reduce or eliminate alcohol withdrawal symptoms.

Campral has been shown to help you avoid alcohol only in combination with a treatment program that includes counseling and support. Discuss treatment program options with your doctor.

Campral should be used with caution in the elderly because they may be more sensitive to its effects.

Patients with kidney impairment may need a dose reduction or, if the impairment is severe, should not use this medication.

Who should not take this medication?

Campral should not be taken by those who have previously exhibited a hypersensitivity to this drug or any of its ingredients.

Campral should not be used in patients with severe kidney impairment.

What should I tell my doctor before I take the first dose of this medication?

Tell your doctor about all prescription, over-the-counter, and herbal medications you are taking before beginning treatment with Campral. Also, talk to your doctor about your complete medical history, especially if you have a history of kidney problems or impairment, sensitivity reactions to Campral or any of its ingredients, depression, or suicidal thoughts or behaviors. In addition, tell your doctor if you are pregnant, planning to become pregnant, or are nursing.

What is the usual dosage?

The information below is based on the dosage guidelines your doctor uses. Depending on your condition and medical history, your doctor may prescribe a different regimen. Do not change the dosage or stop taking your medication without your doctor's approval.

Adults: The recommended dose of Campral is two 333 milligrams (mg) tablets taken 3 times daily. A lower dose may be effective in some patients.

Treatment with Campral should be initiated as soon as possible following the period of alcohol withdrawal, when the patient has achieved abstinence, and should be maintained if the patient relapses.

Patients with kidney problems: For patients with moderate kidney dysfunction, a starting dose of one 333 mg tablet taken 3 times daily is recommended.

The safety and efficacy of Campral have not been established in the pediatric population.

How should I take this medication?

Campral should be taken exactly as prescribed by your doctor. Campral may be taken with or without food. Campral must be swallowed whole. Do not chew, crush, or break Campral before swallowing.

What should I avoid while taking this medication?

Do not drive, operate machinery, or do anything else that could be dangerous until you know how you react to Campral. Using Campral alone, with certain other medicines, or with alcohol may lessen your ability to drive or perform other potentially dangerous tasks.

Do not drink alcohol while you are using Campral. Continue taking Campral even if you begin drinking alcohol again. Discuss any drinking with your doctor.

What are possible food and drug interactions associated with this medication?

Some medicines may interact with Campral; however, no specific interactions with Campral are known at this time.

What are the possible side effects of this medication?

Side effects cannot be anticipated. If any develop or change in intensity, tell your doctor as soon as possible. Only your doctor can determine if it is safe for you to continue taking this drug.

Side effects may include: drowsiness, dizziness, gas, loss of appetite, nausea, trouble sleeping, weakness, anxiety, behavior changes, depression, mental or mood changes, nervousness, panic attacks, severe allergic reactions (such as rash, hives, difficulty breathing, swelling of the mouth, face, lips, or tongue), suicidal thoughts or behaviors

Can I receive this medication if I am pregnant or breastfeeding?

The effects of Campral during pregnancy and breastfeeding are unknown. Tell your doctor immediately if you are pregnant, plan to become pregnant, or are breastfeeding.

This drug should only be used during pregnancy if the benefits clearly outweigh the risks in the judgment of your doctor.

Women receiving Campral should not breastfeed due to the possible excretion of the drug into breast milk.

What should I do if I miss a dose of this medication?
If you miss a dose of Campral, take it as soon as possible. If it is almost time for your next dose, skip the missed dose and go back to your regular dosing schedule. Do not take 2 doses at once.

How should I store this medication?
Store Campral at room temperature.

CELEXA
Generic name: Citalopram hydrobromide

What is this medication?
Celexa is a medication for the treatment of depression that persists nearly every day for at least 2 weeks and interferes with everyday living.

What is the most important information I should know about this medication?
Celexa is not approved for use in children or adolescents.

Antidepressant medicines may increase suicidal thoughts or actions in some children, teenagers, and young adults when the medicine is first started. Depression and other serious mental illnesses are the most important causes of suicidal thoughts and actions. Some people may have a particularly high risk of having suicidal thoughts or actions. These include people who have (or have a family history of) bipolar disorder (also called manic-depressive illness) or suicidal thoughts or actions.

Pay close attention to any changes, especially sudden changes, in mood, behaviors, thoughts, or feelings. This is very important when an antidepressant medicine is first started or when the dose is changed.

Call the doctor right away to report new or sudden changes in mood, behavior, thoughts, or feelings. Signs to watch for include new or worsening depression, new or worsening anxiety, agitation, insomnia, hostility, panic attacks, restlessness, extreme hyperactivity, and suicidal thinking or behavior.

Keep all follow-up visits as scheduled, and call the doctor between visits as needed, especially if you have concerns about symptoms.

Who should not take this medication?
Do not take Celexa if you are taking pimozide or a monoamine oxidase inhibitor (MAOI) or if you have stopped taking an MAOI in the last 14 days.

Do not take if you are allergic to Celexa or any of its components.

What should I tell my doctor before I take the first dose of this medication?

Tell your doctor about all prescription, over-the-counter, and herbal medications you are taking before beginning treatment with Celexa. Also, talk to your doctor about your complete medical history, especially if you are taking MAOIs or other antidepressants, migraine drugs known as triptans, or tramadol. Tell your doctor if you have heart disease, high blood pressure, kidney or liver disease, or have ever had seizures.

What is the usual dosage?

The information below is based on the dosage guidelines your doctor uses. Depending on your condition and medical history, your doctor may prescribe a different regimen. Do not change the dosage or stop taking your medication without your doctor's approval.

Adults: The recommended starting dose of Celexa tablets or oral solution is 20 milligrams (mg) taken once a day. Dosage is usually increased to 40 mg taken once a day after at least a week has passed. The maximum dose is 40 mg a day.

For older adults and individuals with liver problems, the recommended dose is 20 mg taken once a day.

How should I take this medication?

Celexa should be taken once a day. You can take it either in the morning or in the evening with or without food.

What should I avoid while taking this medication?

Use caution when driving or operating dangerous equipment until you are familiar with Celexa's effects.

Do not abruptly discontinue Celexa. Abrupt discontinuation may result in irritability, agitation, dizziness, emotional ups and downs, headache, or sleepiness.

Do not take Lexapro while you are taking Celexa, since the two drugs are similar and could have increased effects.

What are possible food and drug interactions associated with this medication?

If Celexa is taken with certain other drugs, the effects of either could be increased, decreased, or altered. It is especially important to check with your doctor before combining Celexa with any of the following: antidepressants, carbamazepine, cimetidine, digoxin, ketoconazole, lithium, metoprolol, omeprazole, pimozide, sumatriptan, theophylline, triazolam, warfarin.

Never combine Celexa with any drug classified as an MAOI. Drugs in this category include the antidepressants phenelzine and tranylcypromine. Celexa and MAOIs should not be taken together or within 14 days of each other. Combining these drugs with Celexa can cause serious and even fatal reactions such as high body temperature, muscle rigidity, twitching, and agitation leading to delirium and coma.

What are the possible side effects of this medication?
Side effects cannot be anticipated. If any develop or change in intensity, tell your doctor as soon as possible. Only your doctor can determine if it is safe for you to continue taking this drug.

Side effects may include: abdominal pain, agitation, anxiety, diarrhea, drowsiness, dry mouth, ejaculation disorders, fatigue, impotence, indigestion, insomnia, loss of appetite, nausea, painful menstruation, respiratory tract infection, sinus or nasal inflammation, sweating, tremor, vomiting

Can I receive this medication if I am pregnant or breastfeeding?
The effects of Celexa during pregnancy and breastfeeding are unknown. Tell your doctor immediately if you are pregnant, plan to become pregnant, or are breastfeeding.

What should I do if I miss a dose of this medication?
Take it as soon as you remember. If it is almost time for your next dose, skip the dose you missed and go back to your regular schedule. Do not take 2 doses at the same time.

How should I store this medication?
Store Celexa at room temperature.

CHANTIX
Generic name: Varenicline

What is this medication?
Chantix is a prescription medicine to help adults stop smoking.

What is the most important information I should know about this medication?
Your body may undergo changes if you stop smoking (with or without Chantix). These changes may alter the dosage of other medications you are taking. If you experience agitation, depressed mood, or unusual changes in behavior, or if you develop suicidal behavior, stop taking Chantix and notify your doctor immediately.

Tell your doctor if you have or ever had depression before beginning Chantix therapy.

When you try to quit smoking, with or without Chantix, you may experience symptoms that may be due to nicotine withdrawal. These symptoms include the urge to smoke, depressed mood, trouble sleeping, irritability, frustration, weight gain, and others.

Who should not take this medication?

Chantix is not recommended for people under 18 years of age. Do not take Chantix if you are allergic to any of its ingredients.

What should I tell my doctor before I take the first dose of this medication?

Tell your doctor about all prescription, over-the-counter, and herbal medications you are taking before beginning treatment with Chantix. Also, talk to your doctor about your entire medical history, especially if you are using insulin, asthma medicine, or blood thinners. Also tell your doctor if you have ever had depression or other mental health problems, and if you have kidney problems or receive kidney dialysis, since this may require a lower dose.

What is the usual dosage?

The information below is based on the dosage guidelines your doctor uses. Depending on your condition and medical history, your doctor may prescribe a different regimen. Do not change the dosage or stop taking your medication without your doctor's approval.

Adults: From Day 1 to Day 3, the usual dosage of Chantix is 1 white tablet (0.5 milligrams [mg]). From Day 4 to Day 7, dosage increases to 2 white tablets, one in the morning and one at night. Day 8 to the end of treatment consists of 2 blue tablets (1 mg each), once in the morning and once at night.

How should I take this medication?

First, choose a date when you will stop smoking. Start taking Chantix 7 days before your quit date, as this lets Chantix build up in your body. You can keep smoking during this time. Be sure to stop smoking on your quit date, and continue to take Chantix as directed.

Take Chantix after eating and with a full glass of water.

What should I avoid while taking this medication?

Avoid smoking after the seventh day of taking Chantix.

Use caution when driving or operating machinery until you know how quitting smoking while taking Chantix may affect you.

What are the possible side effects of this medication?

Side effects cannot be anticipated. If any develop or change in intensity, tell your doctor as soon as possible. Only your doctor can determine if it is safe for you to continue taking this drug.

Side effects may include: changes in dreaming or sleeping patterns, constipation, gas, nausea, vomiting

Can I receive this medication if I am pregnant or breastfeeding?
The effects of Chantix during pregnancy and breastfeeding are unknown. Tell your doctor immediately if you are pregnant, plan to become pregnant, or are breastfeeding.

What should I do if I miss a dose of this medication?
If you miss a dose, take it as soon as you remember. If it is close to the time for your next dose, wait and take your next regular dose. Do not take a double dose.

How should I store this medication?
Store at room temperature.

CHLORPROMAZINE

What is this medication?
Chlorpromazine has actions at all levels of the central nervous system (CNS). It is used for the treatment of the following conditions: schizophrenia; to control nausea and vomiting; for relief of restlessness and apprehension before surgery; for acute intermittent porphyria (a rare blood disease); an adjunct in the treatment of tetanus; to control the manifestations of the manic type of bipolar disorder; and for relief of intractable hiccups.

What is the most important information I should know about this medication?
Because chlorpromazine can suppress the cough reflex, aspiration vomiting is possible.

Chlorpromazine prolongs and intensifies the action of CNS depressants such as anesthetics, barbiturates and narcotics.

Use with caution if you or your child will be exposed to extreme heat, insecticides, or pesticides.

Who should not take this medication?
Chlorpromazine should not be taken if you or your child has: heart disease; liver or kidney problems; cirrhosis; or bone marrow depression.

Chlorpromazine should not be taken by anyone taking (or who has taken within the past 14 days) a monoamine oxidase inhibitor (MAOI) for depression, or by anyone sensitive to, allergic to, or had a reaction to other medications like chlorpromazine.

What should I tell my doctor before I take the first dose of this medication?
Tell your doctor about all prescription, over-the-counter, and herbal medications you are taking before beginning treatment with chlorpromazine. Also, talk to your doctor about your or your child's complete medical history, including: heart problems, heart defects or a family history of these

problems; liver disease, including cirrhosis; kidney disease; certain eye problems, such as glaucoma; asthma, emphysema and acute respiratory infections, particularly in children.

Tell your doctor if you or your child are pregnant, planning to become pregnant, or breastfeeding.

What is the usual dosage?

The information below is based on the dosage guidelines your doctor uses. Depending on your condition and medical history, your doctor may prescribe a different regimen. Do not change the dosage or stop taking your medication without your doctor's approval.

Adults: The dose will be adjusted by your doctor according to the severity of the condition; it is important to increase the dosage until symptoms are controlled. Dosage should be increased more gradually in debilitated patients. In continued therapy, gradually reducing the dosage to the lowest effective maintenance level is recommended.

Available dosages are 10 milligrams (mg), 25 mg, 50 mg, 100 mg and 200 mg. The 100 mg and 200 mg tablets are for use in severe neuropsychiatric conditions.

Children (6 months to 12 years of age): Chlorpromazine should generally not be used in pediatric patients under 6 months of age. For patients with severe behavioral problems, dose is based on body weight. Your child's doctor will determine the appropriate dose. In severe behavior disorders, higher dosages (50-100 mg daily and in older children, 200 mg daily or more) may be necessary.

How should I take this medication?

Do not exceed the recommended dosage or take this medication for longer than prescribed. Follow dosage instructions provided by your physician.

What should I avoid while taking this medication?

Chlorpromazine may impair mental and/or physical abilities, especially during the first few days of therapy. Therefore, use caution in partaking in activities that require alertness.

Avoid the use of alcohol with this drug.

What are possible food and drug interactions associated with this medication?

If chlorpromazine is taken with certain other drugs, the effects of either could be increased, decreased, or altered. It is especially important to check with your doctor before combining chlorpromazine with the following: blood pressure medicines, blood thinners, propranolol, seizure medicines, thiazide diuretics such as hydrochlorothiazide.

What are the possible side effects of this medication?
Side effects cannot be anticipated. If any develop or change in intensity, tell your doctor as soon as possible. Only your doctor can determine if it is safe for you to continue taking this drug.

Side effects may include: drowsiness, jaundice, dizziness upon standing, spasm of the neck muscle, motor restlessness, tardive dyskinesia (a movement disorder), adverse behavioral effects, changes in vision

Can I receive this medication if I am pregnant or breastfeeding?
Safety of chlorpromazine during pregnancy has not been established. It is not recommended that the drug be taken by pregnant patients. There is evidence that chlorpromazine is secreted in the breast milk of nursing mothers.

What should I do if I miss a dose of this medication?
Take it as soon as you remember. If it is almost time for your next dose, skip the missed dose and return to your regular schedule. Do not take two doses at the same time.

How should I store this medication?
Store in a cool, dry place in a tightly closed light-resistant container.

CLOZARIL
Generic name: Clozapine

What is this medication?
Clozaril belongs to a class of drugs known as atypical antipsychotics. Clozaril is used for the management of treatment-resistant schizophrenia (patients who fail to adequately respond to standard drug treatment for schizophrenia). This is usually due to insufficient effectiveness or inability to achieve an effective dose because of intolerable side effects of standard drug treatment.

Clozaril is also used for reducing the risk of recurrent suicidal behavior in patients with schizophrenia or schizoaffective disorder who are at chronic risk for re-experiencing suicidal behavior. People with schizoaffective disorder have symptoms of both schizophrenia and mood disorders, such as mental or physical mania (overactivity).

What is the most important information I should know about this medication?
Elderly patients with dementia-related psychosis who are on Clozaril are at an increased risk of death. These patients should not take Clozaril.

Although it is extremely rare, a blood disorder called agranulocytosis has been associated with Clozaril. In this disorder, white blood cells are not made in adequate numbers or are not made at all; this reduces the body's resistance to infection. Even though the risk of agranulocytosis is low, people who take Clozaril must have their blood tested on a regular basis. If you experience lethargy, weakness, fever, sore throat, malaise, or any other sign of possible infection contact your doctor immediately as this may a sign of a more serious problem.

Those patients who have an established diagnosis of diabetes and are started on Clozaril should be regularly monitored for signs and symptoms of elevated sugar levels in the blood (increased thirst, hunger, urination, and weakness).

Clozaril has been associated with causing seizures, with dose being an important predictor of this side effect. Caution should be used in patients who have a pre-existing seizure disorder or other predisposing factors.

When initiating Clozaril therapy you should not drive, operate machinery, or participate in any activity where a sudden loss of consciousness could cause serious risk to you or to others (such as swimming or climbing).

Clozaril has been associated with an increased risk of fatal myocarditis (inflammation of the myocardium or the muscular part of the heart) especially during, but not limited to, the first month of therapy. If you are experiencing fatigue, a fast heartbeat, fever, or chest pain, contact your doctor immediately.

Clozaril may cause a drop in your blood pressure, especially when you first start taking this medication or if the dose is increased. If this happens, try not to stand up too quickly and contact your doctor concerning this problem. Sometimes the decrease in blood pressure may be accompanied with loss of consciousness and in rare cases may lead to respiratory and/or cardiac arrest.

Clozaril should be used with caution in patients with known cardiovascular and/or lung disease; a gradual titration of dose and careful monitoring is recommended.

Clozaril should not be taken with other medicines that may cause blood problems. Also, Clozaril may increase the effects of certain drugs used to lower blood pressure, anticholinergic drugs (sometimes used as ophthalmics or in treating an extremely low heart rate), and medicines used for pain relief. Let your doctor know the medication you are currently using or have used in the past.

Clozaril may cause some slowing down or obstruction of your bowel muscles, which may cause constipation or a more serious side effect. On rare occasion these cases may be fatal.

Clozaril should be taken exactly as prescribed by your doctor. It may take a few weeks for Clozaril to work; do not stop taking the drug if you do not see results right away. It may take as long as 6 to 8 weeks to determine the correct dose of Clozaril. Do not take more or less of the medication without speaking to your doctor. If a dose is missed or forgotten for more than 2 days, do not start taking the drug again without speaking to your doctor.

Who should not take this medication?
Do not use if you have exhibited previous sensitivity to Clozaril or any other component of this drug.

Elderly patients with dementia-related psychosis should not take Clozaril due to an increased risk of death.

Do not use Clozaril if you have bone marrow problems.

Do not use Clozaril if you have uncontrolled seizures (epilepsy) or loss of bowel muscle movements.

Clozaril should not be used if you have a history of blood problems caused by Clozaril.

What should I tell my doctor before I take the first dose of this medication?
Tell your doctor about all prescription, over-the-counter, and herbal medications you are taking before beginning treatment with Clozaril. Also, talk to your doctor about your complete medical history, especially if you have a history of liver problems or liver disease, narrow-angle glaucoma, diabetes, prostate enlargement, dementia-related psychosis, known cardiovascular and/or lung disease, a history of loss of bowel muscle movement, history of seizure disorder, prolonged or painful erections in the past, a history of agranulocytosis (inadequate white blood cell production), a history of blood clots or any blood problems, high cholesterol, or have been allergic to Clozaril in the past. In addition, tell your doctor if you are pregnant, planning to become pregnant, or are nursing.

What is the usual dosage?
The information below is based on the dosage guidelines your doctor uses. Depending on your condition and medical history, your doctor may prescribe a different regimen. Do not change the dosage or stop taking your medication without your doctor's approval.

Treatment-Resistant Schizophrenia and Reducing Recurrent Suicidal Behavior in Schizophrenia or Schizoaffective Disorder
Adults: The recommended beginning dose of Clozaril is one-half of a 25 milligram (mg) tablet (12.5mg) once or twice daily, followed by a continued daily dosage increments of 25 to 50 mg daily. If well tolerated, the targeted dose of 300 to 450 mg daily can be achieved by the end of 2 weeks. Dosage increments after that should not be made more than once or twice weekly with increments not exceeding 100 mg. Cautious dosage increase and divided doses are necessary to minimize side effects.

Many patients respond adequately to doses between 300 to 600 mg daily, but it may be necessary to raise the dose within the range of 600 to 900 mg daily to obtain acceptable response. The daily dose should not exceed 900 mg. It may take as long as 6 to 8 weeks to determine the correct dose of Clozaril.

When going off of Clozaril, a gradual reduction over a 1 to 2 week period is recommended. However, if a medical condition requires abrupt discontinuation, careful observation for recurrence of psychotic symptoms as well as symptoms such as headache, nausea, vomiting, and diarrhea is required.

Safety and effectiveness in pediatric patients have not been established.

How should I take this medication?
Clozaril should be taken exactly as prescribed by your doctor. It may take a few weeks for Clozaril to work, do not stop taking the drug if you do not see results right away. It may take as long as 6 to 8 weeks to determine the correct dose of Clozaril. Do not take more or less of the medication without speaking to your doctor. If a dose is missed or forgotten for more than 2 days, do not start taking the drug again without speaking to your doctor.

What should I avoid while taking this medication?
Avoid standing up too quickly when beginning treatment with Clozaril as the drug may cause a drop in your blood pressure, especially when you first start taking this medication or if the dose is increased. Call your doctor if this problem continues or increases in intensity.

You may experience drowsiness when you start this medication. Avoid driving or operating dangerous machinery until you know how this medication affects you.

Avoid taking Clozaril with other medicines which may cause blood problems as well as severe drowsiness. Avoid the consumption of alcohol, a CNS depressant, while on Clozaril due to potential increase in side effects.

What are possible food and drug interactions associated with this medication?
If Clozaril is taken with certain other drugs, the effects of either could be increased, decreased, or altered. It is especially important to check with your doctor before combining Clozaril with the following: alcohol, antiarrhythmics (propafenone, quinidine), anticholinergics (benztropine), barbiturates (phenobarbital), benzodiazepines (lorazepam), carbamazepine, cimetidine, debrisoquin, dextromethorphan, erythromycin, hydantoins (phenytoin), nicotine, phenothiazines (chlorpromazine), quinolone antibiotics (ciprofloxacin), rifampin, risperidone, SSRIs (fluoxetine), and tricyclic antidepressants (amitriptyline).

What are the possible side effects of this medication?
Side effects cannot be anticipated. If any develop or change in intensity, tell your doctor as soon as possible. Only your doctor can determine if it is safe for you to continue taking this drug.

Side effects may include: drowsiness, sedation, seizures, dizziness, decrease in blood pressure, faster heartbeat, headache, tremor, abdominal discomfort, nausea, profuse salivation during sleep, fever, constipation

A rare but serious condition known as neuroleptic malignant syndrome can occur with Clozaril. If you experience a very high fever, rigidity in your muscles, shaking, confusion, sweating, or increased heart rate and blood pressure, contact your doctor immediately; this may be fatal.

Can I receive this medication if I am pregnant or breastfeeding?
The effects of Clozaril during pregnancy and breastfeeding are unknown. Tell your doctor immediately if you are pregnant, plan to become pregnant, or are breastfeeding.

This drug should only be used during pregnancy if it is clearly needed.

Women receiving Clozaril should not breastfeed due to the possible excretion of the drug into breast milk.

What should I do if I miss a dose of this medication?
If you miss a dose of Clozaril, take the dose as soon as possible unless it is almost time for the next dose. If a dose is skipped, you should not double the next dose. If a dose is missed or forgotten for more than 2 days, do not start taking the drug again without speaking to your doctor.

How should I store this medication?
Storage temperature should not exceed 86°F (30°C).

CONCERTA
Generic name: Methylphenidate hydrochloride

What is this medication?
Concerta is used for the treatment of attention-deficit/hyperactivity disorder (ADHD).

What is the most important information I should know about this medication?
When given for ADHD, Concerta should be an integral part of a total treatment program that includes psychological, educational, and social measures. Symptoms of ADHD include continual problems with moderate to severe distractibility, short attention span, hyperactivity, emotional changeability, and impulsiveness.

There are reports of heart and mental problems in patients taking Concerta or other related stimulants. Some of the problems are sudden death in patients with previous heart problems, heart attacks in adults, increased blood pressure and heart rate, new or worsening symptoms of behavior problems, bipolar disorder, and aggressive or hostile behavior. Call your doctor right away if you or child develops signs of heart problems such as chest pain, shortness of breath, or fainting while taking Concerta.

Excessive doses of Concerta over a long period of time may cause addiction. It is also possible to develop tolerance to the drug so that larger doses are needed to produce the original effect. Be sure to check with your doctor before making any change in dosage; and stop the drug only under your doctor's supervision.

There is no information regarding the safety and effectiveness of long-term treatment in children. However, slowing of growth has been seen with the long-term use of stimulants, so your doctor will monitor your child carefully while he or she is taking Concerta.

The use of Concerta in not recommended in children less than 6 years old.

Who should not take this medication?
This medication should not be taken by individuals with glaucoma or those who suffer from tics (repeated, involuntary twitches) or with a family history of Tourette's syndrome (severe and multiple tics).

Concerta should also be avoided if you or your child are taking or have taken antidepressants called monoamine oxidase inhibitors (MAOIs) within the last 14 days, or are allergic to anything in Concerta.

What should I tell my doctor before I take the first dose of this medication?
Tell your doctor about all prescription, over-the-counter, and herbal medications you are taking before beginning treatment with Concerta. Also, talk to your doctor about your complete medical history, especially if you have heart problems, heart defects, high blood pressure, mental problems including psychosis, mania, bipolar disorder or depression, tics (muscle twitches) or Tourette's syndrome, seizures or have had an abnormal brain wave test, stomach or small or large intestine problems, or if pregnant or planning to become pregnant.

What is the usual dosage?
The information below is based on the dosage guidelines your doctor uses. Depending on your condition and medical history, your doctor may prescribe a different regimen. Do not change the dosage or stop taking your medication without your doctor's approval.

Patients New to Methylphenidate
Adults: The recommended starting dose of Concerta for patients who are not currently taking methylphenidate, or for patients who are on stimulants other than methylphenidate, is 18 milligrams (mg) once daily.
Adolescents 13-17 years of age: The usual starting dose is 18 mg daily up to a maximum daily dose of 72 mg.
Children 6-12 years of age: The usual starting dose is 18 mg daily up to a maximum daily dose of 54 mg.

Patients Currently Using Methylphenidate

Adults: Your doctor will determine your exact dose.

Children: Your doctor will determine the exact dose for your child.

How should I take this medication?

Take Concerta exactly as prescribed. Do not chew, crush, or divide the tablets. Swallow Concerta tablets as a whole with water or other liquids. Concerta is usually taken in the morning and can be taken with or without food.

What should I avoid while taking this medication?

Concerta can cause side effects that may impair your vision or reactions. Be careful if you drive or do anything that requires you to be awake and alert until you know how this medication affects you.

What are possible food and drug interactions associated with this medication?

If Concerta is taken with certain other drugs, the effects of either could be increased, decreased, or altered. It is especially important to check with your doctor before combining Concerta with any of the following: antidepressants (including MAOIs), antiseizure medicines, blood thinners, blood pressure medicines, cold or allergy medicines that contain decongestants.

What are the possible side effects of this medication?

Side effects cannot be anticipated. If any develop or change in intensity, tell your doctor as soon as possible. Only your doctor can determine if it is safe for you to continue taking this drug.

Side effects may include: heart and mental problems, slowing of growth (height and weight) in children, eyesight changes or blurred vision, decreased appetite, stomachache, insomnia, headache, and muscle twitches

Can I receive this medication if I am pregnant or breastfeeding?

The effects of Concerta during pregnancy and breastfeeding are unknown. Tell your doctor immediately if you are pregnant, plan to become pregnant, or are breastfeeding.

What should I do if I miss a dose of this medication?

Take the missed dose as soon as you remember. If it is almost time for your next dose, skip the missed dose and take the medicine at your next regularly scheduled time. Do not take extra medicine to make up the missed dose.

How should I store this medication?

Store Concerta at room temperature. Protect from moisture.

CYMBALTA
Generic name: Duloxetine hydrochloride

What is this medication?
Cymbalta is used to treat major depression and diabetic neuropathy, a painful nerve disorder associated with diabetes that affects the hands, legs, and feet. Cymbalta is also used to treat generalized anxiety disorder and fibromyalgia.

What is the most important information I should know about this medication?
Cymbalta is not approved for use in children or adolescents.

Antidepressant medicines may increase suicidal thoughts or actions in some children, teenagers, and young adults when the medicine is first started. Depression and other serious mental illnesses are the most important causes of suicidal thoughts and actions. Some people may have a particularly high risk of having suicidal thoughts or actions. These include people who have (or have a family history of) bipolar disorder (also called manic-depressive illness) or suicidal thoughts or actions.

Individuals being treated with antidepressants and their caregivers can help reduce the risk of suicidal thoughts and actions by doing the following:

Pay close attention to any changes, especially sudden ones, in mood, behavior, thoughts, or feelings. This is very important when an antidepressant medicine is first started or when the dose is changed.

Call the doctor right away to report new or sudden changes in mood, behavior, thoughts, or feelings. Signs to watch for include new or worsening depression, new or worsening anxiety, agitation, insomnia, hostility, panic attacks, restlessness, extreme hyperactivity, and suicidal thinking or behavior.

Keep all follow-up visits as scheduled, and call the doctor between visits as needed, especially if you have concerns about symptoms.

Who should not take this medication?
Do not use Cymbalta if you are allergic to it; if you are taking a monoamine oxidase inhibitor (MAOI) or the drug thioridazine; if you have uncontrolled increased pressure in your eyes (narrow-angle glaucoma); or if you have serious kidney or liver disease or drink alcohol excessively.

What should I tell my doctor before I take the first dose of this medication?
Tell your doctor about all prescription, over-the-counter, and herbal medications you are taking before beginning treatment with Cymbalta. Also, talk to your doctor about your complete medical history, especially if you have liver problems, severe kidney disease, diabetes, glaucoma, high blood pressure, a seizure disorder, bipolar disorder, or if you consume large amounts of alcohol.

What is the usual dosage?

The information below is based on the dosage guidelines your doctor uses. Depending on your condition and medical history, your doctor may prescribe a different regimen. Do not change the dosage or stop taking your medication without your doctor's approval.

Major Depression

Adults: The total daily dose ranges from 40 milligrams (mg) taken as a 20-mg capsule twice a day to 60 mg taken as a 60-mg capsule once a day or as a 30 mg capsule taken twice a day.

Diabetic Peripheral Neuropathy, Generalized Anxiety Disorder, and Fibromyalgia

Adults: The recommended dose is 60 mg taken once daily.

How should I take this medication?

Cymbalta can be taken with or without food. Do not crush, chew, or open the capsule; swallow whole.

What should I avoid while taking this medication?

Cymbalta may cause drowsiness and can affect judgment or motor skills. Avoid driving or operating heavy machinery until you know how this drug affects you.

What are possible food and drug interactions associated with this medication?

Never take Cymbalta with the drug thioridazine.

Due to the possibility of liver damage, do not take Cymbalta if you use alcohol more than occasionally.

If Cymbalta is taken with certain other drugs, the effects of either could be increased, decreased, or altered. It is especially important to check with your doctor before combining Cymbalta with the following: antibiotics known as quinolones, such as ciprofloxacin; antidepressants known as tricyclics, including amitriptyline, nortriptyline, and imipramine; antidepressants such as fluoxetine, paroxetine, sertraline, and venlafaxine; antipsychotic medications known as phenothiazines, including chlorpromazine, fluphenazine, mesoridazine, perphenazine, and prochlorperazine; flecainide; fluvoxamine; narcotic painkillers; propafenone; quinidine; sleep inducers; and tranquilizers.

Never combine Cymbalta with any drug classified as an MAOI. Drugs in this category include the antidepressants phenelzine and tranylcypromine. Cymbalta and MAOIs should not be taken together or within 14 days of each other. Combining these drugs with Cymbalta can cause serious and even fatal reactions such as high body temperature, muscle rigidity, twitching, and agitation leading to delirium and coma.

What are the possible side effects of this medication?
Side effects cannot be anticipated. If any develop or change in intensity, tell your doctor as soon as possible. Only your doctor can determine if it is safe for you to continue taking this drug.

Side effects may include: appetite changes, constipation, diarrhea, dizziness, dry mouth, fatigue, headache, insomnia, nausea, sexual difficulties, sleepiness, sweating, tremor, urinary difficulties, vomiting, weakness

Can I receive this medication if I am pregnant or breastfeeding?
The effects of Cymbalta during pregnancy and breastfeeding are unknown. Talk with your doctor before taking this drug if you are pregnant or plan to become pregnant. Avoid breastfeeding while taking Cymbalta.

What should I do if I miss a dose of this medication?
Take the missed dose as soon as you remember. However, if it is almost time for your next dose, skip the one you missed and return to your regular schedule. Do not take two doses at once.

How should I store this medication?
Store at room temperature.

DALMANE
Generic name: Flurazepam hydrochloride

What is this medication?
Dalmane is a hypnotic agent used to treat insomnia, which includes difficulty falling asleep, waking up frequently at night, or waking up early in the morning. Dalmane is also used to treat patients who have medical conditions requiring restful sleep.

What is the most important information I should know about this medication?
Do not use this medication if you are pregnant.

The failure of insomnia to remit after 7 to 10 days of treatment may indicate the presence of a primary psychiatric and/or medical illness that should be evaluated.

Due to sedative properties, avoid alcohol consumption while on Dalmane.

Tolerance and dependence may occur with the use of Dalmane.

You may experience withdrawal symptoms if you stop using Dalmane abruptly. Discontinue or change your dose only in consultation with your doctor.

Who should not take this medication?
Do not take Dalmane if you are pregnant, under the age of 15, or if you are allergic to it or any of its ingredients.

Elderly patients should use caution, since Dalmane may lead to oversedation, dizziness, and confusion.

What should I tell my doctor before I take the first dose of this medication?

Tell your doctor about all prescription, over-the-counter, and herbal medications you are taking before beginning treatment with Dalmane. Also, talk to your doctor about your complete medical history, especially if you have chronic breathing problems, liver or kidney problems, or if you are depressed or have suicidal thoughts. Advise your doctor if you are pregnant, nursing, or you are planning to become pregnant.

What is the usual dosage?

The information below is based on the dosage guidelines your doctor uses. Depending on your condition and medical history, your doctor may prescribe a different regimen. Do not change the dosage or stop taking your medication without your doctor's approval.

Adults: The usual adult dosage is 30 milligrams (mg) taken before bedtime. In some patients, 15 mg may be sufficient.

How should I take this medication?

Take Dalmane exactly as prescribed.

What should I avoid while taking this medication?

Avoid driving or participating in hazardous activities after taking Dalmane. Avoid other sedatives such as alcohol or sleep aids while taking Dalmane.

What are possible food and drug interactions associated with this medication?

Alcohol intensifies the effects of Dalmane. Do not drink alcohol while taking Dalmane or until several days after discontinuing it.

If Dalmane is taken with certain other drugs, the effects of either could be increased, decreased, or altered. It is especially important to check with your doctor before combining Dalmane with drugs that slow or depress the central nervous system or that have hypnotic properties. Tell your doctor about all medicines you are taking or plan to take, including prescription and nonprescription medications, nutritional supplements, and herbs.

What are the possible side effects of this medication?

Side effects cannot be anticipated. If any develop or change in intensity, tell your doctor as soon as possible. Only your doctor can determine if it is safe for you to continue taking this drug.

Side effects may include: dizziness, drowsiness, light-headedness, staggering, falling, sedation, lethargy, disorientation, headache, heartburn, upset stomach, nausea, vomiting, diarrhea, constipation, stomach pain, nervousness, talkativeness, apprehension, irritability, weakness, palpitations, chest pains, body and joint pain, genital and urinary pain

Withdrawal symptoms may include: convulsions, tremor, abdominal and muscle cramps, vomiting and sweating

Can I receive this medication if I am pregnant or breastfeeding?
Do not take Dalmane if you are pregnant or planning to become pregnant. Dalmane should be discontinued prior to becoming pregnant. Consult with your doctor if you are breastfeeding or planning to breastfeed.

How should I store this medication?
Store at room temperature.

DAYTRANA
Generic name: Methylphenidate

What is this medication?
Daytrana is a central nervous system stimulant used for the treatment of attention-deficit/hyperactivity disorder (ADHD). The active ingredient in Daytrana is delivered via an adhesive skin patch that releases the medication through clean and intact skin areas into the bloodstream.

What is the most important information I should know about this medication?
Daytrana is a stimulant medicine. The following have been reported with the use of Daytrana or other stimulant medicines: heart-related problems including sudden death in patients who have heart problems or heart defects; stroke and heart attack in adults; increased blood pressure and heart rate.

Remove patch immediately and call your doctor right away if your child has any signs of heart problems.

Other potential problems reported with stimulant medicines include new or worsening behavior and thought problems; new or worsening bipolar disorder; new or worsening aggressive behavior or hostility. For children and teenagers: new psychotic symptoms (such as hearing voices, believing things that are not true, becoming suspicious) or new manic symptoms.

Call your doctor right away if you notice any new or worsening mental symptoms.

Abuse of Daytrana can lead to dependence. Daytrana should be given cautiously to patients with a history of drug dependence or alcoholism.

Who should not take this medication?

Daytrana should not be used by anyone who is very anxious, tense, or agitated; has an eye problem called glaucoma; experiences tics or has Tourette's syndrome, or a family history of Tourette's syndrome; is taking or has taken within the past 14 days an antidepressant called a monoamine oxidase inhibitor, or MAOI.

Daytrana is not for use in patients known to be hypersensitive to methylphenidate or other components of the product.

What should I tell my doctor before I take the first dose of this medication?

Tell your doctor about all prescription, over-the-counter, and herbal medications you or your child are taking before beginning treatment with Daytrana. Also, talk to your doctor about the complete medical history, including: heart problems, heart defects, high blood pressure; mental problems including psychosis, mania, bipolar disorder, or depression; tics or Tourette's syndrome; seizures or abnormal brain wave test (EEG); skin problems such as eczema or psoriasis, or any history of skin reactions to soaps, lotions, makeup, or adhesives (glues).

Talk with your doctor especially if you or your child takes antidepressants including MAOIs, antiseizure medications, blood thinners, blood pressure medications, or cold or allergy medications that contain decongestants.

What is the usual dosage?

The information below is based on the dosage guidelines your doctor uses. Depending on your condition and medical history, your doctor may prescribe a different regimen. Do not change the dosage or stop taking your medication without your doctor's approval.

The Daytrana patch should be fixed to the skin once a day for about 9 hours. Daytrana comes in four different strength patches; your doctor may adjust the dose until it is right for you or your child.

How should I take this medication?

Daytrana patches should be fixed to a clean, dry area on the hip. Alternate hips each day, and make sure the application site is free of redness and irritation before applying. When applying Daytrana, press and hold the patch firmly to the skin with the palm of your hand for 30 seconds.

What should I avoid while taking this medication?

Avoid applying heating pads or subjecting the patch to other external sources of heat. Do not touch the sticky part of the patch.

Avoid applying the patch to cuts or to irritated areas of skin.

What are possible food and drug interactions associated with this medication?

If Daytrana is taken with other drugs, the effects of either could be increased, decreased, or altered. It is especially important to check with your doctor before combining Daytrana with a monoamine oxidase inhibitor (MAOI), a class of medications used to treat depression.

What are the possible side effects of this medication?

Side effects cannot be anticipated. If any develop or change in intensity, tell your doctor as soon as possible. Only your doctor can determine if it is safe for you to continue taking this drug.

Side effects may include: decreased appetite, inflammation of the nasal passages, irritation (redness, itching) at site of application, nasal congestion, nausea, sadness/crying, sleeplessness, twitching, vomiting, weight loss

Other side effects of drugs of this type include: allergic reactions, blurred vision, dizziness, drowsiness, fever, growth suppression, headache, increased blood pressure, nervousness, psychosis (abnormal thinking or hallucinations)

Can I receive this medication if I am pregnant or breastfeeding?

If your child is sexually active, pregnant or breastfeeding, talk to your doctor about the effects of Daytrana. It is possible for methylphenidate to pass into breast milk.

What should I do if I miss a dose of this medication?

If you forget to apply Daytrana at the correct time, apply it as soon as you remember. Remove the patch at the normally scheduled time, even if it has been less than 9 hours, to avoid side effects later in the day.

How should I store this medication?

Store at room temperature. Upon removal of Daytrana, fold used patches so that the adhesive side of the patch adheres to itself. Flush used patches down the toilet or dispose of them in a secure container with a lid.

DEPAKOTE

Generic name: Divalproex sodium

What is this medication?

Depakote is used for the prevention of migraine headaches in adults.

Depakote is also used for the treatment of episodes associated with bipolar disorder (manic or mixed episodes with or without psychotic features). A manic episode is a period of abnormally and persistently elevated, unreserved, or irritable mood. A mixed episode is a manic episode with a major depressive episode (depressed mood, loss of interest or pleasure in nearly all activities).

Depakote is also used to treat complex partial seizures, and simple and complex absence seizures in adults and children 10 years and older with epilepsy.

What is the most important information I should know about this medication?

Women who can become pregnant should know Depakote is associated with birth defects such as spina bifida and other neural canal closure problems. Those taking Depakote during pregnancy may develop clotting abnormalities and should be monitored carefully. Additionally, an increased incidence of epilepsy in children born to mothers who took Depakote in their first 12 weeks of pregnancy has been reported. If you become pregnant while taking this drug, contact your doctor immediately.

Some people who take Depakote experience serious liver problems. Your doctor should check your liver function before you start this medication and continue frequently thereafter. If you experience malaise, weakness, tiredness, facial swelling, loss of appetite, or vomiting, inform your doctor immediately; this may be a sign of more serious liver problems.

Some people may experience pancreatitis, a serious and life-threatening inflammation of the pancreas. If you experience stomach pain, nausea, vomiting, and/or loss appetite, contact your doctor immediately; this may be a sign of pancreatitis.

You may experience drowsiness when you start this medication. You should not drive or operate dangerous machinery until you know how this medication will affect you.

Elevated ammonia levels and hypothermia, an unintentional drop in body temperature, have been reported in some patients receiving Depakote. Contact your doctor immediately if you experience abnormal drowsiness and vomiting or changes in mental status.

You should not take this medication if you are allergic to it, or if you have a condition called urea cycle disorder, which may cause too much ammonia to build up in your body. Let your doctor know if you have been diagnosed with these conditions.

Some people taking Depakote may experience low blood platelet counts. Your doctor should order blood tests to check your platelets while you are taking this medication, as well as prior to surgery.

Who should not take this medication?

Women who are pregnant, planning to become pregnant, or are nursing, should not begin treatment with Depakote.

Depakote should not be given to patients with liver disease or significant liver dysfunction.

You should not take this medication if you are allergic to it, or if you have a condition called urea cycle disorder.

What should I tell my doctor before I take the first dose of this medication?

Tell your doctor about all prescription, over-the-counter, and herbal medications you are taking before beginning treatment with Depakote. Also, talk to your doctor about your complete medical history, especially if you have a condition called urea cycle disorder, a history of liver problems or liver disease, or have been allergic to Depakote in the past. In addition, tell your doctor if you are pregnant, planning to become pregnant, or are nursing.

What is the usual dosage?

The information below is based on the dosage guidelines your doctor uses. Depending on your condition and medical history, your doctor may prescribe a different regimen. Do not change the dosage or stop taking your medication without your doctor's approval.

Complex Partial Seizures

Adults and Children ≥10 years: The usual starting dose of Depakote is 10 milligrams (mg) to 15 mg/kg/day. This dosage should be increased by 5 to 10 mg/kg per week until optimal clinical response is achieved. Usually, the optimal clinical response is achieved at a daily dose below 60 mg/kg per day.

Mania

Adults and Children ≥10 years: The recommended starting dose of Depakote is 750 mg daily given in divided doses. The dose should increase as rapidly as possible to achieve the lowest therapeutic dose that produces the desired clinical effect. The maximum recommended dose is 60mg/kg per day.

Migraines

Adults and Children ≥10 years: The recommended starting dose for Depakote is 250 mg two times a day. Some patients may benefit from doses up to 1000 mg daily.

Simple and Complex Absence Seizures

Adults and Children ≥10 years: The recommended initial dose is 15 mg/kg daily, increasing by 5 to 10 mg/kg per day at one week intervals. The maximum recommended dose is 60 mg/kg daily. If the total daily dose exceeds 250 mg, it should be given in divided doses.

Due to an increased sensitivity to Depakote, elderly patients should be started on a lower dose of the drug. Dosage should be increased more slowly with regular monitoring.

How should I take this medication?

Take Depakote only as directed by your doctor. Depakote tablets should be swallowed whole and should not be crushed or chewed. If you experience stomach irritation, you may benefit from taking Depakote with food or by slowly building up the dose from the initial low level. Try to take Depakote at the same time(s) every day.

What should I avoid while taking this medication?

You should avoid combining Depakote with alcohol, a CNS depressant, which may increase the side effects of the drug.

You may experience drowsiness when you start this medication. Avoid driving or operating dangerous machinery until you know how this medication affects you.

What are possible food and drug interactions associated with this medication?

If Depakote is taken with certain other drugs, the effects of either could be increased, decreased, or altered. It is especially important to check with your doctor before combining Depakote with the following: alcohol, amitryptyline, aspirin, carbamazepine, carbapenem antibiotics, diazepam, ethosuximide, lamotrigine, nortryptyline, phenobarbital, phenytoin, primidone, rifampin, topiramate, warfarin, zidovudine.

What are the possible side effects of this medication?

Side effects cannot be anticipated. If any develop or change in intensity, tell your doctor as soon as possible. Only your doctor can determine if it is safe for you to continue taking this drug.

Side effects may include: nausea, drowsiness, dizziness, vomiting, abdominal pain, diarrhea, increased appetite, weight gain, headache, fever, loss of appetite, constipation, flu, infection, sleepiness, nervousness

Can I receive this medication if I am pregnant or breastfeeding?

The use of Depakote during pregnancy has been associated with birth defects such as spina bifida and other defects where the neural canal does not close normally. Women taking Depakote during pregnancy may develop clotting abnormalities and should be monitored carefully. Also, there is an incidence of epilepsy in children born to mothers who took Depakote in their first 12 weeks of pregnancy. If you become pregnant while on Depakote notify your doctor immediately.

Depakote is also secreted in breast milk with potential for adverse reactions in the nursing infant. A decision between you and your doctor should be made on whether to discontinue nursing or consider an alternative drug treatment.

What should I do if I miss a dose of this medication?

If you miss a dose of Depakote, take the dose as soon as possible unless it is almost time for the next dose. If a dose is skipped, you should not double the next dose.

How should I store this medication?

Store Depakote at room temperature.

DEPAKOTE ER

Generic name: Divalproex sodium

What is this medication?

Depakote is used for the prevention of migraine headaches in adults.

Depakote is also used for the treatment of episodes associated with bipolar disorder (manic or mixed episodes with or without psychotic features). A manic episode is a period of abnormally and persistently elevated, unreserved, or irritable mood. A mixed episode is a manic episode with a major depressive episode (depressed mood, loss of interest or pleasure in nearly all activities).

Depakote is also used to treat complex partial seizures, and simple and complex absence seizures in adults and children 10 years and older with epilepsy.

What is the most important information I should know about this medication?

Women who can become pregnant should know Depakote is associated with birth defects such as spina bifida and other neural canal closure problems. Those taking Depakote during pregnancy may develop clotting abnormalities and should be monitored carefully. Additionally, an increased incidence of epilepsy in children born to mothers who took Depakote in their first 12 weeks of pregnancy has been reported. If you become pregnant while taking this drug, contact your doctor immediately.

Some people who take Depakote experience serious liver problems. Your doctor should check your liver function before you start this medication and continue frequently thereafter. If you experience malaise, weakness, tiredness, facial swelling, loss of appetite, or vomiting inform your doctor immediately for this may be a sign of more serious liver problems.

Some people may experience pancreatitis, a serious and life-threatening inflammation of the pancreas. If you experience stomach pain, nausea, vomiting, and/or appetite loss, contact your doctor immediately; this may be a sign of pancreatitis.

You may experience drowsiness when you start this medication. You should not drive or operate dangerous machinery until you know how this medication will affect you.

Elevated ammonia levels and hypothermia, an unintentional drop in body temperature, have been reported in some patients receiving Depakote ER. Contact your doctor immediately if you experience abnormal drowsiness and vomiting or changes in mental status.

You should not take this medication if you are allergic to it, or if you have a condition called urea cycle disorder, which may cause too much ammonia to build up in your body. Let your doctor know if you have been diagnosed with these conditions.

Some people taking Depakote ER may experience low blood platelet counts. Your doctor should order blood tests to check your platelets while you are taking this medication, as well as prior to surgery.

Who should not take this medication?

Women who are pregnant, planning to become pregnant, or are nursing, should not begin treatment with Depakote ER.

Depakote ER should not be given to patients with liver disease or significant liver dysfunction.

You should not take this medication if you are allergic to it, or if you have a condition called urea cycle disorder.

What should I tell my doctor before I take the first dose of this medication?

Tell your doctor about all prescription, over-the-counter, and herbal medications you are taking before beginning treatment with Depakote ER. Also, talk to your doctor about your complete medical history, especially if you have a condition called urea cycle disorder, a history of liver problems or liver disease, or have been allergic to Depakote ER in the past. In addition, tell your doctor if you are pregnant, planning to become pregnant, or are nursing.

What is the usual dosage?

The information below is based on the dosage guidelines your doctor uses. Depending on your condition and medical history, your doctor may prescribe a different regimen. Do not change the dosage or stop taking your medication without your doctor's approval.

Complex Partial Seizures

Adults and Children ≥10 years: The usual starting dose of Depakote is 10 milligrams (mg) to 15 mg/kg/day. This dosage should be increased by 5 to 10 mg/kg per week until optimal clinical response is achieved. Usually, the optimal clinical response is achieved at a daily dose below 60 mg/kg per day.

Mania

Adults and Children ≥10 years: The recommended starting dose of Depakote ER is 25 mg/kg daily given once daily. The dose should increase as rapidly as possible to achieve the lowest therapeutic dose that produces the desired clinical effect. The maximum recommended dose is 60 mg/kg per day.

Migraines

Adults and Children ≥10 years: The recommended starting dose for Depakote ER is 500 mg once a day for one week. After one week, the dose should be increased to 1000 mg daily. The effective dose range for patients with migraines is 500-1000 mg daily.

Simple and Complex Absence Seizures

Adults and Children ≥10 years: The recommended initial dose is 15 mg/kg daily, increasing by 5 to 10 mg/kg per day at one week intervals. The maximum recommended dose is 60 mg/kg daily.

Due to an increased sensitivity to Depakote, elderly patients should be started on a lower dose of the drug. Dosage should be increased more slowly with regular monitoring.

How should I take this medication?

Depakote ER tablets should be swallowed whole and should not be crushed or chewed. If you experience stomach irritation, try taking Depakote ER with food or by slowly building up the dose from the initial low level. Take Depakote ER only as directed by your doctor. Try to take Depakote ER at the same time every day.

What should I avoid while taking this medication?

You should avoid combining Depakote ER with alcohol, a CNS depressant, which may increase the side effects of the drug.

You may experience drowsiness when you start this medication. Avoid driving or operating dangerous machinery until you know how this medication affects you.

What are possible food and drug interactions associated with this medication?

If Depakote ER is taken with certain other drugs, the effects of either could be increased, decreased, or altered. It is especially important to check with your doctor before combining Depakote ER with the following: alcohol, amitryptyline, aspirin, carbamazepine, carbapenem antibiotics, diazepam, ethosuximide, lamotrigine, nortryptyline, phenobarbital, phenytoin, primidone, rifampin, topiramate, warfarin, zidovudine.

What are the possible side effects of this medication?

Side effects cannot be anticipated. If any develop or change in intensity, tell your doctor as soon as possible. Only your doctor can determine if it is safe for you to continue taking this drug.

Side effects may include: nausea, drowsiness, dizziness, vomiting, abdominal pain, diarrhea, increased appetite, weight gain, headache, fever, loss of appetite, constipation, flu, infection, sleepiness, nervousness

Can I receive this medication if I am pregnant or breastfeeding?

The use of Depakote ER during pregnancy has been associated with birth defects such as spina bifida and other defects where the neural canal does not close normally. Women taking Depakote ER during pregnancy may develop clotting abnormalities and should be monitored carefully. Also, there has been a reported incidence of epilepsy in children born to mothers who took Depakote ER in their first 12 weeks of pregnancy If you become pregnant while on Depakote ER, notify your doctor immediately.

Depakote ER is also secreted in breast milk with potential for adverse reactions in the nursing infant. A decision between yourself and your doctor should be made on whether to discontinue nursing or consider an alternative drug treatment.

What should I do if I miss a dose of this medication?

If you missed a dose of Depakote ER, take the dose as soon as possible unless it is almost time for the next dose. If a dose is skipped, you should not double the next dose.

How should I store this medication?

Store Depakote ER at room temperature.

DESOXYN

Generic name: Methamphetamine hydrochloride

What is this medication?

Desoxyn is used to treat attention-deficit/hyperactivity disorder (ADHD). This drug is given as part of a total treatment program that includes psychological, educational, and social measures.

Desoxyn also may be used for a short time as part of an overall diet plan for weight reduction. Desoxyn is given only when other weight loss drugs and weight loss programs have been unsuccessful.

What is the most important information I should know about this medication?

Inform your doctor of any heart problems, heart defects, high blood pressure, or of a family history of these problems. Your doctor may check for any heart problems before prescribing Desoxyn and should monitor blood pressure and heart rate regularly while the medication is being used.

Call your doctor right away if symptoms such as chest pain, shortness of breath, or fainting occur.

Inform your doctor of any mental health problems or a family history of suicide, bipolar disorder, or depression. Call your doctor right away in the event of any new or worsening mental symptoms or problems while taking Desoxyn, especially psychotic symptoms such as visual or audible hallucinations or paranoia.

Excessive doses of this medication can produce addiction. Individuals who stop taking this medication after taking high doses for a long time may suffer withdrawal symptoms, including extreme fatigue, depression, and sleep disorders. Signs of excessive use of Desoxyn include severe skin inflammation, difficulty sleeping, irritability, hyperactivity, personality changes, and psychiatric problems.

Desoxyn is not appropriate for all children with symptoms of ADHD. Your doctor will do a complete history and evaluation before prescribing this medication. The doctor will take into account the duration and severity of the symptoms as well as your child's age.

This type of medication can affect the growth of children, so your doctor will monitor your child carefully while he or she is taking this drug. The long-term effects of this type of medication in children have not been established.

Desoxyn can lose its effectiveness in decreasing the appetite after a few weeks. If this happens, you should stop taking the medication. Do not take more than the recommended dose in an attempt to increase its effect.

Who should not take this medication?

Do not take Desoxyn if you are also taking a monoamine oxidase inhibitor (MAOI) antidepressant such as phenelzine or tranylcypromine. Allow 14 days between stopping an MAOI and beginning therapy with Desoxyn.

Do not take Desoxyn if there is pre-existing glaucoma, advanced hardening of the arteries, heart disease, moderate to severe high blood pressure, thyroid problems, or allergy to this type of drug.

This medication should not be taken by anyone who suffers from tics (repeated, involuntary twitches) or Tourette's syndrome or who has a family history of these conditions.

People who are in an agitated state or who have a history of drug abuse should not take this medication.

Desoxyn should not be used to treat children whose symptoms may be caused by stress or a psychiatric disorder.

Desoxyn is not recommended for use in children younger than 6 years old in the treatment of ADHD.

What should I tell my doctor before I take the first dose of this medication?

Tell your doctor about all prescription, over-the-counter, and herbal medications you are taking before beginning treatment with this drug. Also, talk to your doctor about your complete medical history, especially if you have mild high blood pressure.

What is the usual dosage?

The information below is based on the dosage guidelines your doctor uses. Depending on your condition and medical history, your doctor

may prescribe a different regimen. **Do not change the dosage or stop taking your medication without your doctor's approval.**

Weight Loss

Adults and Children ≥12 years: The usual starting dose for weight loss is 5 milligrams (mg) taken one-half hour before each meal. Treatment should not continue for longer than a few weeks. The safety and effectiveness of Desoxyn for weight loss have not been established in children under age 12.

ADHD

Children >6 years: The usual starting dose for ADHD is 5 mg taken once or twice a day. Your doctor may increase the dose by 5 mg a week until the desired response to the medication is achieved. The typical effective dose is 20 to 25 mg a day, usually divided into two doses.

Your doctor may periodically discontinue this drug in order to reassess the child's condition and see whether therapy is still needed.

Desoxyn should not be given to children under 6 years of age to treat attention deficit disorder; the safety and effectiveness in this age group have not been established.

How should I take this medication?

Follow your doctor's directions carefully. Your doctor will prescribe the lowest effective dose of Desoxyn; never increase it without approval. Do not take this medication late in the evening as it can cause difficulty sleeping.

What should I avoid while taking this medication?

Desoxyn may affect your ability to perform potentially hazardous activities, such as operating machinery or driving a car. Also be aware that Desoxyn should not be used to combat fatigue or to replace rest.

What are possible food and drug interactions associated with this medication?

If Desoxyn is taken with certain other drugs, the effects of either could be increased, decreased, or changed. It is especially important to check with your doctor before combining Desoxyn with the following: antidepressants classified as tricyclics (such as amitriptyline, imipramine, and nortriptyline) or as MAOIs (such as phenelzine or tranylcypromine); phenothiazines (such as the antipsychotic medications chlorpromazine and prochlorperazine); guanethidine; insulin.

What are the possible side effects of this medication?

Side effects cannot be anticipated. If any develop or change in intensity, inform your doctor as soon as possible. Only your doctor can determine if it is safe to continue taking Desoxyn.

Side effects may include: changes in sex drive, constipation, diarrhea, dizziness, dry mouth, euphoria, headache, hives, impaired growth, impotence, increased blood pressure, overstimulation, rapid or irregular heartbeat, restlessness, sleeplessness, stomach or intestinal problems, tremor, unpleasant taste, worsening of tics and Tourette's syndrome (severe twitching)

Can I receive this medication if I am pregnant or breastfeeding?

Infants born to women taking this type of drug have a risk of prematurity and low birth weight. Drug dependence may occur in newborns when the mother has taken this drug prior to delivery. If you are pregnant or plan to become pregnant, tell your doctor immediately. Desoxyn appears in breast milk. Therefore, do not breastfeed while taking this medication.

What should I do if I miss a dose of this medication?

If you miss a dose of this drug, skip it. Do not take an extra dose to make up for missed doses.

How should I store this medication?

Store at room temperature and away from direct light.

DEXEDRINE/DEXTROSTAT

Generic name: Dextroamphetamine sulfate

What is this medication?

Dexedrine, a stimulant drug available as a sustained-release capsule or as a tablet by the trade name DextroStat, is prescribed to help treat narcolepsy (recurrent "sleep attacks") and attention-deficit/hyperactivity disorder (ADHD).

What is the most important information I should know about this medication?

Because it is a stimulant, this drug has high abuse potential. If you habitually take Dexedrine/DextroStat in doses higher than recommended, or if you take it over a long period of time, you may eventually become dependent on the drug and suffer from withdrawal symptoms when it is unavailable.

Avoid activities requiring mental alertness or coordination until you know how this drug affects you.

Who should not take this medication?

Do not take Dexedrine/DextroStat if you are sensitive to or have ever had an allergic reaction to it.

Do not take Dexedrine/DextroStat for at least 14 days after taking a monoamine oxidase inhibitor (MAOI) such as the antidepressants phenelzine and tranylcypromine. Dexedrine/DextroStat and MAOIs interact to cause a sharp, potentially life-threatening rise in blood pressure.

Your doctor will not prescribe Dexedrine/DextroStat for you if you suffer from any of the following conditions: agitation, cardiovascular disease, glaucoma, hardening of the arteries, high blood pressure, overactive thyroid, or substance abuse.

What should I tell my doctor before I take the first dose of this medication?

Tell your doctor about all prescription, over-the-counter, and herbal medications you are taking before beginning treatment with this drug. Also, talk to your doctor about your complete medical history, especially if you have allergies to food coloring. One of the inactive ingredients in Dexedrine/DextroStat is a yellow food coloring called tartrazine (Yellow No. 5). In a few people, particularly those who are allergic to aspirin, tartrazine can cause a severe allergic reaction.

There is some concern that Dexedrine/DextroStat may stunt a child's growth. Children prescribed Dexedrine/DextroStat should have their growth monitored.

What is the usual dosage?

The information below is based on the dosage guidelines your doctor uses. Depending on your condition and medical history, your doctor may prescribe a different regimen. Do not change the dosage or stop taking your medication without your doctor's approval.

Take no more Dexedrine/DextroStat than your doctor prescribes. Intake should be kept to the lowest level that proves effective.

Narcolepsy

Adults: The usual adult dose is 5 to 60 milligrams (mg) per day, divided into smaller, equal doses.

Children 6 to 12 years: The suggested initial dose is 5 mg per day. Your doctor may increase the daily dose in increments of 5 mg at weekly intervals until it becomes effective. For children 12 years and older, the initial dose is usually 10 mg daily. The doctor may increase the daily dose in increments of 10 mg at weekly intervals until it becomes effective.

This drug is not recommended for children under 3 years of age.

ADHD

Children ≥6 years: In children 6 years and older, the usual starting dose is 5 mg once or twice a day. The doctor may raise the dose by 5 mg at weekly intervals as needed. Only in rare cases will the child take more than 40 mg per day.

Children 3 to 5 years: The usual starting dose is 2.5 mg daily, in tablet form. Your doctor may raise the daily dosage by 2.5 mg at weekly intervals until the drug becomes effective.

How should I take this medication?

Take Dexedrine/DextroStat exactly as prescribed. If it is prescribed in tablet form, you may need up to 3 doses a day. Take the first dose when you wake up; take the next 1 or 2 doses at intervals of 4 to 6 hours. You can take the sustained-release capsules only once a day.

Do not take Dexedrine/DextroStat late in the day, since this could cause insomnia. If you experience insomnia or loss of appetite while taking this drug, notify your doctor; you may need a lower dosage.

It is likely that your doctor will periodically take you off Dexedrine/DextroStat to determine whether you still need it.

Do not chew or crush the sustained-release form, Dexedrine/DextroStat Spansules.

Do not increase the dosage, except on your doctor's advice.

Do not use Dexedrine/DextroStat to improve mental alertness or stay awake. Do not share it with others.

What should I avoid while taking this medication?

Dexedrine/DextroStat may impair judgment or coordination. Do not drive or operate dangerous machinery until you know how you react to the medication.

What are possible food and drug interactions associated with this medication?

If Dexedrine/DextroStat is taken with certain foods or drugs, the effects of either could be increased, decreased, or altered. It is especially important to check with your doctor before combining Dexedrine/DextroStat with the following:

Substances that dampen the effects of Dexedrine/DextroStat: ammonium chloride, chlorpromazine, fruit juices, glutamic acid hydrochloride, guanethidine, haloperidol, lithium carbonate, methenamine, reserpine, sodium acid phosphate, vitamin c (as ascorbic acid)

Substances that boost the effects of Dexedrine/DextroStat: acetazolamide, MAO inhibitors such as phenelzine and tranylcypromine, propoxyphene, sodium bicarbonate (baking soda), thiazide diuretics

Substances that have decreased effect when taken with Dexedrine/DextroStat: antihistamines, blood pressure medications such as clonidine, ethosuximide, prazosin, terazosin, veratrum alkaloids (found in certain blood pressure drugs)

Substances that have increased effect when taken with Dexedrine/DextroStat: antidepressants such as desipramine, meperidine, norepinephrine, phenobarbital, phenytoin

What are the possible side effects of this medication?

Side effects cannot be anticipated. If any develop or change in intensity, inform your doctor as soon as possible. Only your doctor can determine if it is safe for you to continue taking Dexedrine/DextroStat.

Side effects may include: excessive restlessness, overstimulation, aggressive behavior, growth suppression, seizures, visual disturbances

Effects of chronic heavy abuse of Dexedrine/DextroStat may include: Hyperactivity, irritability, personality changes, schizophrenia-like thoughts and behavior, severe insomnia, severe skin disease

Can I receive this medication if I am pregnant or breastfeeding?

If you are pregnant or plan to become pregnant, inform your doctor immediately. Babies born to women taking Dexedrine/DextroStat may be premature or have low birth weight. They may also be depressed, agitated, or apathetic due to withdrawal symptoms. Since Dexedrine/DextroStat appears in breast milk, it should not be taken by a nursing mother.

What should I do if I miss a dose of this medication?

If you take 1 dose a day, take it as soon as you remember, but not within 6 hours of going to bed. If you do not remember until the next day, skip the dose you missed and go back to your regular schedule.

If you take 2 or 3 doses a day, take the dose you missed if it is within an hour or so of the scheduled time. Otherwise, skip the dose and go back to your regular schedule. Never take 2 doses at once.

How should I store this medication?

Store at room temperature, away from light.

EFFEXOR

Generic name: Venlafaxine hydrochloride

What is this medication?

Effexor is prescribed for the treatment of depression that interferes with daily functioning. The symptoms usually include changes in appetite, sleep habits, and mind/body coordination, decreased sex drive, increased fatigue, feelings of guilt or worthlessness, difficulty concentrating, slowed thinking, and suicidal thoughts.

What is the most important information I should know about this medication?

Effexor is not approved for use in children or adolescents.

Antidepressants can increase the risk of suicidal thinking and behavior in children and teenagers. Both adult and pediatric patients taking antidepressants should be watched closely for changes in moods or actions, especially when they first start therapy or when their dose is increased or decreased. Patients and their families should contact the doctor immediately if new symptoms develop or seem to get worse. Signs to watch for include anxiety, hostility, insomnia, restlessness, impulsive or dangerous behavior, and thoughts about suicide or dying.

Who should not take this medication?
Never take Effexor while taking other drugs known as monoamine oxidase inhibitors (MAOIs). Also avoid this drug if it has ever given you an allergic reaction.

What should I tell my doctor before I take the first dose of this medication?
Tell your doctor about all prescription, over-the-counter, and herbal medication you are taking before beginning treatment with Effexor. Also, talk to your doctor about your complete medical history, especially if you have high blood pressure; heart, liver, or kidney disease; a history of seizures or mania; glaucoma; or an overactive thyroid.

What is the usual dosage?
The information below is based on the dosage guidelines your doctor uses. Depending on your condition and medical history, your doctor may prescribe a different regimen. Do not change the dosage or stop taking your medication without your doctor's approval.

Adults: The usual starting dose is 75 milligrams (mg) a day, divided into 2 or 3 smaller doses, and taken with food. If needed, your doctor may gradually increase your daily dose up to a maximum of 375 mg per day, generally divided in three divided doses.

If you have kidney or liver disease or are taking other medications, your doctor will adjust your dosage accordingly.

How should I take this medication?
Effexor must be taken 2 or 3 times daily. Take it with food, exactly as prescribed. It may take several weeks before you begin to feel better. Your doctor should check your progress periodically.

What should I avoid while taking this medication?
Effexor may cause you to feel drowsy or less alert and may affect your judgment. Therefore, avoid driving or operating dangerous machinery or participating in any hazardous activity that requires full mental alertness until you know how this drug affects you.

What are possible food and drug interactions associated with this medication?
Effexor should never be combined with MAOIs such as the antidepressants phenelzine and tranylcypromine as this could cause a fatal reaction.

Avoid alcohol while taking this medication.

If you have high blood pressure or liver disease, or are elderly, check with your doctor before combining Effexor with cimetidine.

You should consult your doctor before combining Effexor with other drugs that affect the central nervous system, including lithium, migraine medications known as triptans, narcotic painkillers, sleep aids, weight-loss products such as phentermine, tranquilizers, antipsychotic medicines, and other antidepressants that affect serotonin, such as fluoxetine and paroxetine.

Effexor has been found to reduce blood levels of the HIV drug indinavir.

What are the possible side effects of this medication?
Side effects cannot be anticipated. If any develop or change in intensity, tell your doctor as soon as possible. Only your doctor can determine if it is safe for you to continue taking this drug.

Side effects may include: abnormal ejaculation/orgasm, anxiety, blurred vision, constipation, dizziness, dry mouth, impotence, insomnia, nausea, nervousness, sleepiness, sweating, tremor, vomiting, weakness, weight loss

Can I receive this medication if I am pregnant or breastfeeding?
The effects of Effexor during pregnancy have not been adequately studied. If you are pregnant or are planning to become pregnant, tell your doctor immediately. Effexor should be used during pregnancy only if clearly needed.

If Effexor is taken shortly before delivery, the baby may suffer withdrawal symptoms. Effexor appears in breast milk and could cause serious side effects in a nursing infant. You'll need to choose between nursing your baby or continuing your treatment with Effexor.

What should I do if I miss a dose of this medication?
It is not necessary to make it up. Skip the missed dose and continue with your next scheduled dose. Do not take 2 doses at once.

How should I store this medication?
Store in a tightly closed container at room temperature. Protect from excessive heat and moisture.

EFFEXOR XR
Generic name: Venlafaxine hydrochloride

What is this medication?
Effexor XR is used to treat depression, generalized anxiety disorder, and social anxiety disorder in adults. It may take several weeks for your symptoms to get better with Effexor XR.

What is the most important information I should know about this medication?

Antidepressants can increase the risk of suicidal thinking and behavior in children and teenagers. Both adult and pediatric patients taking antidepressants should be watched closely for changes in moods or actions, especially when they first start therapy or when their dose is increased or decreased. Patients and their families should contact the doctor immediately if new symptoms develop or seem to get worse. Signs to watch for include anxiety, hostility, insomnia, restlessness, impulsive or dangerous behavior, and thoughts about suicide or dying.

Do not take this medication if you are currently taking a drug known as a monoamine oxidase inhibitor (MAOI). MAOIs can cause a very serious reaction or even death if taken at the same time as Effexor XR. You must stop taking your MAOI at least 14 days before beginning treatment with Effexor XR. Similarly, you should wait 7 days after stopping Effexor XR before starting an MAOI.

Effexor XR is not approved for use in pediatric patients.

Who should not take this medication?

Do not take Effexor XR if you are allergic to it or any of its ingredients, or if you are currently taking an MAOI or have taken an MAOI within the last 14 days.

What should I tell my doctor before I take the first dose of this medication?

Tell your doctor about all your medical problems, including suicidal thoughts, high blood pressure, heart disease, liver or kidney problems, glaucoma, seizures, or thyroid problems. Also alert your doctor if you have ever had symptoms of mania or hypomania, such as persistently elevated or irritable mood, a decreased need for sleep, racing thoughts, hyperactivity, and rapid or excessive talking.

What is the usual dosage?

The information below is based on the dosage guidelines your doctor uses. Depending on your condition and medical history, your doctor may prescribe a different regimen. Do not change the dosage or stop taking your medication without your doctor's approval.

Adults: The usual starting dose is 75 milligrams (mg) once a day. If needed, the doctor may increase your daily dose in steps of 75 mg, up to a maximum of 225 mg a day.

How should I take this medication?

Effexor XR should be taken as a single dose with food at about the same time every day, either in the morning or evening. The capsule should be swallowed whole; it should not be divided, crushed, chewed, or placed in water. The capsule can also be carefully opened and its contents sprinkled onto a spoonful of applesauce. This should be swallowed immediately and followed with a glass of water. Do not chew this mixture before swallowing.

What should I avoid while taking this medication?

Until you know how Effexor XR affects you, be careful doing activities that require alertness, such as driving a car or operating machinery. Also, avoid drinking alcohol while taking this drug.

What are possible food and drug interactions associated with this medication?

Do not take Effexor XR if you have taken an MAOI within the last 14 days.

Also, be sure to tell your doctor about all medicines you plan to take, including prescription and nonprescription medications, nutritional supplements, and herbs. Taking Effexor XR with certain drugs or supplements may increase the risk of serious side effects. It is especially important to check with your doctor before combining this drug with the following: Any drug that affects the central nervous system, antidepressants, cimetidine, diazepam, linezolid, lithium, migraine drugs known as triptans, St. John's wort, tramadol, tryptophan supplements.

What are the possible side effects of this medication?

Side effects cannot be anticipated. If any develop or change in intensity, tell your doctor as soon as possible. Only your doctor can determine if it is safe for you to continue taking this drug.

Side effects may include: abnormal ejaculation, abnormal vision, agitation, confusion, constipation, dizziness, dry mouth, gas, loss of appetite, insomnia, nausea, nervousness, rapid heartbeat, sleepiness, sweating, tremor, yawning

Can I receive this medication if I am pregnant or breastfeeding?

The effects of Effexor XR during pregnancy and breastfeeding are unknown. Talk with your doctor before taking this drug if you are pregnant, plan to become pregnant, or are breastfeeding. Newborns whose mothers took Effexor XR late in the third trimester have had problems.

What should I do if I miss a dose of this medication?

If you miss a dose of Effexor XR, it can be taken later that day. Don't try to make up for the missed dose by taking 2 doses the next day.

How should I store this medication?

Store at room temperature.

EMSAM
Generic name: Selegiline

What is this medication?
Emsam is a skin patch prescribed to treat major depression.

What is the most important information I should know about this medication?
Emsam is not approved for use in children or adolescents.

Antidepressant medicines may increase suicidal thoughts or actions in some children, teenagers, and young adults when the medicine is first started. Depression and other serious mental illnesses are the most important causes of suicidal thoughts and actions. Some people may have a particularly high risk of having suicidal thoughts or actions. These include people who have (or have a family history of) bipolar disorder (also called manic-depressive illness) or suicidal thoughts or actions.

Pay close attention to any changes, especially sudden changes, in mood, behaviors, thoughts, or feelings. This is very important when an antidepressant medicine is first started or when the dose is changed.

Call the doctor right away to report new or sudden changes in mood, behavior, thoughts, or feelings. Signs to watch for include new or worsening depression, new or worsening anxiety, agitation, insomnia, hostility, panic attacks, restlessness, extreme hyperactivity, and suicidal thinking or behavior.

Keep all follow-up visits as scheduled, and call the doctor between visits as needed, especially if you have concerns about symptoms.

Emsam is a monoamine oxidase inhibitor (MAOI). This class of drugs, including Emsam, can cause a sudden, large increase in blood pressure (hypertensive crisis) if you consume foods and drinks that contain high amounts of tyramine.

Who should not take this medication?
You should not use Emsam if you are taking another medication that will interact with it, or if you are allergic to any of the ingredients in it. Talk with your doctor to find the best way to treat depression. Do not take Emsam if you have a condition called pheochromocytoma.

What should I tell my doctor before I take the first dose of this medication?
Tell your doctor about all prescription, over-the-counter, and herbal medications you are taking before beginning treatment with Emsam. Also, talk to your doctor about your complete medical history, including heart problems, manic episodes, seizures, fainting, and if you are pregnant or planning to become pregnant. Tell your doctor if you are breastfeeding. Also, tell your doctor all prescribed, over-the-counter and herbal medicines you are taking.

What is the usual dosage?

The information below is based on the dosage guidelines your doctor uses. Depending on your condition and medical history, your doctor may prescribe a different regimen. Do not change the dosage or stop taking your medication without your doctor's approval.

Adults: Emsam patches are available in three different dosage strengths: 6 milligrams (mg)/24hrs, 9 mg/24 hrs, and 12 mg/24hrs. Your doctor will adjust the dose to best fit your needs.

How should I take this medication?

Apply Emsam patch to dry, smooth skin on your upper chest or back (below the neck and above the waist), upper thigh, or to the outer surface of the upper arm. Choose a new site each time you change your patch. Do not use the same site two days in a row.

What should I avoid while taking this medication?

You must not eat foods or drink beverages that contain high amounts of tyramine while using Emsam 9 mg/24hrs and 12 mg/24hrs patches. (You do not have to make any diet changes with the Emsam 6 mg/24hrs patch.)

Do not take other medicines while using Emsam or for 2 weeks after you remove your last patch unless your doctor has told you to do so.

Do not drive or operate dangerous machinery until you know how Emsam affects you. Emsam may impair your judgment, ability to think, or coordination.

Do not drink alcoholic beverages while using Emsam.

What are possible food and drug interactions associated with this medication?

If Emsam is taken with certain other drugs, the effects of either could be increased, decreased, or altered. It is especially important to check with your doctor before combining Emsam with the following: amphetamines; antiseizure medication; all other antidepressants; carbamazepine and oxcarbazepine; cold medicines; Demerol; diet/weight loss pills; pain medication; St. John's wort. Some of these medications need to be stopped for at least a week before you can start using EMSAM.

While on Emsam, avoid tyramine-rich foods such as dried or aged meats (sausages/salami), fava beans, aged cheeses, beer on tap, yeast, sauerkraut, and soybean products.

What are the possible side effects of this medication?

Side effects cannot be anticipated. If any develop or change in intensity, tell your doctor as soon as possible. Only your doctor can determine if it is safe for you to continue taking this drug.

Side effects may include: increase in blood pressure (hypertensive crisis*); increased depression; mania or hypomania in people who have a history of bipolar disorder; low blood pressure

*Symptoms of a hypertensive crisis include the sudden onset of severe headache, nausea, stiff neck, a fast heartbeat or a change in the way your heart beats, excessive sweating, and confusion. If you suddenly have these symptoms, get medical care right away.

Can I receive this medication if I am pregnant or breastfeeding?
The effects of Emsam during pregnancy and breastfeeding are unknown. Talk with your doctor before taking this drug if you are pregnant, plan to become pregnant, or are breastfeeding.

What should I do if I miss a dose of this medication?
If you forget to change your patch after 24 hours, remove the old patch, put on a new patch in a different area and continue to follow your original schedule.

How should I store this medication?
Store at room temperature, in their pouches.

EQUETRO
Generic name: Carbamazepine

What is this medication?
Equetro is used to treat acute manic and mixed episodes of bipolar I disorder. A manic episode is a time of abnormally elevated, unreserved, or irritable mood. A mixed episode is when a manic episode occurs with a major depressive episode (depressed mood, loss of interest or pleasure in nearly all activities).

What is the most important information I should know about this medication?
Patients with a history of adverse hematologic (blood) reaction to any drug may be particularly at risk of bone marrow depression.

Carbamazepine should not be used in patients with a history of hypersensitivity to the drug, or known sensitivity to any of the tricyclic compounds (such as amitriptyline, desipramine, imipramine, protriptyline, and nortriptyline). In rare cases, serious but fatal dermatological reactions may occur. Call your doctor immediately if you develop a rash after staring Equetro therapy.

Do not take Equetro at the same time as class of antidepressant medications called monoamine oxidase inhibitors (MAOIs). Before administration of carbamazepine, discontinue MAOIs for a minimum of 14 days, or longer if the clinical situation permits.

Do not begin treatment with Equetro if you are already being treated with a drug containing carbamazepine.

If stopped abruptly, Equetro may cause a seizure in epileptic people.

If you experience symptoms such as fever, sore throat, ulcers in the mouth, or easy bruising contact your doctor immediately as this may be a sign of a more serious side effect of Equetro.

Do not take Equetro if you are pregnant, plan to become pregnant, or nursing due to serious side effects associated with the drug.

Do not engage in activities that require mental alertness or coordination, such as operating machinery or driving, after taking Equetro until you know how the medication affects you.

Patients with increased intraocular pressure (glaucoma) should be closely observed during therapy.

Who should not take this medication?

Do not use Equetro if you have had problems with your bone marrow, or if you are allergic to any ingredients.

Carbamazepine should not be used in patients with a history of known sensitivity to any of the tricyclic compounds (such as amitriptyline, desipramine, imipramine, protriptyline, and nortriptyline).

Anyone taking an MAOI should not take Equetro.

Do not take Equetro if you are pregnant, plan to become pregnant, or nursing due to serious side effects associated with the drug.

What should I tell my doctor before I take the first dose of this medication?

Tell your doctor about all prescription, over-the-counter, and herbal medications you are taking before beginning treatment with Equetro. Also, talk to your doctor about your complete medical history, especially if you have a history of liver problems, seizure disorder, problems with your blood, increased ocular pressure (glaucoma), or if you are currently pregnant, plan on becoming pregnant, or are breastfeeding. In addition, you should tell your doctor if you are currently on or have been on an MAOI within the last 14 days, or if you have a known sensitivity to any of the tricyclic compounds (such as amitriptyline, desipramine, imipramine, protriptyline, and nortriptyline).

What is the usual dosage?

The information below is based on the dosage guidelines your doctor uses. Depending on your condition and medical history, your doctor may prescribe a different regimen. Do not change the dosage or stop taking your medication without your doctor's approval.

Adults: The usual dosage of Equetro is 400 milligrams (mg) per day usually given in divided doses of 200 mg two times a day. The dosage may be adjusted by 200 mg increments. The maximum dosage of this drug is 1600 mg/day.

How should I take this medication?

Equetro capsules may be swallowed whole, or opened and sprinkled over food such as applesauce. Capsules may be taken with or without food. Do not crush or chew the capsules.

What should I avoid while taking this medication?

Avoid potentially harmful activities, such as driving and operating machinery, until you see how Equetro affects you, as this drug may cause dizziness and blurred vision.

Equetro contains carbamazepine and should not be used in combination with any other medications containing carbamazepine.

What are possible food and drug interactions associated with this medication?

If Equetro is taken with certain other drugs, the effects of either could be increased, decreased, or altered. It is especially important to check with your doctor before combining Equetro with the following: acetaminophen, alprazolam, amitriptyline, bupropion, buspirone, citalopram, clobazam, clonazepam, clozapine, cyclosporine, delavirdine, desipramine, diazepam, dicumarol, doxycycline, ethosuximide, felbamate, felodipine, glucocorticoids, haloperidol, itraconazole, lamotrigine, levothyroxine, lorazepam, methadone, midazolam, mirtazapine, nortriptyline, olanzapine, oral contraceptives, oxcarbazepine, phenytoin, praziquantel, protease inhibitors, quetiapine, risperidone, theophylline, topiramate, tiagabine, tramadol, triazolam, trazodone, valproate, warfarin, ziprasidone, and zonisamide.

What are the possible side effects of this medication?

Side effects cannot be anticipated. If any develop or change in intensity, tell your doctor as soon as possible. Only your doctor can determine if it is safe for you to continue taking this drug.

Side effects may include: blurred vision, dizziness, dry mouth, itchiness, muscle problems, nausea, speech problems, vomiting

Can I receive this medication if I am pregnant or breastfeeding?

Do not take Equetro if you are pregnant, plan to become pregnant, or breastfeeding. This drug may cause severe problems during pregnancy, such as spina bifida (an opening in the fetus's spinal cord). Also, this drug may pass into breast milk and should not be used if you are breastfeeding.

How should I store this medication?

Store at room temperature and keep away from light and moisture.

ESKALITH

Generic name: Lithium carbonate

What is this medication?

Eskalith is used in the treatment of manic episodes of bipolar disorder. A manic episode is a time of abnormally elevated, unreserved, or irritable mood.

What is the most important information I should know about this medication?

While taking Eskalith, it is very important that you follow your doctor's recommendations and make sure you do not miss any appointments or laboratory tests.

Toxic levels of this medication can occur at any dose and frequent blood tests will be required. You should stop taking Eskalith and contact your doctor immediately if you develop symptoms of lithium toxicity such as diarrhea, vomiting, tremor, mild lack of co-ordination, drowsiness, and muscular weakness.

The safety and efficacy of this medication is unknown in children under 12 years of age, and its use is not recommended.

Who should not take this medication?

Do not take this medication if you are allergic to lithium, Eskalith, Eskalith CR, Lithobid or any of their components.

What should I tell my doctor before I take the first dose of this medication?

Tell your doctor about all prescription, over-the-counter, and herbal medications you are taking before beginning treatment with Eskalith. Also, talk to your doctor about your complete medical history, especially if you have a history of kidney or heart disease, severe weakness, dehydration, low sodium levels, and if you are pregnant or planning to become pregnant or are breastfeeding.

What is the usual dosage?

The information below is based on the dosage guidelines your doctor uses. Depending on your condition and medical history, your doctor may prescribe a different regimen. Do not change the dosage or stop taking your medication without your doctor's approval.

Adults: The dosage of Eskalith varies from patient to patient and your doctor will determine your specific dose based on blood tests and how well you respond.

How should I take this medication?

Eskalith should be taken exactly as prescribed by your doctor.

What should I avoid while taking this medication?

You should never stop taking this medication without consulting your doctor first.

What are possible food and drug interactions associated with this medication?

If Eskalith is taken with certain other drugs, the effects of either could be increased, decreased, or altered. It is especially important to check with your doctor before combining this medication with any the following: acetazolamide, antidepressants, blood pressure medications, carbamazepine, desmopressin, monoamine oxidase inhibitors (MAOIs), methyldopa, nonsteroidal anti-inflammatory drugs (NSAIDs), phenytoin, sodium bicarbonate, urea.

What are the possible side effects of this medication?

Side effects cannot be anticipated. If any develop or change in intensity, inform your doctor as soon as possible. Only your doctor can determine if it is safe for you to continue taking this drug.

Side effects may include: hand tremor, frequent urination, temporary and mild nausea, and general discomfort

Serious side effects may include: diarrhea, vomiting, drowsiness, muscular weakness, and lack of coordination may be early signs of lithium intoxication. Contact your doctor immediately if you experience any serious symptoms.

Can I receive this medication if I am pregnant or breastfeeding?

Eskalith should not be used during pregnancy as there is a risk of fetal death. Eskalith is present in breast milk. While its effects in nursing mothers are unknown, its use should also be avoided. If you are pregnant or plan to become pregnant, tell your doctor immediately.

What should I do if I miss a dose of this medication?

If you miss a dose of this drug, skip it. Never take an extra dose to make up for a missed dose.

How should I store this medication?

Eskalith should be stored at room temperature.

FAZACLO
Generic name: Clozapine

What is this medication?

FazaClo is an atypical antipsychotic used for the management of treatment-resistant schizophrenia.

FazaClo is also used for reducing the risk of recurrent suicidal behavior in patients with schizophrenia or schizoaffective disorder who are at chronic risk for re-experiencing suicidal behavior. People with schizoaffective disorder have symptoms of both schizophrenia and mood disorders, such as mental or physical mania (overactivity).

What is the most important information I should know about this medication?

FazaClo is not approved for use in children.

Elderly patients with dementia-related psychosis who are on FazaClo are at an increased risk of death. These patients should not be taking FazaClo.

A rare but serious and potentially fatal condition known as neuroleptic malignant syndrome can occur with FazaClo. If you experience a very high fever, rigidity in your muscles, shaking, confusion, sweating, or increased heart rate and blood pressure, contact your doctor immediately.

Although it is extremely rare, a blood disorder called agranulocytosis (a reduction or depletion of white blood cells that can reduce the body's resistance to infection) has been associated with FazaClo. People who take FazaClo must have their blood tested on a regular basis. If you experience lethargy, weakness, fever, sore throat, malaise, or any other sign of possible infection, contact your doctor immediately as this may be a sign of a more serious problem.

Phenylketonuric patients should know that FazaClo contains phenylalanine (a component of aspartame). Each 12.5-mg, orally disintegrating tablet contains 0.87 mg phenylalanine. Each 25-mg, orally disintegrating tablet contains 1.74 mg phenylalanine. Each 100-mg, orally disintegrating tablet contains 6.96 mg phenylalanine.) Those patients who have an established diagnosis of diabetes and are started on FazaClo should be regularly monitored for signs and symptoms of elevated sugar levels in the blood (increased thirst, hunger, urination, and weakness).

FazaClo has been associated with causing seizures, with the size of dose being an important predictor of this side effect. Caution should be used in patients who have a pre-existing seizure disorder or other predisposing factors.

When you first start FazaClo therapy, do not drive, operate machinery, or participate in any activity where a sudden loss of consciousness could cause serious risk to you or to others (such as swimming or climbing).

FazaClo has been associated with an increased risk of fatal myocarditis (inflammation of the myocardium or the muscular part of the heart) especially during the first month of therapy (but it could occur at any time). If you are experiencing fatigue, a fast heartbeat, fever, or chest pains, contact your doctor immediately.

FazaClo may cause a drop in your blood pressure, especially when you first start taking this medication or if the dose is increased. If this happens, try not to stand up too quickly and contact your doctor concerning this problem. Sometimes the decrease in blood pressure may be accompanied with loss of consciousness and in rare cases may lead to respiratory and/or cardiac arrest.

FazaClo should be used with caution in patients with known cardiovascular and/or pulmonary disease; a gradual increase of your dose and careful monitoring is recommended.

See "**What are possible food and drug interactions associated with this medication?**" for drugs that you should not take with FazaClo.

FazaClo may cause some slowing down or obstruction of your bowel muscles, which may cause constipation or a more serious side effect. On rare occasions, these cases may be fatal.

Who should not take this medication?

FazaClo should not be used by patients with previous sensitivity to Clozaril or any other component of this drug.

Do not take FazaClo if you have bone marrow problems.

Do not use FazaClo if you have uncontrolled seizures (epilepsy) or loss of bowel muscle movements.

FazaClo should not be used if you have a history of blood problems caused by FazaClo.

What should I tell my doctor before I take the first dose of this medication?

Tell your doctor about all prescription, over-the-counter, and herbal medications you are taking before beginning treatment with FazaClo. Also, talk to your doctor about your complete medical history, especially if you have a history of liver disease, narrow-angle glaucoma, diabetes, prostate enlargement, dementia-related psychosis, known cardiovascular and/or pulmonary disease, a history of loss of bowel muscle movement, history of seizure disorder, prolonged or painful erections, a history of agranulocytosis (inadequate white blood cell production), a history of blood clots or any blood problems, high cholesterol, if you are a phenylketonuric or are allergic to FazaClo. In addition, tell your doctor if you are pregnant, planning to become pregnant, or are breastfeeding.

What is the usual dosage?

The information below is based on the dosage guidelines your doctor uses. Depending on your condition and medical history, your doctor may prescribe a different regimen. Do not change the dosage or stop taking your medication without your doctor's approval.

Adults: The recommended beginning dose of FazaClo is one-half of a 25-milligram (mg) tablet (12.5 mg) once or twice daily, followed by a continued daily dosage increments of 25 to 50 mg daily. If well tolerated, the targeted dose of 300 to 450 mg daily can be achieved by the end of 2 weeks. Dosage increments after that should not be made more than once or twice weekly, with increments not to exceed 100 mg. Cautious dosage increases and divided doses are necessary to minimize side effects. Many patients respond adequately to doses between 300 and 600 mg daily, but it may be necessary to raise the dose within the range of 600 and 900 mg daily to obtain acceptable response. The daily dose should not exceed 900 mg. It may take as long as 6 to 8 weeks to determine the correct dose of FazaClo.

When terminating treatment with FazaClo, a gradual reduction over a 1- to 2-week period is recommended.

How should I take this medication?

FazaClo rapidly disintegrating tablets are dispensed in a blister pack which should be left unopened until the time of use. Do not push the tablet through the blister foil. When you are about to take FazaClo, peel the foil from the blister and gently remove the orally disintegrating tablet. Immediately place the tablet in your mouth. Allow it to disintegrate and then swallow with saliva. No water is needed when taking FazaClo.

FazaClo should be taken exactly as prescribed by your doctor. It may take a few weeks for FazaClo to work; do not stop taking the drug if you do not see results right away. It may take as long as 6 to 8 weeks to determine the correct dose of FazaClo.

Do not take more or less of the medication without speaking to your doctor. If a dose is missed or forgotten for more than 2 days, do not start taking the drug again without speaking to your doctor.

What should I avoid while taking this medication?

Avoid standing up too quickly when beginning treatment with FazaClo as the drug may cause a drop in your blood pressure, especially when you first start taking this medication or if the dose is increased. Call your doctor if this problem continues or increases in intensity.

You may experience drowsiness when you start this medication. Avoid driving or operating machinery until you know how this medication affects you.

Avoid alcohol while on FazaClo due to a potential increase in side effects.

What are possible food and drug interactions associated with this medication?

If FazaClo is taken with certain other drugs, the effects of either could be increased, decreased, or altered. It is especially important to check with your doctor before combining FazaClo with the following: alcohol, antiarrhythmics, anticholinergics, barbiturates such as phenobarbital, benzodiazepines, carbamazepine, cimetidine, debrisoquin, dextromethorphan, erythromycin, hydantoins, nicotine, phenothiazines, quinolone antibiotics such as ciprofloxacin, rifampin, risperidone, SSRIs and tricyclic antidepressants.

What are the possible side effects of this medication?

Side effects cannot be anticipated. If any develop or change in intensity, tell your doctor as soon as possible. Only your doctor can determine if it is safe for you to continue taking this drug.

Side effects may include: drowsiness, sedation, seizures, dizziness, decrease in blood pressure, faster heartbeat, headache, tremor, constipation, abdominal discomfort, nausea, profuse salivation during sleep, fever, constipation

Can I receive this medication if I am pregnant or breastfeeding?

The effects of FazaClo during pregnancy and breastfeeding are unknown. Tell your doctor immediately if you are pregnant, plan to become pregnant, or are breastfeeding.

This drug should only be used during pregnancy or nursing if it is clearly needed.

What should I do if I miss a dose of this medication?

If you missed a dose of FazaClo, take the dose as soon as possible unless it is almost time for the next dose. If a dose is skipped, you should not double the next dose. If a dose is missed or forgotten for more than two days, do not start taking the drug again without speaking to your doctor.

Where should I keep my supply of this medication?

Store at room temperature (not to exceed 86°F).

FLUPHENAZINE HYDROCHLORIDE

What is this medication?

Fluphenazine is used in the management of psychotic disorders.

What is the most important information I should know about this medication?

Fluphenazine may cause tardive dyskinesia, a potentially irreversible condition that causes involuntary muscle spasms and twitches in the face and body. Elderly women seem to be at a higher risk of developing the condition. Tell your doctor immediately if you begin to have any involuntary movement of the mouth, tongue, cheeks, jaw, arms, or legs.

Neuroleptic malignant syndrome (NMS) is a potentially fatal syndrome that can be caused by fluphenazine. Symptoms may include fever, stiff muscles, confusion, abnormal thinking, fast or irregular heartbeat, and sweating. Contact your doctor at once if you have any of these symptoms.

Use caution when driving, operating machinery, or performing other hazardous activities until you know how you respond to fluphenazine; this drug may cause dizziness or drowsiness.

When taking fluphenazine, dizziness may be more likely to occur when you rise from a sitting or lying position. Rise slowly to prevent dizziness and a possible fall.

Do not stop taking fluphenazine without first talking to your doctor. It may be several weeks before you begin to feel better, and you may require continuous treatment for quite some time. Talk to your doctor before you stop taking this medication.

Who should not take this medication?

Fluphenazine should not be used in patients with suspected or established subcortical brain damage, those receiving large doses of hypnotics, and those in comatose or severely depressed states. Fluphenazine should not be used in patients who have shown hypersensitivity to fluphenazine.

What should I tell my doctor before I take the first dose of this medication?

Tell your doctor about all prescription, over-the-counter, and herbal medications you are taking before beginning treatment with fluphenazine. Also, talk to your doctor about your complete medical history, especially if you have bone marrow disease, glaucoma, seizures, Parkinson's disease, an enlarged prostate or difficulty urinating, and liver or kidney disease. In addition, tell your doctor if you are pregnant, plan to become pregnant, or are breastfeeding.

What is the usual dosage?

The information below is based on the dosage guidelines your doctor uses. Depending on your condition and medical history, your doctor may prescribe a different regimen. Do not change the dosage or stop taking your medication without your doctor's approval.

The smallest amount that will produce the desired results must be carefully determined for each individual, since optimal dosage levels of this potent drug vary from patient to patient.

Adults: Elixir: The recommended total daily dosage may range initially from 2.5 milligrams (mg) to 10 mg and should be divided and given at 6- to 8-hour intervals.

Tablets: The desired effect is often achieved with doses under 20 mg daily. Patients remaining severely disturbed or inadequately controlled may require a slow increase in dose. Daily doses up to 40 mg may be necessary.

Injection: Patients who have been stabilized on a fixed daily dose of orally administered fluphenazine may be converted to the long-acting injectable form. Fluphenazine Injection is useful when patients are unable or unwilling to take oral therapy.

Elderly: The suggested starting dose is 1 to 2.5 mg daily, adjusted according to the patient's response.

How should I take this medication?

Take fluphenazine exactly as directed by your doctor.

Inspect fluphenazine Elixir prior to use. Some separation may occur. Gently shake the container to redisperse the contents. Do not use the solution if it is not clear.

Take each dose with a full glass (8 ounces) of water. Mix the concentrate with 4 ounces of water, orange juice, or grapefruit juice. Throw away any discolored liquid.

Fluphenazine can be taken with or without food.

Do not stop taking fluphenazine without first talking to your doctor. It may be several weeks before you begin to feel better, and you may require continuous treatment for quite some time.

What should I avoid while taking this medication?

Do not drive or perform other possibly unsafe tasks until you know how you react to fluphenazine; this drug may cause dizziness, drowsiness, or blurred vision.

Avoid sitting or standing up too quickly when you take fluphenazine. Rise slowly to prevent dizziness and a possible fall.

Use alcohol cautiously as it may increase drowsiness and dizziness while taking fluphenazine.

Avoid prolonged exposure to sunlight. Fluphenazine may increase the sensitivity of the skin to sunlight. Use sunscreen and wear protective clothing when sun exposure is unavoidable.

Do not stop taking fluphenazine without first talking to your doctor. It may be several weeks before you begin to feel better, and you may require continuous treatment for quite some time.

Take antacids at least 2 hours before or 2 hours after a dose of fluphenazine.

What are possible food and drug interactions associated with this medication?

If fluphenazine is taken with certain other drugs, the effects of either could be increased, decreased, or altered. It is especially important to check with your doctor before combining fluphenazine with the following: antacids, anticoagulants such as warfarin, clonidine, methyldopa, phenytoin, propranolol.

What are the possible side effects of this medication?

Side effects cannot be anticipated. If any develop or change in intensity, tell your doctor as soon as possible. Only your doctor can determine if it is safe for you to continue taking this drug.

Side effects may include: decreased sweating, dry mouth or stuffy nose, constipation, blurred vision, mild restlessness, drowsiness, tremor, difficulty urinating, dark urine, decreased sex drive, dizziness, increased appetite, menstrual irregularities, swollen breasts, muscle spasms, fainting, and severe allergic reactions (rash, difficulty breathing, hives, selling of the lips, tongue, or face)

Neuroleptic malignant syndrome (NMS) is a potentially fatal syndrome that can be caused by Prolixin (see "**What is the most important information I should know about this medication?**").

Can I receive this medication if I am pregnant or breastfeeding?

The safety of fluphenazine during pregnancy has not been established. If you become pregnant, contact your doctor. You will need to discuss the benefits and risks of using fluphenazine while you are pregnant.

What should I do if I miss a dose of this medication?

If you take one dose of Prolixin a day, take the missed dose as soon as you remember, then go back to your regular schedule the next day. If you do not remember until the next day, skip the dose you missed and take only your next regularly scheduled dose. Do not take a double dose of this medication.

If you are taking fluphenazine on a regular schedule several times a day, take the missed dose as soon as you remember. If it is almost time for the next dose, skip the missed dose and take only the next regularly scheduled dose. Do not take a double dose of this medication.

How should I store this medication?

Store at room temperature in a tightly closed container. Protect from light and heat. Keep the elixir in a light-resistant container and protect from freezing.

FLUVOXAMINE MALEATE

What is this medication?

Fluvoxamine is used to treat obsessive-compulsive disorder. It is also available as the brand name Luvox.

What is the most important information I should know about this medication?

Antidepressants can increase the risk of suicidal thinking and behavior in children and teenagers. Adult and pediatric patients taking antidepressants should be watched closely for changes in moods or actions, especially when they first start therapy or when their dose is increased or decreased. Patients and their families should contact the doctor immediately if new symptoms develop or seem to get worse. Signs to watch for include anxiety, hostility, insomnia, restlessness, impulsive or dangerous behavior, and thoughts about suicide or dying.

Never take fluvoxamine if you are taking another class of antidepressant drugs called monoamine oxidase inhibitors (MAOIs) or if you have stopped taking an MAOI in the last 14 days. MAOI drugs include phenelzine, tranylcypromine, and isocarboxazid. Taking fluvoxamine in close proximity or concurrently with an MAOI can result in serious—sometimes fatal—reactions, including high body temperature, coma, and seizures.

A life-threatening condition called serotonin syndrome (serious changes in how your brain, muscles, and digestive system work) can occur when you take fluvoxamine with medicines known as triptans, which are used to treat migraine headaches. Signs and symptoms of serotonin syndrome include restlessness, diarrhea, hallucinations, coma, loss of coordination, nausea, fast heartbeat, vomiting, increased body temperature, rapid changes in blood pressure, and overactive reflexes. Serotonin syndrome may be more likely to occur when starting or increasing the dose of fluvoxamine or a triptan.

Who should not take this medication?

Do not take fluvoxamine if you are sensitive to the drug. Never take fluvoxamine if you are taking alosetron, astemizole, cisapride, MAOIs, terfenadine, thioridazine, or tizanidine.

What should I tell my doctor before I take the first dose of this medication?

Tell your doctor about all prescription, over-the-counter, and herbal medications you are taking before beginning treatment with fluvoxamine. Also, talk to your doctor about your complete medical history, especially if you have liver disease, a history of seizure disorders, suffer from mania, or experience worsening symptoms of depression and/or suicidal thoughts.

What is the usual dosage?

The information below is based on the dosage guidelines your doctor uses. Depending on your condition and medical history, your doctor may prescribe a different regimen. Do not change the dosage or stop taking your medication without your doctor's approval.

Adults: The usual starting dose is 50 milligrams (mg) taken daily at bedtime. The dose may be increased depending upon your response. The maximum daily dose is 300 mg. If you take more than 100 mg a day, your doctor will divide the total amount into 2 doses. If the doses are not equal, you should take the larger dose at bedtime.

Elderly patients, or patients with impaired liver function, might require a lower starting dose.

Children 8-17 years of age: The recommended starting dose is 25 mg taken at bedtime. The dose may be increased to a maximum of 200 mg daily for children under 11, and 300 mg for children aged 11-17. Larger daily dosages are divided in two, as for adults.

How should I take this medication?

Take fluvoxamine with or without food, exactly as prescribed by your doctor.

What should I avoid while taking this medication?

Do not stop taking fluvoxamine without first talking to your doctor. An abrupt decrease in dose could cause withdrawal symptoms such as mood problems, tiredness, insomnia, and tingling sensations.

Use caution when driving, operating machinery, or performing hazardous activities. Fluvoxamine can cause dizziness or drowsiness.

Use alcohol cautiously. Alcohol may increase drowsiness and dizziness while taking fluvoxamine or affect your condition.

What are possible food and drug interactions associated with this medication?

If fluvoxamine is taken with certain other drugs, the effects of either could be increased, decreased, or altered. It is especially important to check with your doctor before combining fluvoxamine with the following: antidepressants such as amitriptyline, clomipramine, or imipramine, blood pressure medications known as beta-blockers, including metoprolol and propranolol; blood thinners such as aspirin and aspirin-related products, or warfarin; carbamazepine; clozapine; diltiazem; lithium; methadone; mexiletine; migraine headache drugs such as almotriptan and sumatriptan; nonsteroidal anti-inflammatory drugs such as ibuprofen or naproxen; phenytoin; pimozide; quinidine; tacrine; theophylline; thioridazine; tranquilizers and sedatives such as alprazolam, diazepam, midazolam, and triazolam; tryptophan.

What are the possible side effects of this medication?
Side effects cannot be anticipated. If any develop or change in intensity, tell your doctor as soon as possible. Only your doctor can determine if it is safe for you to continue taking this drug.

Side effects may include: abnormal ejaculation, agitation, anxiety, diarrhea, difficulty falling or staying asleep, dizziness, dry mouth, headache, indigestion, nausea, nervousness, sleepiness, sweating, tremor, vomiting, weakness, weight loss

Can I receive this medication if I am pregnant or breastfeeding?
The effects of fluvoxamine during pregnancy and breastfeeding are unknown. Tell your doctor immediately if you are pregnant, plan to become pregnant, or are breastfeeding. Do not breastfeed while taking fluvoxamine.

What should I do if I miss a dose of this medication?
If you are taking 1 dose a day, skip the missed dose and go back to your regular schedule. If you are taking 2 doses a day, take the missed dose as soon as possible, then go back to your regular schedule. Never take 2 doses at the same time.

How should I store this medication?
Store at room temperature and protect from moisture.

FOCALIN
Generic name: Dexmethylphenidate hydrochloride

What is this medication?
Focalin is a central nervous stimulant used to treat attention-deficit/hyperactivity disorder (ADHD) in children.

What is the most important information I should know about this medication?
Excessive doses of Focalin over a long period of time can produce addiction. It is also possible to develop tolerance to the drug, so that larger doses are needed to produce the original effect. Because of these dangers,

be sure to check with your doctor before making any change in dosage. Do not stop the drug without your doctor's supervision.

Who should not take this medication?

Do not take Focalin if you are sensitive to the drug, or have marked anxiety, tension, and agitation. Focalin can make your symptoms worse.

Do not take Focalin if you have motor tics (repeated, uncontrollable twitches) or a family history or diagnosis of Tourette's syndrome (severe and multiple tics).

Do not take Focalin if you are taking monoamine oxidase inhibitors (MAOIs) such as phenelzine or tranylcypromine or within 14 days after stopping this type of medication.

Do not take this drug if you have glaucoma (elevated pressure in the eye).

Focalin should not be used in children less than 6 years of age because it has not been studied in this age group.

What should I tell my doctor before I take the first dose of this medication?

Tell your doctor about all prescription, over-the-counter, and herbal medications you are taking before beginning treatment with Focalin. Also, talk to your doctor about your complete medic al history, especially if you have any mental or physical problems. Also, inform your doctor of any drug or alcohol abuse, depression, psychosis, epilepsy/seizures, high blood pressure, heart conditions, glaucoma, or if you or any of your family has a history of tics/Tourette's syndrome.

Also tell your doctor if you or your child is pregnant, planning to become pregnant, or is breastfeeding.

What is the usual dosage?

The information below is based on the dosage guidelines your doctor uses. Depending on your condition and medical history, your doctor may prescribe a different regimen. Do not change the dosage or stop taking your medication without your doctor's approval.

Focalin has not been studied in children under 6 years of age.

Children ≥6 years: If you have never taken Focalin before, the usual starting dose is 5 milligrams (mg) a day. For those who are switching from Ritalin, the starting Focalin dose is half the amount of the Ritalin dose. In either case, the total daily dose of Focalin should be divided into 2 doses taken at least 4 hours apart.

Depending on the response, your doctor may increase the dose by 2.5-5 mg a day, up to a maximum of 20 mg (10 mg 2 times a day). Increases are usually made at weekly intervals.

How should I take this medication?

Focalin can be taken with or without food. The drug is usually taken 2 times a day, at least 4 hours apart, but your doctor may adjust the schedule depending on your child's response. Take Focalin exactly as prescribed.

What should I avoid while taking this medication?

Use caution when driving, operating machinery, or performing other hazardous activities. Focalin may cause dizziness, drowsiness, or blurred vision. This drug may interfere with your ability to concentrate.

Do not share Focalin with anyone else. Focalin should not be used to prevent or treat normal fatigue.

What are possible food and drug interactions associated with this medication?

If Focalin is taken with certain other drugs, the effects of either could be increased, decreased, or altered. It is especially important to check with your doctor before combining Focalin with the following: antiseizure drugs such as phenobarbital, phenytoin, primidone; antidepressant drugs, including MAOIs (phenelzine, tranylcypromine), serotonin reuptake inhibitors (fluoxetine, paroxetine), and tricyclics (amitriptyline, imipramine); blood pressure drugs such as clonidine; cold or allergy medicines that contain decongestants; blood thinners such as warfarin or aspirin; ephedra, St. John's wort.

What are the possible side effects of this medication?

Side effects cannot be anticipated. If any develop or change in intensity, tell your doctor as soon as possible. Only your doctor can determine if it is safe for you to continue taking this drug.

Side effects may include: decreased appetite, fever, nausea, stomach pain, increased blood pressure and heart rate, new or worsening behavior and thought problems, aggressive behavior, new psychotic symptoms, slowing of growth

Can I receive this medication if I am pregnant or breastfeeding?

The effects of Focalin during pregnancy and breastfeeding are unknown. Tell your doctor immediately if you are pregnant, plan to become pregnant, or are breastfeeding.

What should I do if I miss a dose of this medication?

Take it as soon as you remember. If it is almost time for your next dose, skip the missed dose and return to your regular schedule. Never take 2 doses at the same time.

How should I store this medication?

Store in a cool, dry place in a tightly closed, light-resistant container.

FOCALIN XR
Generic name: Dexmethylphenidate hydrochloride

What is this medication?
Focalin XR is a once-daily treatment for attention-deficit/hyperactivity disorder (ADHD).

What is the most important information I should know about this medication?
Dexmethylphenidate, the active ingredient in Focalin XR, helps increase attention and decrease impulsiveness and hyperactivity in patients with ADHD.

Who should not take this medication?
You should not take Focalin XR if you have significant anxiety, tension or agitation. This drug may make these symptoms worse. Also, do not take Focalin XR if you have glaucoma, tics from Tourette's syndrome (or a family history of Tourette's syndrome), if you are taking MAOIs, or if you are allergic to any of the ingredients in this drug.

What should I tell my doctor before I take the first dose of this medication?
Tell your doctor about all prescription, over-the-counter, and herbal medications you are taking before beginning treatment with Focalin XR. Also, talk to your doctor about your complete medical history, especially if you have any mental or physical problems. Also, inform your doctor of any drug or alcohol abuse, depression, psychosis, epilepsy/seizures, high blood pressure, heart conditions, glaucoma, or if you or any of your family has a history of tics/Tourette's syndrome.

What is the usual dosage?
The information below is based on the dosage guidelines your doctor uses. Depending on your condition and medical history, your doctor may prescribe a different regimen. Do not change the dosage or stop taking your medication without your doctor's approval.

Focalin XR is available in 5, 10, and 20 milligram (mg) extended-release capsules, and should be taken once each morning.

How should I take this medication?
Focalin XR capsules may be taken at the same time each day, with or without food. The capsules may be swallowed whole, or opened and sprinkled over a spoon of applesauce. The capsule should not be crushed, chewed, nor have its contents divided.

What should I avoid while taking this medication?
Use caution when driving, operating heavy machinery, or performing other activities that require alertness. Focalin may cause dizziness,

drowsiness, or blurred vision. This drug may interfere with your ability to concentrate.

What are possible food and drug interactions associated with this medication?

If Focalin XR is taken with certain other drugs, the effects of either could be increased, decreased, or altered. It is especially important to check with your doctor before combining Focalin XR with the following: antidepressants (MAOIs or SSRIs), antiseizure medications, blood thinners (Coumarin), clomipramine, desipramine, imipramine, phenobarbital, phenytoin, primidone, cold and allergy preparations containing decongestants.

What are the possible side effects of this medication?

Side effects cannot be anticipated. If any develop or change in intensity, tell your doctor as soon as possible. Only your doctor can determine if it is safe for you to continue taking this drug.

Side effects may include: anxiety, dependence, dizziness, dry mouth, jitteriness, slowed growth (in both weight and height) in children, throat pain, upset stomach

Also, if you have blurred vision see your doctor immediately—this may be a sign of a more serious problem.

Can I receive this medication if I am pregnant or breastfeeding?

The effects of Focalin XR during pregnancy and breastfeeding are unknown. Talk with your doctor before taking this drug if you are pregnant, plan to become pregnant, or are breastfeeding.

How should I store this medication?

Store at room temperature in a clean, dry place.

GEODON

Generic name: Ziprasidone hydrochloride

What is this medication?

Geodon is a psychotropic medicine used in the treatment of both schizophrenia and bipolar mania (both manic and mixed episodes). A manic episode is a period of abnormally and persistently elevated, unreserved, or irritable mood. A mixed episode is a manic episode with a major depressive episode (depressed mood, loss of interest or pleasure in nearly all activities).

What is the most important information I should know about this medication?

Geodon should not be used in patients who have psychosis due to dementia (such as Alzheimer's disease). Using this drug in a person with dementia may lead to an increased risk of death.

It may take a few weeks for Geodon to work; do not stop taking the drug if you do not see results right away.

Call your doctor immediately if you feel faint or feel a change in the way that your heart beats as this may be a sign of an abnormal heart rhythm.

Avoid potentially hazardous activities, such as driving or operating machinery, until you know the affect Geodon has on you. This drug has been shown to cause sleepiness.

Geodon may cause a drop in your blood pressure, especially when you first start taking this medication or if the dose is increased. If this happens, try not to stand up too quickly and contact your doctor concerning this problem.

It is unknown if Geodon directly causes high blood glucose levels or diabetes, but when taking this drug you should monitor for symptoms of hyperglycemia (such as frequent thirst, urination, and/or hunger, fatigue, weight loss, blurred vision, dry mouth, or poor wound healing).

Who should not take this medication?
Do not take Geodon if you are allergic to any of its ingredients. This drug should not be taken if you have heart problems (such as a recent heart attack, severe heart failure or heart rhythm irregularities), even if you are taking anti-arrhythmic medication.

What should I tell my doctor before I take the first dose of this medication?
Tell your doctor about all prescription, over-the-counter, and herbal medications you are taking before beginning treatment with Geodon. Also, talk to your doctor about you complete medical history, especially if you have diabetes, a history of heart disease in your family, any problems with your heart beat, fainting or dizziness, or if are pregnant, expecting to become pregnant, or breastfeeding. Also, inform your doctor if you have previously been allergic to Geodon or any of its ingredients and if you have a known history of low potassium or magnesium levels in your blood.

What is the usual dosage?
The information below is based on the dosage guidelines your doctor uses. Depending on your condition and medical history, your doctor may prescribe a different regimen. Do not change the dosage or stop taking your medication without your doctor's approval.

Bipolar Mania
Adults: The usual dose of Geodon capsules is 40 milligrams (mg) twice per day on the first day of treatment. On the second day, the dose should be increased to 60-80 mg twice per day. Dose adjustments should be within the range of 40-80 mg twice daily, based on tolerability and the how well the drug is working for you.

If taken through injection, the maximum dosage allowed is 40 mg per day, in 10-20 mg injections (10 mg injections can be given every 2 hours while 20 mg injections may be given every 4 hours.)

Schizophrenia
Adults: The usual dosage of Geodon capsules is 20 mg twice per day. This daily dose may be adjusted in certain individuals based on clinical status to up to 80 mg twice a day. The dosing adjustment, if indicated, should occur at intervals of no less than 2 days.

Geodon has not been shown to be safe or effective in the treatment of those under the age of 18 years old.

How should I take this medication?
Take Geodon only as directed by your doctor. Geodon capsules should be swallowed whole with food. It is best to take Geodon at the same time every day. It may take a few weeks for Geodon to work; do not stop taking the drug or change the dose if you do not see results right away.

What should I avoid while taking this medication?
Avoid potentially hazardous activities, such as driving or operating machinery, until you know the affect Geodon has on you. This drug has been shown to cause sleepiness.

Since medications of the same drug class as Geodon may interfere with the ability of the body to adjust to heat, it is best to avoid situations involving high temperature or humidity.

Avoid consuming alcoholic beverages while taking Geodon.

What are possible food and drug interactions associated with this medication?
If Geodon is taken with certain other drugs, the effects of either could be increased, decreased, or altered. It is especially important to check with your doctor before combining Geodon with the following: arsenic, carbamazepine, chlorpromazine, dofetilide, dolasetron, droperidol, gatifloxacin, halofantrine, ketoconazole, levomethadyl, mefloquine, mesoridazine, moxifloxacin, pentamidine, pimozide, probucol, quinidine, sotalol, sparfloxacin, tacrolimus, thioridazine.

What are the possible side effects of this medication?
Side effects cannot be anticipated. If any develop or change in intensity, tell your doctor as soon as possible. Only your doctor can determine if it is safe for you to continue taking this drug.

Side effects may include: anxiety, back pain, diarrhea, dizziness, dry mouth, flu, headache, injection site pain, nausea, sleepiness, stomach pain/upset stomach, vomiting, weakness

A rare but serious condition known as neuroleptic malignant syndrome can occur with Geodon. If you experience a very high fever, rigidity in your muscles, shaking, confusion, sweating, or increased heart rate and blood pressure, contact your doctor immediately for this may be fatal.

Can I receive this medication if I am pregnant or breastfeeding?

The effects of Geodon during pregnancy and breastfeeding are unknown. Tell your doctor immediately if you are pregnant, plan to become pregnant, or are breastfeeding. Geodon should only be used during pregnancy if the potential benefit justifies the risk to the fetus.

How should I store this medication?

Store Geodon at room temperature. If Geodon is mixed into injection solution, it will last for 24 hours at room temperature, or 7 days if kept refrigerated.

HALCION

Generic name: Triazolam

What is this medication?

Halcion is used in adults for the short-term treatment of insomnia.

What is the most important information I should know about this medication?

Halcion is not indicated for use in children.

After taking Halcion, you may get out of bed without being fully awake and perform an activity that you do not know you are doing (such as sleep-driving a car, making or eating food, talking on the phone, having sex, or sleep-walking). The next morning you may not have any recollection of this. Drinking alcohol or taking other medications that make you sleepy increases the chances of doing these activities.

You make have withdrawal symptoms for 1 to 2 days if you stop taking Halcion suddenly. These symptoms may include trouble sleeping, unpleasant feelings, stomach and muscle cramps, vomiting, sweating, shakiness and seizures.

Who should not take this medication?

Do not take Halcion if you are allergic to it or any of its components, if you drink alcohol, cannot guarantee a full night's sleep, or are pregnant or considering becoming pregnant.

What should I tell my doctor before I take the first dose of this medication?

Tell your doctor about all prescription, over-the-counter, and herbal medications you are taking before beginning treatment with Halcion. Also, talk to your doctor about your complete medical history, especially if you have a history of depression, mental illness, suicidal thoughts, drug or alcohol abuse or addiction, kidney or liver disease, lung disease or breathing problems, and if you are pregnant, plan to become pregnant, or are breastfeeding.

What is the usual dosage?

The information below is based on the dosage guidelines your doctor uses. Depending on your condition and medical history, your doctor may prescribe a different regimen. Do not change the dosage or stop taking your medication without your doctor's approval.

Adults: The recommended dose for most adults is 0.25 milligrams (mg). In some patients, a lower dose may be prescribed and the maximum daily dose should not exceed 0.5 mg.

How should I take this medication?

Halcion should be taken right before you go to bed or after you have gone to bed and have had trouble falling asleep. Do not take Halcion with or right after a meal. Try to get a full night's sleep before you must be active again.

What should I avoid while taking this medication?

You should never stop taking this medication without consulting your doctor first. Driving or operating dangerous machinery or participating in any hazardous activity is not recommended after taking Halcion until you are fully awake.

What are possible food and drug interactions associated with this medication?

If Halcion is taken with certain other drugs, the effects of either could be increased, decreased, or altered. It is especially important to check with your doctor before combining this medication with any the following: flumazenil, grapefruit juice, itraconazole, isoniazid, ketoconazole, macrolide antibiotics, nefazodone, other sleep medications, oral contraceptives, ranitidine.

What are the possible side effects of this medication?

Side effects cannot be anticipated. If any develop or change in intensity, inform your doctor as soon as possible. Only your doctor can determine if it is safe for you to continue taking this drug.

Side effects may include: coordination difficulties, drowsiness, dizziness, headache, pins and needles sensations

Serious side effects may include: severe allergic reactions, getting out of bed while not being fully awake and performing an activity that you do not know you are doing, memory loss, anxiety, and abnormal thoughts or behavior. If you experience any of these serious side effects, contact your doctor immediately.

Can I receive this medication if I am pregnant or breastfeeding?

There is a risk of potential fetal harm and an increased risk of congenital malformations; therefore, Halcion should not be used during pregnancy. Since the effects of Halcion during breastfeeding are unknown, its use should be avoided. If you are pregnant or planning to become pregnant, tell your doctor immediately.

What should I do if I miss a dose of this medication?

If you missed a dose, skip it. Never take an extra dose to make up for a missed dose. Keep in mind that this medication is to just to help you sleep.

How should I store this medication?

Halcion should be stored at room temperature and protected from light.

HALOPERIDOL

What is this medication?

Haloperidol is an antipsychotic drug used to treat schizophrenia. It is also used to control tics and vocal utterances of Tourette's disorder in adults and children. Additionally, it is also used to treat children with severe aggressive behavior or hyperactive children with aggression after other treatments proven ineffective.

What is the most important information I should know about this medication?

Patients with a condition known as severe toxic central nervous system depression or those who have Parkinson's disease should not take Haloperidol. Since Haloperidol may cause heart-related side effects, your doctor will monitor heart function while on this medication.

If you experience muscle stiffness, high body temperature, or irregular heartbeat, contact your doctor immediately as these may be signs of a serious side effect.

Caution should be used in patients with heart problems, receiving antiseizure medications, or receiving blood thinners, since Haloperidol has the potential to interfere with the effect of these drugs.

Patients receiving Haloperidol and Lithium should be monitored closely, since the combined use of these medications may affect the brain.

Who should not take this medication?

Patients with Parkinson's disease or a condition known as severe toxic central nervous system depression should not take Haloperidol.

Haloperidol should not be given to anyone in a comatose state.

What should I tell my doctor before I take the first dose of this medication?

Tell your doctor about all prescription, over-the-counter, and herbal medications you are taking before beginning treatment with Haloperidol. Also, talk to your doctor about your complete medical history, especially if you have heart problems, are receiving antiseizure medications, blood thinners, or any other agent that affects the brain.

What is the usual dosage?

The information below is based on the dosage guidelines your doctor uses. Depending on your condition and medical history, your doctor may prescribe a different regimen. Do not change the dosage or stop taking your medication without your doctor's approval.

Adults: Usual dosages for adults with moderate symptoms are from 0.5 milligrams (mg) to 2 mg twice daily or three times daily. For severe symptoms, 3 mg to 5 mg twice or three times daily.

Children 3-12 years: Haloperidol is given according to the child's weight and may start at 0.5 mg daily. The dosage may be increased for effect according to your doctor. Doses may be given twice or three times daily.

How should I take this medication?

Take this medication exactly as directed by your physician.

What should I avoid while taking this medication?

Avoid alcohol use, as well as other agents that affect the brain, since they may cause more sedative effects.

Haloperidol may impair the mental and/or physical abilities required for the performance of hazardous tasks such as operating machinery or driving a motor vehicle. Use caution when performing such tasks.

What are possible food and drug interactions associated with this medication?

If Haloperidol is used with certain other drugs, the effects of either could be increased, decreased, or altered. It is especially important to check with your doctor before combining Haloperidol with the following: alcohol, antiseizure drugs, blood thinners, heart medications.

What are the possible side effects of this medication?

Side effects cannot be anticipated. If any develop or change in intensity, tell your doctor as soon as possible. Only your doctor can determine if it is safe for you to continue taking this drug.

Side effects may include: fast heartbeat, Parkinson's-like symptoms, neck spasms/involuntary muscle spasms, insomnia, restlessness, agitation, headache, confusion

Can I receive this medication if I am pregnant or breastfeeding?
The effects of Haloperidol during pregnancy and breastfeeding are unknown. Tell your doctor immediately if you are pregnant, plan to become pregnant, or are breastfeeding.

What should I do if I miss a dose of this medication?
Skip the dose and continue with your normal dosing schedule.

How should I store this medication?
Store at room temperature.

INVEGA

Generic name: Paliperidone

What is this medication?
Invega is used to treat schizophrenia and is known as an "atypical antipsychotic" medicine.

What is the most important information I should know about this medication?
Elderly patients with dementia (such as that seen in Alzheimer's disease) who are treated with atypical antipsychotics have a higher chance for death; Invega is not approved to treat dementia.

In rare cases, Invega may cause neuroleptic malignant syndrome (NMS), a life-threatening nervous system condition that causes a high fever, stiff muscles, sweating, a fast or irregular heart beat, change in blood pressure, and confusion. NMS can also affect your kidneys. NMS is a medical emergency. Call your doctor right away if you experience any of these symptoms.

Invega may also cause tardive dyskinesia, a movement disorder characterized by slow or jerky facial or body movements. Call your doctor right away if you experience uncontrollable muscle movements.

Antipsychotic therapy has induced hyperglycemia (high blood sugar) and diabetes that has progressed to coma or death in extreme cases. Patients with diabetes or those at risk for diabetes should have their blood sugar monitored often.

Overheating and dehydration may occur due to Invega therapy. Take precautions when exercising or doing activities in the heat and stay hydrated.

Take care when driving or using machinery until you know how Invega affects you as you may experience impaired judgment, thinking, and motor skills.

Dizziness and fainting caused by a drop in blood pressure may occur during Invega therapy, especially when you first start taking Invega or when the dose is increased. Get up slowly after sitting or lying down.

Who should not take this medication?

You should not take Invega if you are allergic to paliperidone, risperidone, or to any of the ingredients in Invega.

You should not take Invega if you have pre-existing severe gastrointestinal narrowing (trouble swallowing, inflammation of the small bowel, "short gut syndrome," peritonitis, cystic fibrosis, chronic intestinal pseudo-obstruction, or Meckel's diverticulum).

Invega tablets should only be used in patients who are able to swallow the tablet whole.

What should I tell my doctor before I take the first dose of this medication?

Tell your doctor about all prescription, over-the-counter, and herbal medications you are taking before beginning treatment with Invega. Also, talk to your doctor about your complete medical history, especially past or current heart problems, seizures, diabetes or elevated blood sugar, liver disease, and if you regularly drink alcohol. Tell your doctor if you have or have had problems with your esophagus, stomach or small or large intestine. Inform your doctor if you are pregnant, trying to become pregnant, or are breastfeeding.

What is the usual dosage?

The information below is based on the dosage guidelines your doctor uses. Depending on your condition and medical history, your doctor may prescribe a different regimen. Do not change the dosage or stop taking your medication without your doctor's approval.

Adults: The usual dose is 6 milligrams (mg) daily. Some patients may benefit from either higher doses up to 12 mg/day or a lower dose of 3 mg/day. If needed, the dose can be increased in increments of 3 mg/day at intervals of at least 5 days.

The maximum recommended daily dose is 12 mg/day.

Adults with moderate to severe kidney disease: The maximum recommended dose is 3 mg once daily.

How should I take this medication?

Take Invega once a day in the morning. Swallow Invega tablets whole with water or another liquid. Do not chew, divide, or crush Invega tablets. Invega can be taken with or without food.

What should I avoid while taking this medication?

Avoid drinking alcohol while taking Invega. Be careful not to overexert yourself; be cautious of excessive sweating and keep yourself fully hydrated.

What are possible food and drug interactions associated with this medication?

If Invega is taken with certain other drugs, the effects of either could be increased, decreased, or altered. It is especially important to check with your doctor before combining Invega with the following: alcohol and other central nervous system drugs, amiodarone, chlorpromazine, gatifloxacin, levodopa and other dopamine agonists, moxifloxacin, procainamide, quinidine, sotalol, thioridazine.

What are the possible side effects of this medication?

Side effects cannot be anticipated. If any develop or change in intensity, tell your doctor as soon as possible. Only your doctor can determine if it is safe for you to continue taking this drug.

Side effects may include: abdominal pain, anxiety, back pain, visual disturbances, cough, disturbed digestion, excessive salivary secretions, fainting, fast heartbeat, fatigue, pain in the extremities, headache, high blood pressure, high blood sugar and diabetes, impaired judgment or thinking, involuntary movements, dizziness upon standing, muscle stiffness, nausea, overheating and dehydration, restlessness, seizures, drowsiness, suicidal thoughts, trouble swallowing, upset stomach, weakness

Can I receive this medication if I am pregnant or breastfeeding?

The effects of Invega during pregnancy and breastfeeding are unknown. Tell your doctor immediately if you are pregnant, plan to become pregnant, or are breastfeeding. Taking Invega while breastfeeding is not recommended.

What should I do if I miss a dose of this medication?

If you miss a dose, take it as soon as you remember. If it is almost time for your next dose (less than 12 hours away), skip that dose and resume your normal dosing schedule. Do not take two doses together.

How should I store this medication?

Store Invega at room temperature, away from moisture.

KLONOPIN
Generic name: Clonazepam

What is this medication?

Klonopin is used alone or with other drugs to treat seizure disorders. It is also used to treat panic disorder, which is characterized by unexpected attacks of overwhelming panic along with fear of having additional future attacks.

What is the most important information I should know about this medication?

Physical and/or psychological dependence can occur with Klonopin.

Withdrawal effects are possible if the medication is stopped suddenly after long-term use or after high-dose treatment. Do not stop taking

Klonopin suddenly without first talking to your doctor. Your doctor may want to gradually reduce the dose.

When you start Klonopin, you may experience impaired judgment, thinking, or motor skills. You should not drive or operate dangerous machinery until you know how this medication will affect you. Consuming alcohol, a CNS depressant, may intensify or worsen the side effects of Klonopin.

When on Klonopin, your doctor should monitor your blood liver function during long-term therapy due to possible side effects.

When used in patients with several different types of seizure disorders, Klonopin may increase the incidence or onset of generalized tonic-clonic seizures. These patients may require the addition of appropriate anticonvulsants or an increase in their dosage.

When Klonopin is used in conjunction with valproic acid, there is a risk of absence status (a continual series of seizures).

Who should not take this medication?

Do not use Klonopin if you are sensitive to or have ever had an allergic reaction to it or similar drugs, such as chlordiazepoxide and diazepam.

Do not take Klonopin if you have severe liver disease or the eye condition known as acute narrow-angle glaucoma (increased pressure in the eye). Patients with open-angle glaucoma who are receiving appropriate treatment may use Klonopin.

What should I tell my doctor before I take the first dose of this medication?

Tell your doctor about all prescription, over-the-counter, and herbal medication you are taking before beginning treatment with Klonopin. Also, talk to your doctor about your complete medical history, especially if you have kidney or liver disease, seizures, are depressed or have suicidal thoughts, are on valproic acid or any other anticonvulsants, have several different types of coexisting seizure disorders, have a history of sensitivity to Klonopin or other benzodiazepines, or have a history of substance abuse. In addition, tell your doctor if you are pregnant, planning on becoming pregnant, or breastfeeding.

What is the usual dosage?

The information below is based on the dosage guidelines your doctor uses. Depending on your condition and medical history, your doctor may prescribe a different regimen. Do not change the dosage or stop taking your medication without your doctor's approval.

Panic Disorder

Adults: The usual starting dose is 0.25 milligrams (mg) taken twice a day. The dose may be increased by 1 mg per day after 3 days. Some people may need as much as 4 mg per day; for these patients the dose should be incrementally increased by 0.125 to 0.25 mg twice a day every 3 days until the panic disorder is controlled or until the side effects become too bothersome.

Klonopin therapy should be stopped slowly, with a decrease of 0.125 mg twice a day every 3 days, until the drug is completely withdrawn.

Elderly: There is no clinical trial experience with the use of Klonopin in patients ≥65 years of age. In general, elderly patients should be started on a low dose of Klonopin and observed closely.

Children: The safety and effectiveness of Klonopin to treat panic disorder have not been established in children under age 18.

Seizure Disorders

Adults: The usual starting dose is 1.5 mg per day divided into 3 doses. The dose may be increased by 0.5-1 mg every 3 days until seizures are controlled or the side effects become too bothersome. The maximum daily dose is 20 mg.

Elderly: There is no clinical trial experience with the use of Klonopin is patients 65 years of age and older. In general, elderly patients should be started on a low dose of Klonopin and observed closely.

Children: The starting dose for infants and children up to 10 years old or up to 66 pounds should be 0.01-0.03 mg per 2.2 pounds of body weight per day. Do not give more than 0.05 mg per 2.2 pounds of body weight per day. The dose may be increased by 0.25-0.5 mg every 3 days, up to 0.1-0.2 mg per 2.2 pounds of body weight a day, until seizures are controlled or the side effects become too bothersome.

How should I take this medication?

Take Klonopin exactly as prescribed. Klonopin is available as a tablet or as a wafer that melts in your mouth. Take Klonopin tablets with water and swallow the tablet whole. The wafers can be taken with or without water. With dry hands, peel back the foil on the blister pack. Do not push the wafer through the foil. Immediately after opening the blister, remove the wafer and place it on your tongue. You must take the wafer right after opening the blister. It will melt rapidly in your mouth.

What should I avoid while taking this medication?

Klonopin will cause drowsiness and may cause dizziness. Use caution when driving, operating machinery, or performing other hazardous activities. Avoid using Klonopin with other drugs that may cause drowsiness or dizziness. Use alcohol cautiously. Alcohol may increase drowsiness and dizziness while taking Klonopin. Alcohol may also increase the risk of having a seizure.

Klonopin can be habit-forming and can lose its effectiveness as you build up a tolerance to it. You may experience withdrawal symptoms, such as convulsions, hallucinations, tremor, and abdominal and muscle cramps, if you stop using Klonopin suddenly. You should only stop or change your dose only after first talking to your doctor.

What are possible food and drug interactions associated with this medication?

If Klonopin is taken with certain other drugs, the effects of either could be increased, decreased, or altered. It is especially important to check with your doctor before combining Klonopin with the following: amphotericin, antidepressants (imipramine, phenelzine, and tranylcypromine), barbiturates, carbamazepine, chlorpromazine, diazepam, haloperidol, narcotic pain relievers (meperidine and morphine), nystatin, other anticonvulsants (phenytoin and divalproex), and sedatives (triazolam).

What are the possible side effects of this medication?

Side effects cannot be anticipated. If any develop or change in intensity, tell your doctor as soon as possible. Only your doctor can determine if it is safe for you to continue taking this drug.

Side effects may include: depression, dizziness, fatigue, flu, inflamed sinuses or nasal passages, lack of coordination, memory problems, menstrual problems, nervousness, sleepiness, upper respiratory tract infection

Klonopin can also cause aggressive behavior, agitation, anxiety, excitability, hostility, irritability, nervousness, nightmares, sleep disturbances, and vivid dreams.

Can I receive this medication if I am pregnant or breastfeeding?

Do not take Klonopin if you are pregnant or planning on becoming pregnant. Talk to your doctor first. Do not take Klonopin while breastfeeding. There have been suggested associations between the use of anticonvulsants by women with epilepsy and an elevated incidence of birth defects in children born to these women. The use of Klonopin in women of childbearing potential should be weighed carefully by the patient and her doctor.

What should I do if I miss a dose of this medication?

If it is within an hour after the missed time, take the dose as soon as you remember. If you do not remember until later, skip the missed dose and go back to your regular schedule. Never take two doses at the same time.

How should I store this medication?

Store Klonopin at room temperature. Keep away from heat, light, and moisture.

LAMICTAL

Generic name: Lamotrigine

What is this medication?

Lamictal is used to treat epilepsy, a seizure disorder. It is also used to help prevent the extreme mood swings associated with bipolar disorder.

What is the most important information I should know about this medication?

All patients who are currently taking or are about to start drugs for epilepsy should be closely monitored for changes in behavior that indicate the emergence or worsening of suicidal thoughts or behavior or depression.

Rarely, serious and possibly fatal rashes have been reported with the use of Lamictal. Although most patients who develop rash while receiving Lamictal have mild to moderate symptoms, some individuals may develop a serious skin reaction that requires hospitalization. Because of this risk, it's important to contact your doctor immediately if you develop any of the following: fever, hives, painful sores in your mouth or around your eyes, skin rash, swelling of your lips or tongue, swollen lymph glands.

These serious skin reactions are most likely to happen within the first 8 weeks of treatment and occur more often in children than adults. They are also more likely to happen if you take Lamictal with the anticonvulsant valproate (Depakene or Depakote); if you take a higher starting dose of Lamictal than your doctor prescribed; or if you increase your dose of Lamictal faster than prescribed.

Who should not take this medication?

Do not take Lamictal if you are allergic to the medication or any of its ingredients.

Lamictal is not approved for treating children or teenagers with mood disorders such as bipolar disorder or depression.

What should I tell my doctor before I take the first dose of this medication?

Tell your doctor about all prescription, over-the-counter, and herbal medications you are taking before beginning treatment with Lamictal. Also, talk to your doctor about your complete medical history, especially if you have kidney, liver, or heart problems; or if you have thoughts of harming yourself or committing suicide.

What is the usual dosage?

The information below is based on the dosage guidelines your doctor uses. Depending on your condition and medical history, your doctor may prescribe a different regimen. Do not change the dosage or stop taking your medication without your doctor's approval.

There are very specific calculations for your starting dose and dosage increase schedule based on your age, weight, medical condition, and other medications you're taking. The dose of Lamictal must be increased slowly, generally every 1 to 2 weeks. It may take several weeks or months before your final dosage can be determined by your doctor.

How should I take this medication?

Lamictal tablets should be swallowed whole; chewing them may leave a bitter taste.

Lamictal also comes as Chewable Dispersible Tablets that may be swallowed whole, chewed, or mixed in water or diluted fruit juice. If chewing them, drink some water to aid in swallowing. To mix in liquid, add the tablets to a small amount of water or juice (1 teaspoon or enough to cover the tablets) in a glass. Approximately 1 minute later, mix the solution and take the entire amount at once.

What should I avoid while taking this medication?

Do not abruptly stop taking Lamictal without consulting your doctor first. Do not start or stop estrogen-containing birth control pills while taking Lamictal unless you have discussed with your doctor any dosage adjustments that might be necessary. Use caution before driving a car or operating complex, hazardous machinery until you know if Lamictal affects your ability to perform these tasks.

What are possible food and drug interactions associated with this medication?

If Lamictal is taken with certain other drugs, the effects of either could be increased, decreased, or altered. It is especially important to check with your doctor before combining Lamictal with the following: carbamazepine, estrogen-containing birth control pills, medicines that inhibit folic acid metabolism, oxcarbazepine, phenobarbital, phenytoin, primidone, rifampin, topiramate, valproate.

What are the possible side effects of this medication?

Side effects cannot be anticipated. If any develop or change in intensity, tell your doctor as soon as possible. Only your doctor can determine if it is safe for you to continue taking this drug.

Side effects may include: blurred or double vision, coordination problems, dizziness, headache, insomnia, nausea, rash, sleepiness, vomiting

The most serious side effect of Lamictal is a rash that can be life-threatening. See "**What is the most important information I should know about this medication?**" above.

Can I receive this medication if I am pregnant or breastfeeding?

The effects of Lamictal during pregnancy are not known. Lamictal can pass into breast milk, and the effects on the infant are unknown. Tell your doctor immediately if you are pregnant, plan to become pregnant, or are breastfeeding.

What should I do if I miss a dose of this medication?

Never double your dose of Lamictal if you miss a dose. Skip the missed dose and return to your regular schedule.

How should I store this medication?
Store at room temperature away from heat and light.

LAMICTAL CD
Generic name: Lamotrigine

What is this medication?
Lamictal is used to treat epilepsy, a seizure disorder. It may also be used to help prevent the extreme mood swings associated with bipolar disorder.

What is the most important information I should know about this medication?
All patients who are currently taking or are about to start drugs for epilepsy should be closely monitored for changes in behavior that indicate the emergence or worsening of suicidal thoughts or behavior or depression.

Rarely, serious and possibly fatal rashes have been reported with the use of Lamictal. Although most patients who develop rash while receiving Lamictal have mild to moderate symptoms, some individuals may develop a serious skin reaction that requires hospitalization. Because of this risk, it's important to contact your doctor immediately if you develop fever, hives, painful sores in your mouth or around the eyes, skin rash, swelling of lips of tongue or swollen lymph glands.

These serious skin reactions are most likely to happen within the first 8 weeks of treatment and occur more often in children than adults. They are also more likely to happen if you take Lamictal in combination with valproate (Depakene or Depakote); take a higher starting dose of Lamictal than your doctor prescribed; or if you increase your dose of Lamictal faster than prescribed.

Lamictal is intended to be used alone or in combination with other seizure medications in patients aged 2 years or older.

Who should not take this medication?
Do not take Lamictal if you are allergic to the medication or any of its ingredients.

Lamictal is not approved for treating children or teenagers with mood disorders such as bipolar disorder or depression.

What should I tell my doctor before I take the first dose of this medication?
Tell your doctor about all prescription, over-the-counter, and herbal medications you are taking before beginning treatment with Lamictal. Also, talk to your doctor about your complete medical history, especially if you have kidney, liver, or heart problems; or if you have thoughts of harming yourself or committing suicide.

What is the usual dosage?

The information below is based on the dosage guidelines your doctor uses. Depending on your condition and medical history, your doctor may prescribe a different regimen. Do not change the dosage or stop taking your medication without your doctor's approval.

There are very specific calculations for your starting dose and dosage increase schedule based on your age, weight, medical condition, and other medications you're taking. The dose of Lamictal must be increased slowly, generally every 1 to 2 weeks. Based on how well you respond, it may take several weeks or months before your final dosage can be determined by your doctor.

How should I take this medication?

Lamictal Chewable Dispersible Tablets may be swallowed whole, chewed, or mixed in water or diluted fruit juice. If chewing them, drink some water to aid in swallowing. To mix in liquid, add the tablets to a small amount of water or juice (1 teaspoon or enough to cover the tablets) in a glass or spoon. After approximately 1 minute later, mix the solution and take the entire amount at once.

Lamictal also come in tablets and should be swallowed whole; chewing them may leave a bitter taste.

What should I avoid while taking this medication?

Do not abruptly stop taking Lamictal without consulting your doctor first. Do not start or stop estrogen-containing birth control pills while taking Lamictal unless you have discussed with your doctor any dosage adjustments that might be necessary. Use caution before driving a car or operating complex, hazardous machinery until you know if Lamictal affects your ability to perform these tasks.

What are possible food and drug interactions associated with this medication?

If Lamictal is taken with certain other drugs, the effects of either could be increased, decreased, or altered. It is especially important to check with your doctor before combining Lamictal with the following: carbamazepine, estrogen-containing birth control pills, medicines that inhibit folic acid metabolism, oxcarbazepine, phenobarbital, phenytoin, primidone, rifampin, topiramate, valproate.

What are the possible side effects of this medication?

Side effects cannot be anticipated. If any develop or change in intensity, tell your doctor as soon as possible. Only your doctor can determine if it is safe for you to continue taking this drug.

Side effects may include: Blurred or double vision, coordination problems, dizziness, headache, insomnia, nausea, rash, sleepiness, and vomiting

The most serious side effect of Lamictal is a rash that can be life-threatening. See "**What is the most important information I should know about this medication?**".

Can I receive this medication if I am pregnant or breastfeeding?

The effects of Lamictal during pregnancy are not known. Lamictal can pass into breast milk, and the effects on the infant are unknown. Tell your doctor immediately if you are pregnant, plan to become pregnant, or are breastfeeding.

What should I do if I miss a dose of this medication?

Never double your dose of Lamictal if you miss a dose. Skip the missed dose and return to your regular schedule.

How should I store this medication?

Store at room temperature away from heat and light.

LEXAPRO

Generic name: Escitalopram oxalate

What is this medication?

Lexapro is used to treat major depression, a persistently low mood that interferes with daily functioning. Lexapro is also used to treat generalized anxiety disorder, a condition marked by excessive worry and anxiety that is hard to control and interferes with daily life.

What is the most important information I should know about this medication?

Lexapro is not approved for use in children or adolescents.

Antidepressant medicines may increase suicidal thoughts or actions in some children, teenagers, and young adults when the medicine is first started. Depression and other serious mental illnesses are the most important causes of suicidal thoughts and actions. Some people may have a particularly high risk of having suicidal thoughts or actions. These include people who have (or have a family history of) bipolar disorder (also called manic-depressive illness) or suicidal thoughts or actions.

Pay close attention to any changes, especially sudden ones, in mood, behaviors, thoughts, or feelings. This is very important when an antidepressant medicine is first started or when the dose is changed.

Call your doctor right away to report new or sudden changes in mood, behavior, thoughts, or feelings. Signs to watch for include new or worsening depression, new or worsening anxiety, agitation, insomnia, hostility, panic attacks, restlessness, extreme hyperactivity, and suicidal thinking or behavior.

Keep all follow-up visits as scheduled, and call the doctor between visits as needed, especially if you have concerns about symptoms.

Abrupt discontinuation of this drug or any antidepressant could cause side effects such as irritability, agitation, dizziness, headache, insomnia, and many others. Do not stop taking this medication without first consulting your physician.

Taking Lexapro at the same time you are taking aspirin, aspirin-related products, or any other blood thinner or anticoagulant increases the risk of bleeding.

Who should not take this medication?
Do not use Lexapro if you are taking pimozide or a monoamine oxidase inhibitor (MAOI), if you are allergic to Lexapro, or if you are sensitive to any component of the drug.

What should I tell my doctor before I take the first dose of this medication?
Tell your doctor about all prescription, over-the-counter, and herbal medications you are taking before beginning treatment with Lexapro. Also, talk to your doctor about your complete medical history, especially if you have a bleeding disorder, kidney or liver disease, a history of seizure disorders, suffer from mania, or experience worsening symptoms of depression and/or suicidal thoughts.

What is the usual dosage?
The information below is based on the dosage guidelines your doctor uses. Depending on your condition and medical history, your doctor may prescribe a different regimen. Do not change the dosage or stop taking your medication without your doctor's approval.

Adults: The recommended starting dose is 10 milligrams (mg) once daily. If necessary, your doctor may increase the dose to 20 mg after a minimum of 1 week. The higher dose is not recommended for most older adults and people with liver problems.

How should I take this medication?
Lexapro is available in tablet and liquid forms and can be taken with or without food in the morning or evening. Although improvement usually begins within 1-4 weeks, treatment typically continues for several months.

What should I avoid while taking this medication?
Do not stop taking Lexapro without first talking to your doctor. An abrupt decrease in dose could cause withdrawal symptoms such as mood problems, fatigue, insomnia, and tingling sensations.

Because Lexapro can cause dizziness or drowsiness, use caution when driving, operating machinery, or performing hazardous activities until you know how the drug affects you. It's also best to avoid alcohol while taking Lexapro.

Do not take Celexa (citalopram) while you are taking Lexapro, since the two drugs are related.

What are possible food and drug interactions associated with this medication?

If Lexapro is taken with certain other drugs, the effects of either could be increased, decreased, or altered. It is especially important to check with your doctor before combining Lexapro with the following: antidepressants, painkillers, sedatives, and tranquilizers and other drugs that act on the brain; aspirin and other blood thinners such as warfarin; carbamazepine; cimetidine; citalopram; ketoconazole; lithium; metoprolol; migraine drugs known as triptans, such as sumatriptan and zolmitriptan; nonsteroidal anti-inflammatory drugs such as ibuprofen and naproxen; narcotic painkillers such as oxycodone; tryptophan.

Never combine Lexapro with any drug classified as an MAOI. Drugs in this category include the antidepressants phenelzine and tranylcypromine. Lexapro and MAOIs should not be taken together or within 14 days of each other. Combining these drugs with Lexapro can cause serious and even fatal reactions such as high body temperature, muscle rigidity, twitching, and agitation leading to delirium and coma.

What are the possible side effects of this medication?

Side effects cannot be anticipated. If any develop or change in intensity, tell your doctor as soon as possible. Only your doctor can determine if it is safe for you to continue taking this drug.

Side effects may include: decreased sex drive and inability to have an orgasm, difficulty falling or staying asleep, ejaculation problems, fatigue, increased sweating, nausea, sleepiness

Can I receive this medication if I am pregnant or breastfeeding?

The effects of Lexapro during pregnancy and breastfeeding are unknown. Tell your doctor immediately if you are pregnant, plan to become pregnant, or are breastfeeding. If you decide to breastfeed, Lexapro is not recommended.

What should I do if I miss a dose of this medication?

Take it as soon as you remember. If it is almost time for your next dose, skip the missed dose and go back to your regular schedule. Never take two doses at the same time.

How should I store this medication?

Store at room temperature, away from moisture and heat.

LIBRIUM
Generic name: Chlordiazepoxide hydrochloride

What is this medication?

Librium is used to treat anxiety disorders. It is also prescribed for short-term relief of the symptoms of anxiety, symptoms of withdrawal in acute alcoholism, and anxiety and apprehension before surgery.

What is the most important information I should know about this medication?

Librium has the potential to cause dependence.

You could experience withdrawal symptoms if you stop taking Librium abruptly. Do not discontinue the drug or change your dose without your doctor's approval.

Who should not take this medication?

Do not use Librium if you are allergic to any of its ingredients.

What should I tell my doctor before I take the first dose of this medication?

Tell your doctor about all prescription, over-the-counter, and herbal medications you are taking before beginning treatment with Librium. Also, talk to your doctor about your complete medical history, especially if you have kidney or liver disease, porphyria (a rare metabolic disorder), or suffer from depression or have suicidal thoughts.

What is the usual dosage?

The information below is based on the dosage guidelines your doctor uses. Depending on your condition and medical history, your doctor may prescribe a different regimen. Do not change the dosage or stop taking your medication without your doctor's approval.

Mild to Moderate Anxiety

Adults: The usual dose is 5 or 10 milligrams (mg), 3-4 times a day.
Children ≥6 years: The usual dose is 5 mg, 2-4 times per day. Some children may need to take 10 mg, 2-3 times per day.

The drug is not recommended for children under 6 years of age.

Severe Anxiety

Adults: The usual dose is 20 or 25 mg, 3-4 times a day.

Apprehension and Anxiety before Surgery

Adults: On days before surgery, the usual dose is 5-10 mg, 3-4 times a day.

Withdrawal Symptoms of Acute Alcoholism

Adults: The injectable form is usually used initially. Following this is the oral medication starting at doses from 50 to 100 mg, to be followed by repeated doses as needed up to 300 mg per day. The doctor will repeat this dose, up to a maximum of 300 mg per day, until agitation is controlled. The dose will then be reduced as much as possible.

In elderly patients, your doctor may limit the dose to the smallest effective amount in order to avoid over-sedation or lack of coordination. The usual dose is 5 mg, 2-4 times per day.

How should I take this medication?

Take Librium exactly as prescribed.

What should I avoid while taking this medication?

Librium may cause you to become drowsy or less alert. Do not drive or operate dangerous machinery or participate in any hazardous activity that requires full mental alertness until you know how you react to Librium.

Avoid alcohol while taking Librium as it may increase drowsiness and dizziness caused by Librium.

What are possible food and drug interactions associated with this medication?

If Librium is taken with certain other drugs, the effects of either could be increased, decreased, or altered. It is especially important to check with your doctor before combining Librium with the following: antacids, antidepressant drugs known as MAO inhibitors, including phenelzine and tranylcypromine, antihistamines, antipsychotic drugs such as chlorpromazine and trifluoperazine, antiseizure drugs such as carbamazepine and phenytoin, barbiturates, blood-thinners, cimetidine, disulfiram, levodopa, muscle relaxants such as cyclobenzaprine, narcotic pain relievers, tranquilizers and sedatives such as alprazolam, diazepam, midazolam, and triazolam.

What are the possible side effects of this medication?

Side effects cannot be anticipated. If any develop or change in intensity, tell your doctor as soon as possible. Only your doctor can determine if it is safe for you to continue taking this drug.

Side effects may include: confusion, constipation, drowsiness, fainting, increased or decreased sex drive, liver problems, lack of muscle coordination, minor menstrual irregularities, nausea, skin rash or eruptions, swelling due to fluid retention, yellow eyes and skin

Side effects due to rapid decrease or abrupt withdrawal from Librium may include: abdominal and muscle cramps, convulsions, exaggerated feeling of depression, sleeplessness, sweating, tremors, vomiting

Can I receive this medication if I am pregnant or breastfeeding?

Do not take Librium if you are pregnant or planning to become pregnant. There may be an increased risk of birth defects. Do not breastfeed while you are taking Librium.

What should I do if I miss a dose of this medication?

Take it as soon as you remember if it is within an hour or of your scheduled time. If you do not remember until later, skip the dose you missed and go back to your regular schedule. Do not take two doses at once.

How should I store this medication?

Store away from heat, light, and moisture.

LIMBITROL
Generic name: Chlordiazepoxide and Amitriptyline

What is this medication?
Limbitrol is a combination of an antianxiety drug (chlordiazepoxide) and an antidepressant (amitriptyline). It is used to treat moderate to severe depression associated with moderate to severe anxiety.

What is the most important information I should know about this medication?
Children, teenagers, and young adults who take Limbitrol may be at an increased risk for suicidal thoughts or actions. The patients' family and/ or caregivers should closely observe the individual who is on Limbitrol. Contact the doctor at the onset of new, worsened, or sudden symptoms such as depressed mood; anxious, restless, or irritable behavior; panic attacks; or any unusual change in mood or behavior occur.

Contact the doctor right away if any signs of suicidal thoughts or actions occur. The risk of suicidal actions may be especially high in patients with bipolar disorder (also called manic-depressive illness), a family history of bipolar disorder, and a personal or family history of suicide attempt. After starting your child on an antidepressant, regular visits with your doctor should be set up.

When using Limbitrol for long periods of time or at high doses, tolerance may develop; you may require higher doses to obtain the same effect as when you first started taking this drug. Talk with your doctor if Limbitrol stops working well. Do not take more than prescribed.

Some people who use Limbitrol over an extended period of time may develop dependence or a need to continue taking it. If you stop taking Limbitrol suddenly, you may have withdrawal symptoms which may include convulsions, tremor, stomach and muscle cramps, vomiting, or sweating. Contact your doctor if you experience any of these symptoms or if you wish to alter your Limbitrol dose; do not change your dose independently.

Do not drive or perform other possibly unsafe tasks until you know how you react to Limbitrol; this drug may cause dizziness, drowsiness, or blurred vision. These effects may be worse if you take it with alcohol or certain medicines.

Do not drink alcohol or use medicines that may cause drowsiness (such as sleep aids and muscle relaxers) while you are using Limbitrol; it may add to their effects.

Limbitrol may cause dizziness, lightheadedness, or fainting; alcohol, hot weather, exercise, or fever may increase these effects. To prevent them, sit up or stand slowly, especially in the morning. Sit or lie down at the first sign of any of these effects.

Limbitrol may affect your blood sugar. Check blood sugar levels closely. Ask your doctor before you change the dose of your diabetes medicine.

Limbitrol may cause you to become sunburned more easily. Avoid the sun, sunlamps, or tanning booths until you know how you react to Limbitrol. Use sunscreen or wear protective clothing if you must be outside for more than a short time.

Do not become overheated in hot weather or while you are being active; heatstroke may occur.

Separate Limbitrol and monoamine oxidase inhibitors (MAOIs by a minimum of 14 days. Do not start Limbitrol therapy if you are currently on an MAOI.

If your symptoms do not get better within 4 weeks or if they get worse, check with your doctor.

This drug should be used with caution in patients with a history of seizures.

Close supervision is required when Limbitrol is given to patients with an overactive thyroid or those on thyroid medication.

Tell your doctor or dentist that you take Limbitrol before you receive any medical or dental care, emergency care, or surgery.

Who should not take this medication?
Limbitrol should not be used in patients with hypersensitivity to either benzodiazepines or tricyclic antidepressants, both components of Limbitrol.

Limbitrol should not be given concomitantly with an MAOI due to serious side effects that may occur. Limbitrol and MAOIs must be separated by a minimum of 14 days.

Limbitrol should not be used during the acute recovery phase following myocardial infarction (heart attack).

What should I tell my doctor before I take the first dose of this medication?
Tell your doctor about all prescription, over-the-counter, and herbal medications you are taking before beginning treatment with Limbitrol. Also, talk to your doctor about your complete medical history, especially if you have a history of bipolar disorder, considered or attempted suicide, have a history of alcohol or other substance abuse or dependence, an irregular heart beat, heart disease, chest pain, liver or kidney problems, thyroid disease, lung or breathing problems, muscle problems (myasthenia gravis), glaucoma, seizures, blood problems, or if you unable to urinate (urinary retention).

What is the usual dosage?
The information below is based on the dosage guidelines your doctor uses. Depending on your condition and medical history, your doctor may prescribe a different regimen. Do not change the dosage or stop taking your medication without your doctor's approval.

Optimum dosage varies with the severity of the symptoms and the response of the individual patient. When a satisfactory response is obtained, dosage should be reduced to the smallest amount needed to maintain the remission. The larger portion of the total daily dose may be taken at bedtime. In some patients, a single dose at bedtime may be sufficient. In general, lower dosages are recommended for elderly patients.

Adults: Limbitrol tablets contain 5 milligrams (mg) chlordiazepoxide and 12.5 mg amitriptyline. The recommended starting dose of Limbitrol tablets is 3 or 4 tablets taken daily in divided doses may be satisfactory in patients who do not tolerate higher doses.

Limbitrol DS (double strength) tablets contain 10 mg chlordiazepoxide and 25 mg amitriptyline. The recommended starting dose is 3 or 4 tablets taken daily in divided doses. This may increase to 6 tablets daily if required. Some patients may respond to smaller doses and can be maintained on 2 tablets daily.

How should I take this medication?

Limbitrol can be swallowed with or without food daily. Withdrawal symptoms may occur if you decrease your dose or suddenly stop taking Limbitrol. Talk with your doctor about any changes to your dose.

Do not eat grapefruit or drink grapefruit juice while using Limbitrol without first contacting your doctor.

What should I avoid while taking this medication?

Do not start Limbitrol therapy if you are currently on an MAOI.

Do not take more than prescribed or suddenly stop taking Limbitrol.

Do not drive or perform other possibly unsafe tasks until you know how you react to Limbitrol; this drug may cause dizziness, drowsiness, or blurred vision.

Do not drink alcohol or use medicines that may cause drowsiness (such as sleep aids and muscle relaxers) while you are using Limbitrol; it may add to their effects.

Avoid sitting or standing up too quickly, especially in the morning and when you start treatment with Limbitrol. Sit or lie down at the first sign of any dizziness or lightheadedness.

Avoid the sun, sunlamps, or tanning booths until you know how you react to Limbitrol. Use sunscreen or wear protective clothing if you must be outside for more than a short time. Limbitrol may cause you to become sunburned more easily.

Do not become overheated in hot weather or while you are being active; heatstroke may occur.

Do not eat grapefruit or drink grapefruit juice while using Limbitrol without first contacting your doctor.

What are possible food and drug interactions associated with this medication?

If Limbitrol is taken with certain other drugs, the effects of either could be increased, decreased, or altered. It is especially important to check with your doctor before combining Limbitrol with the following: antiarrhythmics, anticholinergics such as scopolamine, anticoagulants/blood thinners, antifungals, antidepressants (including MAOIs, SSRIs, and SNRIs), bupropion, carbamazepine, cimetidine, clonidine, clozapine, disulfiram, fluconazole, guanethidine, guanfacine, H1 antagonists such as astemizole and terfenadine, ketolide antibiotics, macrolide antibiotics, MAOIs such as phenelzine and selegiline, omeprazole, phenothiazines such as chlorpromazine, pimozide, rifampin, sodium oxybate GHB, quinupristin/dalfopristin, sympathomimetics such as albuterol and pseudoephedrine, terbinafine, valproic acid.

What are the possible side effects of this medication?
Side effects cannot be anticipated. If any develop or change in intensity, tell your doctor as soon as possible. Only your doctor can determine if it is safe for you to continue taking this drug.

Side effects may include: abnormal skin sensations, bloating, blurred vision, constipation, diarrhea, disturbed concentration, dizziness, drowsiness, dry mouth, headache, loss of appetite, nausea, restlessness, tiredness, upset stomach, vomiting, weakness, weight gain or loss, chest pain, confusion, decreased sexual ability, delusions, disorientation, decreased or increased urination, fast or irregular heartbeat, fever, chills, persistent sore throat, involuntary movements of the tongue, face, mouth, or jaw (such as protrusion of tongue, puffing of cheeks, puckering of mouth, chewing movements), involuntary movements of the arms and legs

Can I receive this medication if I am pregnant or breastfeeding?
Limbitrol has been shown to cause fetal harm. If you think you may be pregnant, contact your doctor. You will need to discuss the benefits and risks of using Limbitrol while you are pregnant.

Limbitrol is found in breast milk. Do not breastfeed while taking Limbitrol.

What should I do if I miss a dose of this medication?
If you miss a dose of Limbitrol, take it as soon as possible. If it is almost time for your next dose, skip the missed dose and go back to your regular dosing schedule. Do not take two doses at once.

How should I store this medication?
Store Limbitrol at room temperature in a tightly closed container. Store away from heat, moisture, and light. Do not store in the bathroom.

LITHIUM CARBONATE

What is this medication?
Lithium carbonate is used in the treatment of manic episodes of patients with bipolar disorder. A manic episode is a time of abnormally elevated, unreserved, or irritable mood.

Lithium carbonate is also used in the maintenance treatment of patients diagnosed with bipolar disorder.

What is the most important information I should know about this medication?

It may take up to 3 weeks before you see any improvement in your symptoms.

While taking lithium carbonate, it is very important that you follow your doctor's recommendations and make sure you do not miss any appointments or laboratory tests.

Toxic levels of this medication can occur at any dose and frequent blood tests will be required. You should stop taking lithium carbonate and contact your doctor immediately if you develop signs of lithium toxicity such as diarrhea, vomiting, tremor, mild lack of coordination, drowsiness, and muscular weakness.

The safety and efficacy of this medication is unknown in children under 12 years of age, and its use is not recommended.

Who should not take this medication?

Do not take this medication if you are allergic to lithium, Lithobid, Eskalith, Eskalith CR or any of their components.

What should I tell my doctor before I take the first dose of this medication?

Tell your doctor about all prescription, over-the-counter, and herbal medications you are taking before beginning treatment with lithium carbonate. Also, talk to your doctor about your complete medical history, especially if you have a history of kidney or heart disease, thyroid problems, severe debilitation, dehydration, low sodium levels, and if you are pregnant, plan to become pregnant, or are breastfeeding.

What is the usual dosage?

The information below is based on the dosage guidelines your doctor uses. Depending on your condition and medical history, your doctor may prescribe a different regimen. Do not change the dosage or stop taking your medication without your doctor's approval.

Acute Mania in Bipolar Disorder

Adults: The optimal dose is 1800 milligrams (mg) daily and taken as 600 mg capsules three times daily. This medication is also available in liquid form and the optimal dose is 30 mL daily and it consists of 2 full teaspoons taken three times daily.

Maintenance Therapy for Bipolar Disorder

Adults: The optimal dose is different from one individual to another, however, the usual dose is 900 to 1200 mg daily taken as 300 mg tablets three or four times daily. If you are taking the liquid form, the recommended dose is 1 full teaspoon taken three or four times daily.

How should I take this medication?

Lithium carbonate capsules or tablets should be swallowed whole and should never be chewed or crushed. If you are taking the liquid form, do not take more than your recommended dose.

What should I avoid while taking this medication?

You should never stop taking this medication without consulting your doctor first. Driving or operating dangerous machinery or participating in any hazardous activity that requires full mental alertness should be avoided until you know how this drug affects you.

What are possible food and drug interactions associated with this medication?

If lithium carbonate is taken with certain other drugs, the effects of either could be increased, decreased, or altered. It is especially important to check with your doctor before combining this medication with any the following: acetazolamide, antidepressants, blood pressure medications, carbamazepine, desmopressin, haloperidol, methyldopa, metronidazole, monoamine oxidase inhibitors (MAOIs), methyldopa, nonsteroidal anti-inflammatory drugs (NSAIDs), phenytoin, potassium iodide, sodium bicarbonate, urea.

What are the possible side effects of this medication?

Side effects cannot be anticipated. If any develop or change in intensity, inform your doctor as soon as possible. Only your doctor can determine if it is safe for you to continue taking this drug.

Side effects may include: fine hand tremor, frequent urination, temporary and mild nausea, and general discomfort

Serious side effects may include: diarrhea, vomiting, drowsiness, muscular weakness, and lack of coordination may be early signs of lithium intoxication. Contact your doctor immediately if you experience any serious symptoms

Can I receive this medication if I am pregnant or breastfeeding?

Lithium carbonate should not be used during pregnancy as there is a risk of fetal death. Lithium carbonate is present in breast milk. Since its effects are unknown, its use should also be avoided. If you are pregnant or plan to become pregnant, tell your doctor immediately.

What should I do if I miss a dose of this medication?

If you miss a dose of this drug, skip it. Never take an extra dose to make up for a missed dose.

How should I store this medication?

Lithium carbonate should be stored at room temperature in a dry place and protected from light.

LITHOBID
Generic name: Lithium carbonate

What is this medication?
Lithobid is used in the treatment of manic episodes of patients with bipolar disorder. A manic episode is a time of abnormally elevated, unreserved, or irritable mood.

Lithobid is also used in the maintenance treatment of patients diagnosed with bipolar disorder.

What is the most important information I should know about this medication?
It may take up to 3 weeks before you see any improvement in your symptoms.

While taking Lithobid, it is very important that you follow your doctor's recommendations and make sure you do not miss any appointments or laboratory tests.

Toxic levels of this medication can occur at any dose and frequent blood tests will be required. You should stop taking Lithobid and contact your doctor immediately if you develop signs of lithium toxicity such as diarrhea, vomiting, tremor, mild lack of coordination, drowsiness, and muscular weakness.

The safety and efficacy of this medication is unknown in children under 12 years of age, and its use is not recommended.

Who should not take this medication?
Do not take this medication if you are allergic to lithium, Lithobid, Eskalith, Eskalith CR or any of their components.

What should I tell my doctor before I take the first dose of this medication?
Tell your doctor about all prescription, over-the-counter, and herbal medications you are taking before beginning treatment with Lithobid. Also, talk to your doctor about your complete medical history, especially if you have a history of kidney or heart disease, thyroid problems, severe debilitation, dehydration, low sodium levels, and if you are pregnant, plan to become pregnant, or are breastfeeding.

What is the usual dosage?
The information below is based on the dosage guidelines your doctor uses. Depending on your condition and medical history, your doctor may prescribe a different regimen. Do not change the dosage or stop taking your medication without your doctor's approval.

Acute Mania of Bipolar Disorder
Adults: The optimal dose is 1800 milligrams (mg) daily usually taken as three 300-mg tablets in the morning and three 300-mg tablets at night. Lithobid can also be taken in doses of 600 mg or 2 tablets three times daily.

Maintenance Treatment of Bipolar Disorder

Adults: The optimal dose is 900 to 1200 mg daily usually taken as two 300-mg tablets taken in the morning and two 300-mg tablets at night. Lithobid can also be taken three times daily up to a maximum daily dose of 1200 mg.

How should I take this medication?

Lithobid tablets should be swallowed whole. Never chew or crush this medication.

What should I avoid while taking this medication?

You should never stop taking this medication without consulting your doctor first. Driving or operating dangerous machinery or participating in any hazardous activity that requires full mental alertness should be avoided until you know how this drug affects you.

What are possible food and drug interactions associated with this medication?

If Lithobid is taken with certain other drugs, the effects of either could be increased, decreased, or altered. It is especially important to check with your doctor before combining this medication with any the following: acetazolamide, antidepressants, blood pressure medications, carbamazepine, desmopressin, monoamine oxidase inhibitors (MAOIs), methyldopa, metronidazole, nonsteroidal anti-inflammatory drugs (NSAIDs), phenytoin, potassium iodide, sodium bicarbonate, urea.

What are the possible side effects of this medication?

Side effects cannot be anticipated. If any develop or change in intensity, inform your doctor as soon as possible. Only your doctor can determine if it is safe for you to continue taking this drug.

Side effects may include: hand tremor, frequent urination, temporary and mild nausea, and general discomfort

Serious side effects may include: diarrhea, vomiting, drowsiness, muscular weakness, and lack of coordination may be early signs of lithium intoxication

Contact your doctor immediately if you experience any serious symptoms.

Can I receive this medication if I am pregnant or breastfeeding?

Lithobid should not be used during pregnancy as there is a risk of fetal death. Lithobid is present in breast milk. While its effects in nursing mothers are unknown, its use should also be avoided. If you are pregnant or plan to become pregnant, tell your doctor immediately.

What should I do if I miss a dose of this medication?

If you miss a dose of this drug, skip it. Never take an extra dose to make up for a missed dose.

How should I store this medication?

Lithobid should be stored at room temperature in a dry place and protected from light.

LUNESTA

Generic name: Eszopiclone

What is this medication?

Lunesta is a sleep medication known as a hypnotic. It is used to help if you have trouble falling asleep or staying asleep.

What is the most important information I should know about this medication?

If you do not experience an improvement after 7-10 days, contact your doctor to rule out other causes for your sleeping problems.

Inform your doctor immediately if you experience any changes in your behavior or mood, including aggression, agitation, hallucinations, depression, or suicidal thinking.

Lunesta works quickly, and can affect your ability to drive or operate heavy machinery, including the day after you take Lunesta. Do not engage in any activities that require mental alertness right after you take Lunesta or the next day until you know how Lunesta will affect you.

Rarely, Lunesta can cause short-term memory loss, which may be avoided if you are able to devote an entire night to sleep after taking Lunesta.

If you take Lunesta for more than several weeks, you may experience a dependence on Lunesta in order to fall asleep, or a decrease in Lunesta's ability to help you fall asleep.

Withdrawal symptoms may occur if you suddenly stop taking Lunesta, even after taking it for 1 week, but it is more likely to occur with long-term Lunesta therapy.

What should I tell my doctor before I take the first dose of this medication?

Tell your doctor about all prescription, over-the-counter, and herbal medications you are taking before beginning treatment with Lunesta. Also, talk to your doctor about your complete medical history, especially if you are over 65 years old, you are depressed or have a history of depression, or you have liver impairment or any disease that makes it difficult to breathe.

What is the usual dosage?

The information below is based on the dosage guidelines your doctor uses. Depending on your condition and medical history, your doctor may prescribe a different regimen. Do not change the dosage or stop taking your medication without your doctor's approval.

Adults: The usual starting dose of Lunesta is 2 milligrams (mg) taken once daily. Your doctor may increase your individual dose to 3 mg daily depending on how Lunesta affects you.

If you are over 65, you have liver impairment, or you are taking certain medications that interact with Lunesta, the usual starting dose is 1 mg daily, and may be increased by your doctor to 2 mg daily.

How should I take this medication?
Lunesta should be taken immediately before going to bed. Do not take Lunesta with or right after a meal, and do not take Lunesta unless you are able to get a full night's sleep (7 to 8 hours) before returning to your normal activities.

What should I avoid while taking this medication?
Avoid drinking alcohol while taking Lunesta. Also avoid operating an automobile or heavy machinery until you know how Lunesta will affect you.

What are possible food and drug interactions associated with this medication?
If Lunesta is taken with certain other drugs, the effects of either could be increased, decreased, or altered. It is especially important to check with your doctor before combining Lunesta with the following: alcohol, clarithromycin, itraconazole, ketoconazole, nefazodone, nelfinavir, olanzapine, other sleep-inducing drugs, ritonavir, rifampicin, troleandomycin.

What are the possible side effects of this medication?
Side effects cannot be anticipated. If any develop or change in intensity, tell your doctor as soon as possible. Only your doctor can determine if it is safe for you to continue taking this drug.

Side effects may include: lightheadedness, dizziness, headache, unpleasant taste, drowsiness, difficulty with coordination

Can I receive this medication if I am pregnant or breastfeeding?
Sleep medicines may cause sedation or other potential effects in the unborn baby when used during the last weeks of pregnancy. Be sure to tell your doctor if you are pregnant, if you are planning to become pregnant, or if you become pregnant while taking Lunesta. A very small amount of Lunesta may be present in breast milk after use of the medication. The effects of very small amounts of Lunesta on an infant are not known. Therefore, as with all other prescription sleep medicines, it is recommended that you not take Lunesta if you are breastfeeding a baby.

What should I do if I miss a dose of this medication?
If you forget to take a dose of Lunesta, do not double your next dose when you do remember. Take Lunesta as soon as you remember before you go to bed, as long as you can devote a full night to sleep.

How should I store this medication?
Store at room temperature.

LUVOX CR
Generic Name: Fluvoxamine maleate

What is this medication?
Luvox CR is used to treat social anxiety disorder, also known as social phobia. It is also used to treat obsessions and compulsions in patients with obsessive-compulsive disorder (OCD).

What is the most important information I should know about this medication?
Luvox CR is not approved for use in children.

Antidepressant medicines may increase suicidal thoughts or actions in some children, teenagers, and young adults when the medicine is first started. Depression and other serious mental illnesses are the most important causes of suicidal thoughts and actions. Some people may have a particularly high risk of having suicidal thoughts or actions. These include people who have (or have a family history of) bipolar disorder (also called manic-depressive illness) or suicidal thoughts or actions.

Pay close attention to any changes, especially sudden changes, in mood, behaviors, thoughts, or feelings. This is very important when an antidepressant medicine is first started or when the dose is changed.

Call the doctor right away to report new or sudden changes in mood, behavior, thoughts, or feelings. Signs to watch for include new or worsening depression, new or worsening anxiety, agitation, insomnia, hostility, panic attacks, restlessness, extreme hyperactivity, and suicidal thinking or behavior.

Keep all follow-up visits as scheduled, and call the doctor between visits as needed, especially if you have concerns about symptoms.

Who should not take this medication?
Luvox CR should not be taken if you have an allergy to fluvoxamine maleate or any of its ingredients.

What should I tell my doctor before I take the first dose of this medication?
Tell your doctor about all prescription, over-the-counter, and herbal medications you are taking before beginning treatment with Luvox CR. Also, talk to your doctor about your complete medical history, especially if you have a history of mental health problems. You need to inform your doctor if you are pregnant or planning to become pregnant or are breastfeeding.

What is the usually dosage?
The information below is based on the dosage guidelines your doctor uses. Depending on your condition and medical history, your doctor

may prescribe a different regimen. Do not change the dosage or stop taking your medication without your doctor's approval.

Adults: The recommended starting dose for Luvox CR is 100 milligrams (mg) once daily.

How should I take this medication?
Luvox CR can be taken with or without food as a single daily dose at bedtime. Do not crush or chew capsules

What should I avoid while taking this medication?
Avoid driving or operating machinery until you are certain how this medication affects you.

Avoid drugs that affect the brain as they may impair judgment, thinking, or motor skills when taken with Luvox CR.

What are possible food and drug interactions associated with this medication?
If Luvox CR is taken with certain drugs, the effects of either could be increased, decreased, or altered. It is important to check with your doctor before combining Luvox CR with the following: alcohol, antidepressants (such as amitriptyline, clomipramine, or imipramine), antipsychotics (such as clozapine and thioridazine), aspirin, beta-blockers, carbamazepine, clozapine, diltiazem, lithium, lorazepam, MAOIs, methadone, NSAIDs (such as such as ibuprofen or naproxen), propranolol, ramelteon, serotonergic drugs, sumatriptan, tacrine, thioridazine, tizanidine, tranquilizers and sedatives (such as alprazolam, diazepam, midazolam, and triazolam), triptans, tryptophan, warfarin.

You should also not take Luvox CR with drugs that are metabolized by a certain liver enzyme (CYP450). Your doctor will check for this interaction.

What are the possible side effects of this medication?
Side effects cannot be anticipated. If any develop or change in intensity, tell your doctor as soon as possible. Only your doctor can determine if it is safe for you to continue taking this drug.

Side effects may include: sleepiness, sweating, tremor, abnormal ejaculation, loss of appetite, weakness, diarrhea, nausea, stomach upset, dizziness, sleeplessness, yawning, anxiety, decreased libido, vomiting, and muscle pain

Can I receive this medication if I am pregnant or breastfeeding?
Notify your doctor if you become pregnant or intend to become pregnant during therapy with Luvox CR. Fluvoxamine is secreted in human breast milk. Because of the potential for serious adverse reactions in nursing infants from Luvox CR, a decision should be made whether to discontinue nursing or discontinue the drug, taking into account the importance of the drug to the mother.

How should I store this medication?

Luvox CR should be protected from high humidity and stored at room temperature. Avoid exposure to temperatures above 30°C (86°F).

MAPROTILINE HYDROCHLORIDE

What is this medication?

Maprotiline hydrochloride tablets are used to treat depression. Maprotiline is also used for the relief of anxiety associated with depression.

What is the most important information I should know about this medication?

Antidepressant medicines may increase suicidal thoughts or actions in some children, teenagers, and young adults when the medicine is first started. Depression and other serious mental illnesses are the most important causes of suicidal thoughts and actions. Some people may have a particularly high risk of having suicidal thoughts or actions. These include people who have (or have a family history of) bipolar disorder (also called manic-depressive illness) or suicidal thoughts or actions.

Pay close attention to any changes, especially sudden changes, in mood, behaviors, thoughts, or feelings. This is very important when an antidepressant medicine is first started or when the dose is changed.

Call the doctor right away to report new or sudden changes in mood, behavior, thoughts, or feelings. Signs to watch for include new or worsening depression, new or worsening anxiety, agitation, insomnia, hostility, panic attacks, restlessness, extreme hyperactivity, and suicidal thinking or behavior.

Keep all follow-up visits as scheduled, and call the doctor between visits as needed, especially if you have concerns about symptoms.

Who should not take this medication?

You should not take maprotiline if you are allergic to any of its components.

You should not take maprotiline if you have a known or suspected seizure disorder.

Do not take maprotiline with a monoamine oxidase inhibitor (MAOI) or within 14 days after discontinuing an MAOI.

What should I tell my doctor before I take the first dose of this medication?

Tell your doctor about all prescription, over-the-counter, and herbal medications you are taking before beginning treatment with maprotiline. Talk to your doctor about your complete medical history, especially past or current heart problems, seizures, history of depression or suicidality, or history or family history of psychiatric illness, such as bipolar disorder. Tell your doctor if you have glaucoma, an enlarged prostate, bladder problems, or an overactive thyroid.

Tell your doctor if you are planning to have surgery, or plan to have it while taking maprotiline.

What is the usual dosage?

The information below is based on the dosage guidelines your doctor uses. Depending on your condition and medical history, your doctor may prescribe a different regimen. Do not change the dosage or stop taking your medication without your doctor's approval.

Adults: The usual starting dose for patients with mild to moderate depression is 75 milligrams (mg) daily. In elderly patients, maprotiline may be started at a lower dosage, such as 25 mg until the drug's effects are known.

The initial dose should be maintained for 2 weeks and may be gradually increased in increments of 25 mg as required and as tolerated.

In most patients, a maximum dose is 150 mg daily.

How should I take this medication?

Take maprotiline as directed by your physician.

What should I avoid while taking this medication?

Avoid drinking alcohol while taking maprotiline; once you speak with your doctor about your individual case, he or she may tell you to avoid other medications and/or foods.

What are possible food and drug interactions associated with this medication?

If maprotiline is taken with certain other drugs, the effects of either could be increased, decreased, or altered. It is especially important to check with your doctor before combining maprotiline with the following: barbiturates, benzodiazepines (such as Xanax and Valium), cimetidine, electroshock therapy, fluoxetine, phenytoin, thyroid medications.

What are the possible side effects of this medication?

Side effects cannot be anticipated. If any develop or change in intensity, tell your doctor as soon as possible. Only your doctor can determine if it is safe for you to continue taking this drug.

Side effects may include: fluctuations in blood pressure, shortness of breath, nervousness, insomnia, nightmares, dizziness, drowsiness, dry mouth, decreased urination, nausea, sexual dysfunction

Can I receive this medication if I am pregnant or breastfeeding?

The effects of maprotiline are not known during pregnancy. There are no adequate and well-controlled studies in pregnant women. Discuss with your doctor if you are pregnant or plan on becoming pregnant. Also, maprotiline is secreted in breast milk, so consult with your physician before breastfeeding.

What should I do if I miss a dose of this medication?
If you miss a dose, take it as soon as you remember. If it is almost time for your next dose, skip the missed dose, and resume your normal dosage schedule.

How should I store this medication?
Store maprotiline at room temperature; away from heat, light, and moisture.

MEBARAL
Generic name: Mephobarbital

What is this medication?
Mebaral is used as a sedative for the relief of anxiety, tension, and apprehension, and as an anticonvulsant to prevent seizures (epilepsy). Mebaral is a barbiturate and works by depressing the central nervous system.

What is the most important information I should know about this medication?
Mebaral may decrease the effectiveness of your birth control pills. To prevent pregnancy, use an additional form of birth control while you are using Mebaral and for a month after stopping it.

When using Mebaral for long periods of time or at high doses, tolerance may develop; you may require higher doses to obtain the same effect as when you first started taking this drug. Talk with your doctor if Mebaral stops working well.

Some people who use Mebaral for an extended period may develop dependence or a need to continue taking it. If you stop taking Mebaral suddenly, you may have withdrawal symptoms that may include anxiety, nausea, sleeplessness, and body aches. Contact your doctor if you experience any of these symptoms.

Do not stop taking Mebaral suddenly or change the dose without asking your doctor.

Do not drive or perform other possibly unsafe tasks until you know how you react to Mebaral; this drug may cause dizziness, drowsiness, or blurred vision. These effects may be worse if you take it with alcohol or certain medicines.

Do not drink alcohol or use medicines that may cause drowsiness (such as sleep aids and muscle relaxants) while you are using Mebaral; it may add to their effects.

Tell your doctor or dentist that you take Mebaral before you receive any medical or dental care, emergency care, or surgery.

Who should not take this medication?
Do not use Mebaral if you are allergic to it or any other ingredient found in this product. Do not use Mebaral if you have the blood disorder porphyria.

What should I tell my doctor before I take the first dose of this medication?

Tell your doctor about all prescription, over-the-counter, and herbal medications you are taking before beginning treatment with Mebaral. Also, talk to your doctor about your complete medical history, especially if you have depression, pain, lung or breathing problems, heart problems, myasthenia gravis (muscle problems), a history of substance abuse or dependence, and suicidal thoughts or behaviors.

What is the usual dosage?

The information below is based on the dosage guidelines your doctor uses. Depending on your condition and medical history, your doctor may prescribe a different regimen. Do not change the dosage or stop taking your medication without your doctor's approval.

Epilepsy

Adults: The average recommended dose is 400 milligrams (mg) to 600 mg daily.

Children >5 years: The average recommended dose is 32 mg to 64 mg three or four times a day for children >5 years of age.

Children <5 years: The average recommended dose is 16 mg to 32 mg three or four times a day for children <5 years of age.

Sedation

Adults: The average recommended dose is 32 mg to 100 mg. The optimum dose is 50 mg three to four times daily.

Children: The average recommended dose is 16 mg to 32 mg three to four times a day.

Dosage should be reduced in the elderly or debilitated because these patients may be more sensitive to Mebaral. Dosage should be reduced for patients with impaired kidney function or liver disease.

How should I take this medication?

Mebaral is best taken at bedtime if seizures generally occur at night and during the day if attacks are during the day. Treatment should be started with a small dose which is gradually increased over four or five days until the optimum dosage is determined. If the patient has been taking another antiepileptic drug, it should be tapered off as the doses of Mebaral are increased. This is to prevent any seizures that may occur when any treatment for epilepsy is changed abruptly. Similarly, when the dose is lowered to a maintenance level or to be discontinued, the amount should be reduced gradually over four or five days.

Mebaral is taken by mouth with or without food daily.

Take Mebaral at the same time each day to receive the most benefit from this drug.

What should I avoid while taking this medication?

Do not stop taking Mebaral suddenly or change the dose without asking your doctor.

Do not drive or perform other possibly unsafe tasks until you know how you react to Mebaral; this drug may cause dizziness, drowsiness, or blurred vision.

Do not drink alcohol or use medicines that may cause drowsiness (such as sleep aids and muscle relaxants) while you are using Mebaral; it may add to their effects.

What are possible food and drug interactions associated with this medication?

If Mebaral is taken with certain other drugs, the effects of either could be increased, decreased, or altered. It is especially important to check with your doctor before combining Mebaral with the following: anticoagulants such as warfarin, beta-blockers such as propranolol, clozapine, corticosteroids, cyclosporine, doxorubicin, doxycycline, estrogens such as estradiol, griseofulvin, hydantoins such as phenytoin, imatinib, metronidazole, monoamine oxidase inhibitors (MAOIs) such as phenelzine and selegiline, oral contraceptives, quinidine, quinine, sodium oxybate (GHB), stiripentol, theophylline, valproic acid, voriconazole.

What are the possible side effects of this medication?

Side effects cannot be anticipated. If any develop or change in intensity, tell your doctor as soon as possible. Only your doctor can determine if it is safe for you to continue taking this drug.

Side effects may include: clumsiness, dizziness, drowsiness, excessive daytime drowsiness ("hangover effect"), fatigue, feeling like things are whirling, headache, lightheadedness, nausea, tired feeling, vomiting, weak bones, confusion, difficulty sleeping, fainting, very slow breathing and severe allergic reactions (rash, hives, difficulty breathing, tightness in the chest, swelling of the mouth, face, lips, or tongue)

Can I receive this medication if I am pregnant or breastfeeding?

Mebaral has been shown to cause fetal harm. If you think you may be pregnant, contact your doctor. You will need to discuss the benefits and risks of using Mebaral while you are pregnant.

Mebaral is found in breast milk. Do not breastfeed while taking Mebaral.

What should I do if I miss a dose of this medication?

If you miss a dose of Mebaral, take it as soon as possible. If it is almost time for your next dose, skip the missed dose and go back to your regular dosing schedule. Do not take two doses at once.

How should I store this medication?
Store Mebaral at room temperature in a tightly closed container. Store away from heat, moisture, and light. Do not store in the bathroom.

MEPROBAMATE

What is this medication?
Meprobamate is used in the treatment of anxiety disorders or for the short-term relief of the symptoms of anxiety.

What is the most important information I should know about this medication?
Meprobamate should not be used in children under age six.

The effectiveness of this medication for long-term use or more than 4 months is not known, therefore, your doctor may periodically reassess your condition to see if this drug is working for you.

There have been reports of addiction or becoming physically and/or psychologically dependent to this medication. If you take more than prescribed, you may experience symptoms that include lack of coordination, slurred speech, and dizziness.

Meprobamate may occasionally precipitate seizures in patients with epilepsy.

Who should not take this medication?
Do not take if you are allergic to meprobamate or related compounds such as carisoprodol, mebutamate, tybamate, or carbromal.

What should I tell my doctor before I take the first dose of this medication?
Tell your doctor about all prescription, over-the-counter, and herbal medications you are taking before beginning treatment with meprobamate. Also, talk to your doctor about your complete medical history, especially if you have a history of alcohol or drug abuse, kidney or liver problems, and if you are pregnant, planning to become pregnant, or are breastfeeding.

What is the usual dosage?
The information below is based on the dosage guidelines your doctor uses. Depending on your condition and medical history, your doctor may prescribe a different regimen. Do not change the dosage or stop taking your medication without your doctor's approval.

Adults: The usual adult daily dose is 1200 milligrams (mg) to 1600 mg, in three or four divided doses. The maximum daily dose is 2400 mg.
Children >6 years: The usual daily dose for children ages 6 to 12 is 200 mg to 600 mg, in two to three divided doses. Meprobamate is not recommended in children under age 6.

How should I take this medication?
Take this medication exactly as indicated by your doctor.

What should I avoid while taking this medication?
You should never stop taking this medication without consulting your doctor first.

Driving or operating dangerous machinery or participating in any hazardous activity that requires full mental alertness should be avoided until you know how this drug affects you.

Avoid drinking alcohol while taking meprobamate.

What are possible food and drug interactions associated with this medication?
If meprobamate is taken with certain other drugs, the effects of either could be increased, decreased, or altered. It is especially important to check with your doctor before combining this medication with alcohol or other antidepressants.

What are the possible side effects of this medication?
Side effects cannot be anticipated. If any develop or change in intensity, inform your doctor as soon as possible. Only your doctor can determine if it is safe for you to continue taking this drug.

Side effects may include: euphoria, palpitations, increased heart rate, drowsiness, dizziness, headache, nausea

Can I receive this medication if I am pregnant or breastfeeding?
Meprobamate should not be used during pregnancy as there is an increased risk of fetal harm, especially during the first trimester. The effects of meprobamate in nursing mothers are unknown; however, studies have shown that it is present in breast milk and its use should be avoided. If you are pregnant or planning to become pregnant, tell your doctor immediately.

What should I do if I miss a dose of this medication?
If you miss a dose, skip it. Never take an extra dose to make up for a missed dose.

How should I store this medication?
Store at room temperature.

METADATE CD/METADATE ER
Generic name: Methylphenidate hydrochloride

What is this medication?
Metadate and other brands of methylphenidate are medications known as stimulants and are used in the treatment of attention-deficit/hyperactivity disorder (ADHD).

What is the most important information I should know about this medication?

Metadate should be an integral part of a total treatment program for ADHD that includes psychological, educational, and social measures. Symptoms of ADHD include continual problems with moderate to severe distractibility, short attention span, hyperactivity, emotional changeability, and impulsiveness.

There are reports of heart and mental problems in patients taking Metadate or other related stimulants. Some of the problems are sudden death in patients with previous heart problems, heart attacks in adults, increased blood pressure and heart rate. Metadate can also cause new or worsening symptoms of behavior problems, bipolar illness, and aggressive or hostile behavior. Call your doctor right away if you or child develops signs of heart problems such as chest pain, shortness of breath, or fainting while taking Metadate.

Excessive doses of Metadate over a long period of time may cause addiction. It is also possible to develop tolerance to the drug, so that larger doses are needed to produce the original effect. Be sure to check with your doctor before making any change in dosage; and stop the drug only under your doctor's supervision.

There is no information regarding the safety and effectiveness of long-term treatment in children. However, slowing of growth has been seen with the long-term use of stimulants, so your doctor will monitor your child carefully while he or she is taking Metadate.

The use of Metadate in children less than 6 years old is not recommended.

Who should not take this medication?

Metadate should not be taken if you or your child are very anxious, tense, or agitated, have glaucoma, experience tics or have Tourette's syndrome.

Do not take Metadate within 14 days of taking antidepressants called monoamine oxidase inhibitors (MAOIs), or if you are allergic to anything in Metadate.

What should I tell my doctor before I take the first dose of this medication?

Tell your doctor about all prescription, over-the-counter, and herbal medications you are taking before beginning treatment with Metadate, especially if you are currently taking or have recently taken MAOIs. Also, talk to your doctor about your complete medical history, especially if you have a history of heart problems such as congenital heart defects, heart failure, heart rhythm disorder or recent heart attack, high blood pressure, a personal or family history of mental illness, psychotic disorder, bipolar disorder, depression, suicide attempt, seizures or other convulsion disorders, a history of drug or alcohol addiction, glaucoma, a personal or family history of tics (muscle twitches) or Tourette's syndrome, severe anxiety, tension, or agitation.

What is the usual dosage?
The information below is based on the dosage guidelines your doctor uses. Depending on your condition and medical history, your doctor may prescribe a different regimen. Do not change the dosage or stop taking your medication without your doctor's approval.

Metadate CD
Adults: The recommended starting dose is 20 milligrams (mg) once daily. Your doctor may increase your dose in 10- to 20-mg increments at weekly intervals up to a maximum daily dose of 60 mg.
Children ≥6 years: The recommended starting dose is 20 mg once daily. At weekly intervals, your doctor may increase your child's dose in 10 to 20 mg increments up to a maximum daily dose of 60 mg.

Metadate ER
Adults: These are extended-release tablets that keep working for 8 hours. Your doctor will determine your exact dose.
Children ≥6 years: These tablets keep working for 8 hours, and your doctor will determine the exact dose for your child.

This drug should not be given to children under 6 years of age.

How should I take this medication?
Follow your doctor's directions carefully. Metadate CD may also be given by sprinkling the contents of the capsule on a tablespoon of cool applesauce and administering immediately, followed by a drink of water. Do not crush or chew the capsule contents.

Metadate ER tablets must be swallowed whole and never chewed or crushed.

What should I avoid while taking this medication?
Some people have had visual disturbances such as blurred vision while being treated with Metadate. Be careful if you drive or do anything that requires you to be awake and alert until you know how this medication affects you.

What are possible food and drug interactions associated with this medication?
If Metadate is taken with certain other drugs, the effects of either could be increased, decreased, or altered. It is especially important to check with your doctor before combining Metadate with any of the following: antidepressants, antiseizure drugs, blood pressure drugs, blood thinners such as warfarin, clonidine, guanethidine, MAOIs, phenylbutazone.

What are the possible side effects of this medication?

Side effects cannot be anticipated. If any develop or change in intensity, tell your doctor as soon as possible. Only your doctor can determine if it is safe for you to continue taking this drug.

Side effects may include: inability to fall or stay asleep, nervousness

These side effects can usually be controlled by reducing the dosage and omitting the drug in the afternoon or evening.

More common side effects in children may include: loss of appetite, abdominal pain, weight loss during long-term therapy, inability to fall or stay asleep, abnormally fast heartbeat

Can I receive this medication if I am pregnant or breastfeeding?

The effects of Metadate during pregnancy and breastfeeding are unknown. Tell your doctor immediately if you are pregnant, plan to become pregnant, or are breastfeeding.

What should I do if I miss a dose of this medication?

Take the missed dose as soon as you remember. If it is almost time for your next dose, skip the missed dose and take the medicine at your next regularly scheduled time. Do not take a double dose to make up for the missed dose.

How should I store this medication?

Store at room temperature in a tightly closed, light-resistant container, and protect from moisture.

METHYLIN/METHYLIN ER

Generic name: Methylphenidate hydrochloride

What is this medication?

Methylin and other brands of methylphenidate are medications known as stimulants and are used in the treatment of attention-deficit/hyperactivity disorder (ADHD). Methylin may help increase attention and decrease impulsiveness and hyperactivity in ADHD patients.

Methylin is also prescribed for the treatment of narcolepsy.

What is the most important information I should know about this medication?

Methylin should be an integral part of a total treatment program for ADHD that includes psychological, educational, and social measures. Symptoms of ADHD include continual problems with moderate to severe distractibility, short attention span, hyperactivity, emotional changeability, and impulsiveness.

There are reports of heart and mental problems in patients taking Methylin or other related stimulants. Some of the problems are sudden death in patients with previous heart problems, heart attacks in adults, increased blood pressure and heart rate. Methylin can also cause new or worsening symptoms of behavior problems, bipolar disorder, and aggressive or hostile behavior. Call your doctor right away if you or child develops signs of heart problems such as chest pain, shortness of breath, or fainting while taking Methylin.

Excessive doses of Methylin over a long period of time may cause addiction. It is also possible to develop tolerance to the drug, so that larger doses are needed to produce the original effect. Be sure to check with your doctor before making any change in dosage; and stop the drug only under your doctor's supervision.

There is no information regarding the safety and effectiveness of long-term treatment in children. However, slowing of growth has been seen with the long-term use of stimulants, so your doctor will monitor your child carefully while he or she is taking Methylin.

The use of Methylin in children less than 6 years old is not recommended.

Who should not take this medication?

Methylin should not be taken if you or your child are very anxious, tense, or agitated, have glaucoma, thyroid problems, heart problems or recent heart attack, or experience tics or have Tourette's syndrome.

Do not take Methylin within 14 days of taking antidepressants called monoamine oxidase inhibitors (MAOIs), or if you are allergic to anything in Methylin.

What should I tell my doctor before I take the first dose of this medication?

Tell your doctor about all prescription, over-the-counter, and herbal medications you are taking before beginning treatment with Methylin, especially if you are currently taking or have recently taken MAOIs. Also, talk to your doctor about your complete medical history, especially if you have a history of heart problems such as congenital heart defects, heart failure, heart rhythm disorder or recent heart attack, high blood pressure, a personal or family history of mental illness, psychotic disorder, bipolar disorder, depression, suicide attempt, epilepsy or other seizure disorders, a history of drug or alcohol addiction, glaucoma, a personal or family history of tics (muscle twitches) or Tourette's syndrome, severe anxiety, tension, or agitation.

What is the usual dosage?

The information below is based on the dosage guidelines your doctor uses. Depending on your condition and medical history, your doctor may prescribe a different regimen. Do not change the dosage or stop taking your medication without your doctor's approval.

Methylin

Adults: The average dosage is 20 to 30 milligrams (mg) a day, divided into 2 or 3 doses, preferably taken 30 to 45 minutes before meals. Some people may need 40 to 60 mg daily, others only 10 to 15 mg. Your doctor will determine the best dose.

Children ≥6 years: The usual starting dose is 5 mg taken twice a day, before breakfast and lunch; your doctor may increase the dose by 5 to 10 mg a week. Your child should not take more than 60 mg in a day. If you do not see any improvement over a period of one month, check with your doctor.

Methylin ER

Adults: These are extended-release tablets that keep working for 8 hours. They may be used in place of Methylin tablets and your doctor will determine the best dose.

Children ≥6 years: Your child's doctor will decide if these extended-release tablets should be used in place of the regular tablets.

This drug should not be given to children under 6 years of age.

How should I take this medication?

Follow your doctor's directions carefully. Methylin tablets should be taken 30 to 45 minutes before meals. Methylin ER tablets must be swallowed whole and never chewed or crushed.

What should I avoid while taking this medication?

Some people have had visual disturbances such as blurred vision while being treated with Methylin. Be careful if you drive or do anything that requires you to be awake and alert.

What are possible food and drug interactions associated with this medication?

If Methylin is taken with certain other drugs, the effects of either could be increased, decreased, or altered. It is especially important to check with your doctor before combining Methylin with any of the following: antidepressants, antiseizure drugs, blood pressure drugs, blood thinners such as warfarin, clonidine, guanethidine, MAOIs, phenylbutazone.

What are the possible side effects of this medication?

Side effects cannot be anticipated. If any develop or change in intensity, tell your doctor as soon as possible. Only your doctor can determine if it is safe for you to continue taking this drug.

Side effects may include: inability to fall or stay asleep, nervousness

These side effects can usually be controlled by reducing the dosage and omitting the drug in the afternoon or evening.

More common side effects in children may include: loss of appetite, abdominal pain, weight loss during long-term therapy, inability to fall or stay asleep, abnormally fast heartbeat

Can I receive this medication if I am pregnant or breastfeeding?
The effects of Methylin during pregnancy and breastfeeding are unknown. Tell your doctor immediately if you are pregnant, plan to become pregnant, or are breastfeeding.

What should I do if I miss a dose of this medication?
Take the missed dose as soon as you remember. If it is almost time for your next dose, skip the missed dose and take the medicine at your next regularly scheduled time. Do not take a double dose to make up the missed dose.

How should I store this medication?
Store at room temperature in a tightly closed, light-resistant container, and protect from moisture.

MOBAN
Generic name: Molindone hydrochloride

What is this medication?
Moban is used to treat the symptoms of schizophrenia.

What is the most important information I should know about this medication?
Moban can cause tardive dyskinesia, a serious sometimes irreversible movement disorder that causes involuntary movements of muscles. The risk for tardive dyskinesia is higher in the elderly and for women. Tell your doctor immediately if you experience any involuntary muscle movements while taking Moban.

Moban can also cause another serious, sometime fatal, disorder known as neuroleptic malignant syndrome, characterized by muscle stiffness, increased body temperature, sweating, changes in mood or consciousness, and a rapid or irregular heartbeat. If you experience any of these symptoms while taking Moban, seek emergency medical attention immediately.

Moban is not to be used with other agents that cause central nervous system depression, such as alcohol, barbiturates, or narcotic pain killers.

Moban should not be used in elderly patients with dementia-related psychosis, since this puts them at an increased risk of serious side effects, including death.

Who should not take this medication?
Do not take Moban if you are allergic to molindone or any other ingredient in Moban.

Moban should not be administered to anyone in a comatose state.

Elderly patients with dementia-related psychosis should not receive Moban due to an increased risk of death.

What should I tell my doctor before I take the first dose of this medication?

Tell your doctor about all prescription, over-the-counter, and herbal medication you are taking before beginning treatment with Moban. Also, talk to your doctor about your complete medical history, especially if you have a history of tardive dyskinesia, neuroleptic malignant syndrome, or have been previously diagnosed with breast cancer.

What is the usual dosage?

The information below is based on the dosage guidelines your doctor uses. Depending on your condition and medical history, your doctor may prescribe a different regimen. Do not change the dosage or stop taking your medication without your doctor's approval.

Adults and Children ≥12: The usual starting dose is 50 milligrams (mg) to 75 mg per day. Your doctor may increase your dose to 100 mg after 3-4 days of treatment. Based on your individual condition, your dose may be further increased up to 225 mg per day. The dose is usually divided in three to four intervals.

How should I take this medication?

Moban can be taken with or without food. It should be taken at the same time every day.

What should I avoid while taking this medication?

You should not drink alcohol while taking Moban. Moban may cause you to feel drowsy, so you should not operate an automobile or heavy machinery until you know how this medication will affect you. Exercise caution when participating in activities that require alertness.

What are possible food and drug interactions associated with this medication?

If Moban is taken with certain other drugs, the effects of either could be increased, decreased, or altered. It is especially important to check with your doctor before combining Moban with alcohol, barbiturates, or narcotic medications.

Also, be aware that Moban tablets contain calcium, which may interfere with the absorption of tetracycline medications and phenytoin.

What are the possible side effects of this medication?

Side effects cannot be anticipated. If any develop or change in intensity, tell your doctor as soon as possible. Only your doctor can determine if it is safe for you to continue taking this drug.

Side effects may include: dizziness, drowsiness, immobility, involuntary muscle contractions, involuntary muscle movements, muscle restlessness, muscle stiffness, muscle tremors

Can I receive this medication if I am pregnant or breastfeeding?
The effects of Moban during pregnancy and breastfeeding are unknown. Tell your doctor immediately if you are pregnant, plan to become pregnant, or are breastfeeding.

What should I do if I miss a dose of this medication?
If you miss a dose, take it as soon as you remember. If it is almost time for your next dose, skip the dose you missed and take your next regular dose. Do not double your dose to make up for a missed dose.

How should I store this medication?
Moban should be stored at room temperature in a tightly-closed container and away from light.

NARDIL
Generic name: Phenelzine sulfate

What is this medication?
Nardil is a prescription medication known as an MAOI (monoamine oxidase inhibitor) that is used to treat a serious medical disorder known as depression. Nardil is often used in the treatment of depression associated with anxiety, phobias, or other neurotic behaviors.

What is the most important information I should know about this medication?
Antidepressant medicines may increase suicidal thoughts or actions in some children, teenagers, and young adults when the medicine is first started. Depression and other serious mental illnesses are the most important causes of suicidal thoughts and actions. Some people may have a particularly high risk of having suicidal thoughts or actions. These include people who have (or have a family history of) bipolar disorder (also called manic-depressive illness) or suicidal thoughts or actions.

Pay close attention to any changes, especially sudden changes, in mood, behaviors, thoughts, or feelings. This is very important when an antidepressant medicine is first started or when the dose is changed.

Call the doctor right away to report new or sudden changes in mood, behavior, thoughts, or feelings. Signs to watch for include new or worsening depression, new or worsening anxiety, agitation, insomnia, hostility, panic attacks, restlessness, extreme hyperactivity, and suicidal thinking or behavior.

Keep all follow-up visits as scheduled, and call the doctor between visits as needed, especially if you have concerns about symptoms.

Nardil is a monoamine oxidase inhibitor (MAOI). This class of drugs, including Nardil, can cause a sudden, large increase in blood pressure (hypertensive crisis) if you consume foods and drinks that contain high amounts of tyramine.

You should use caution when taking Nardil if you have diabetes, schizophrenia, or epilepsy.

Nardil may also cause low blood pressure, which can lead to dizziness, lightheadedness, or fainting.

Nardil should be discontinued at least 10 days before undergoing any type of surgery that requires anesthesia or numbing agents.

You should wait at least 14 days between the discontinuation of Nardil and starting therapy with another antidepressant of any class.

Who should not take this medication?
You should not take Nardil if you are allergic or sensitive to phenelzine sulfate or any other ingredient in Nardil; if you have a condition known as "pheochromocytoma," congestive heart failure, severe kidney impairment or disease, liver disease, or abnormal liver function tests.

What should I tell my doctor before I take the first dose of this medication?
Tell your doctor about all prescription, over-the-counter, and herbal medications you are taking before beginning treatment with Nardil. Also, talk to your doctor about your complete medical history, especially if you have a history or family history of suicide or suicidal thoughts, bipolar disorder, liver or kidney disease, heart disease, epilepsy, or schizophrenia.

What is the usual dosage?
The information below is based on the dosage guidelines your doctor uses. Depending on your condition and medical history, your doctor may prescribe a different regimen. Do not change the dosage or stop taking your medication without your doctor's approval.

Adults: The usual starting dose is 15 milligrams (mg) taken three times a day. Your doctor will likely increase your daily dose over the course of several weeks to 60 mg to 90 mg per day in divided daily doses. After maximum benefit from Nardil is achieved, dosage should be reduced slowly over several weeks. Maintenance dose may be as low as one tablet, 15 mg, a day or every other day, and should be continued for as long as required.

How should I take this medication?
Nardil can be taken with or without food (see list of foods to avoid below) and should be taken at the same time every day.

What should I avoid while taking this medication?
While on Nardil, avoid tyramine-rich foods such as dried or aged meats (sausages/salami), fava beans, aged cheeses, beer on tap, yeast, sauerkraut, and soybean products.

Avoid taking any cold and cough preparations (including those containing dextromethorphan); nasal decongestants (tablets, drops, or spray); allergy, sinus, and asthma medications; weight-loss, or L-tryptophan-containing preparations.

Avoid the concurrent use of "sympathomimetic" drugs (including amphetamines, cocaine, methylphenidate, dopamine, epinephrine, and norepinephrine) or related compounds (including methyldopa, L-dopa, L-tryptophan, L-tyrosine, and phenylalanine).

What are possible food and drug interactions associated with this medication?

If Nardil is taken with certain other drugs, the effects of either could be increased, decreased, or altered. It is especially important to check with your doctor before combining Nardil with the following: allergy medicines, amitriptyline, amoxapine, appetite suppressants, asthma medicines, carbamazepine, citalopram, clomipramine, cold and cough preparations, cyclobenzaprine, decongestants, desipramine, dexfenfluramine, dextromethorphan, doxepin, fluoxetine, fluvoxamine, guanethidine, imipramine, L-tryptophan-containing preparations, maprotiline, meperidine, mirtazapine, nortriptyline, paroxetine, perphenazine and amitriptyline, protriptyline, rauwolfia alkaloids, sertraline, trimipramine, venlafaxine.

Nardil should be used with caution in combination with antihypertensive drugs, including thiazide diuretics and beta blockers, since low blood pressure may result.

What are the possible side effects of this medication?

Side effects cannot be anticipated. If any develop or change in intensity, tell your doctor as soon as possible. Only your doctor can determine if it is safe for you to continue taking this drug.

Side effects may include: dizziness, headache, drowsiness, trouble sleeping, fatigue, muscle twitching, trouble balancing, psychosis, decreased sexual ability, dry mouth, constipation, weight gain, trouble urinating, rash, itching skin, weakness, blurred vision, glaucoma, sweating, liver injury

Can I receive this medication if I am pregnant or breastfeeding?

The effects of Nardil during pregnancy and breastfeeding are unknown. Tell your doctor immediately if you are pregnant, plan to become pregnant, or are breastfeeding.

What should I do if I miss a dose of this medication?

You should not double your dose of Nardil. Skip the missed dose and return to your normal dosing schedule.

How should I store this medication?

Store at room temperature.

NAVANE
Generic name: Thiothixene

What is this medication?
Navane is an antipsychotic medication that affects certain receptors in the brain and is used to treat schizophrenia.

What is the most important information I should know about this medication?
Navane can cause tardive dyskinesia, a serious, sometimes irreversible movement disorder that causes involuntary movements of muscles. The risk for tardive dyskinesia is higher in the elderly and for women. Tell your doctor immediately if you experience any involuntary muscle movements while taking Navane.

Navane can also cause another serious sometime fatal disorder known as neuroleptic malignant syndrome, characterized by muscle stiffness, increased body temperature, sweating, changes in mood or consciousness, and a rapid or irregular heartbeat. If you experience any of these symptoms while taking Navane, seek emergency medical attention immediately.

Navane should be used with caution in patients who might be exposed to extreme heat or who are receiving atropine. Navane should also be used with caution in patients with cardiovascular disease. Careful adjustment of dosage is indicated when Navane is used with other CNS depressants.

Who should not take this medication?
You should not take Navane if you are sensitive or allergic to any ingredient in Navane.

Navane should not be administered to anyone in a comatose state.

Do not take Navane if you are taking a sleep aid or any other substance that slows your central nervous system.

If you have had circulatory system collapse or if you have an abnormal bone marrow or blood condition, you should not take Navane.

What should I tell my doctor before I take the first dose of this medication?
Tell your doctor about all prescription, over-the-counter, and herbal medications you are taking before beginning treatment with Navane. Also, talk to your doctor about your complete medical history, especially if you have a history of tardive dyskinesia or neuroleptic malignant syndrome (see "**What is the most important information I should know about this medication?**") Let your doctor know if you have liver disease, breast cancer, seizures, high or low blood pressure, depression, lupus, heart disease, or if you are or have been alcohol dependent. Also, let your doctor know if you are pregnant, plan to become pregnant, or are breastfeeding.

What is the usual dosage?
The information below is based on the dosage guidelines your doctor uses. Depending on your condition and medical history, your doctor may prescribe a different regimen. Do not change the dosage or stop taking your medication without your doctor's approval.

The use of Navane in children under 12 years of age is not approved.

The usual daily dose is 20-30 milligrams (mg) once daily. Dosage is individually adjusted depending on the severity of the patient's disease state. Initially, small doses are used. Further gradual increase is based on patient response and the optimal effect of the drug.

For Milder Conditions
Adults and Children ≥12 years: The usual starting dosage is 2 mg taken 3 times a day. Your doctor may increase the dose to a total of 15 mg a day.

For More Severe Conditions
Adults and Children ≥12 years: The usual starting dosage is 5 mg taken two times a day. Your doctor may increase this dose to a total of 60 mg a day. Exceeding a total daily dose of 60 mg rarely increases the beneficial response.

How should I take this medication?
Navane can be taken with or without food and should be taken at the same time(s) every day. Take Navane as prescribed by your doctor.

What should I avoid while taking this medication?
You should not drive a car or operate heavy machinery until you know how Navane will affect you.

When taking Navane, avoid becoming dehydrated and exposing yourself to very hot environments.

When taking Navane, you should avoid consumption of alcohol as it may intensify the side effects of the drug.

What are possible food and drug interactions associated with this medication?
If Navane is taken with certain other drugs, the effects of either could be increased, decreased, or altered. It is especially important to check with your doctor before combining Navane with the following: anticholinergic-type medications such as atropine, antihistamines, barbiturates, blood pressure medications, carbamazepine, opiates, tricyclic antidepressants.

What are the possible side effects of this medication?
Side effects cannot be anticipated. If any develop or change in intensity, tell your doctor as soon as possible. Only your doctor can determine if it is safe for you to continue taking this drug.

Side effects may include: allergic rash, blurred vision, dizziness, drowsiness, dry mouth, immobility, increased heart rate, involuntary muscle contractions, involuntary muscle movements, liver damage, low blood pressure, menstrual irregularities, muscle restlessness, muscle stiffness, muscle tremors, and hematological effects

Navane may cause damage to your liver or your eyes. Some of the warning signs of liver damage include nausea, vomiting, fatigue, loss of appetite, itching, yellow coloring of skin or eyes (jaundice), "flu-like" symptoms, and dark urine. If you experience any of these symptoms, call your doctor right away. Also, contact your doctor right away if you experience any changes in your vision.

Can I receive this medication if I am pregnant or breastfeeding?
The effects of Navane during pregnancy and breastfeeding are unknown. Tell your doctor immediately if you are pregnant, plan to become pregnant, or are breastfeeding.

What should I do if I miss a dose of this medication?
You should not double your dose of Navane. Skip the missed dose and return to your normal dosing schedule.

How should I store this medication?
Store Navane at room temperature.

NEFAZODONE HYDROCHLORIDE

What is this medication?
Nefazodone is used to treat depression, a low mood that persists nearly every day for at least two weeks and interferes with everyday living.

What is the most important information I should know about this medication?
Antidepressant medicines may increase suicidal thoughts or actions in some children, teenagers, and young adults when the medicine is first started. Depression and other serious mental illnesses are the most important causes of suicidal thoughts and actions. Some people may have a particularly high risk of having suicidal thoughts or actions. These include people who have (or have a family history of) bipolar disorder (also called manic-depressive illness) or suicidal thoughts or actions.

Pay close attention to any changes, especially sudden ones, in mood, behaviors, thoughts, or feelings. This is very important when an antidepressant medicine is first started or when the dose is changed.

Call the doctor right away to report new or sudden changes in mood, behavior, thoughts, or feelings. Signs to watch for include new or worsening depression, new or worsening anxiety, agitation, insomnia, hostility, panic attacks, restlessness, extreme hyperactivity, and suicidal thinking or behavior.

Keep all follow-up visits as scheduled, and call the doctor between visits as needed, especially if you have concerns about symptoms.

Although rare, there have been severe cases of liver damage in patients taking nefazodone. Call your doctor immediately if you develop symptoms such as yellowing of the skin or white eyes, unusually dark urine, loss of appetite that lasts for several days, nausea or lower stomach pain while taking nefazodone. People with liver problems should not take nefazodone.

It may take several weeks before you see an improvement of your symptoms while taking nefazodone.

Who should not take this medication?
Do not take this medication if you are allergic to nefazodone or Desyrel.

You should also avoid taking this medication if you have any liver problems.

Do not take nefazodone within 14 days of taking a monoamine oxidase inhibitor (MAOI) such as Nardil or Parnate.

What should I tell my doctor before I take the first dose of this medication?
Tell your doctor about all prescription, over-the-counter, vitamin supplements, and herbal medications you are taking before beginning treatment with nefazodone. Also, talk to your doctor about your complete medical history, especially if you have a history of liver disease, heart problems, extreme agitation or excitability episodes, suicide attempts, convulsions, or are pregnant or breastfeeding.

What is the usual dosage?
The information below is based on the dosage guidelines your doctor uses. Depending on your condition and medical history, your doctor may prescribe a different regimen. Do not change the dosage or stop taking your medication without your doctor's approval.

Adults: The usual recommended starting dose for nefazodone hydrochloride tablets is 200 milligrams (mg) per day, taken twice daily. Your doctor may increase your dose in increments of 100 mg to 200 mg daily up to a maximum daily dose of 600 mg.

In elderly or weak patients, the usual dose is 100 mg per day, taken twice daily.

How should I take this medication?
Take nefazodone at the same time every day as prescribed by your doctor. You can take it with or without food.

What should I avoid while taking this medication?
Never stop taking this medication without consulting your doctor first.

Driving or operating dangerous machinery or participating in any hazardous activity that requires full mental alertness should be avoided until you know how this drug affects you.

Do not drink alcoholic beverages while taking this medication.

What are possible food and drug interactions associated with this medication?

If nefazodone is taken with certain other drugs, the effects of either could be increased, decreased, or altered. It is especially important to check with your doctor before combining this medication with any the following: alprazolam, astemizole, carbamazepine, cisapride, monoamine oxidase inhibitors (MAOIs), pimozide, terfenadine, triazolam.

What are the possible side effects of this medication?

Side effects cannot be anticipated. If any develop or change in intensity, inform your doctor as soon as possible. Only your doctor can determine if it is safe for you to continue taking this drug.

Side effects may include: sleepiness, vision problems, weakness, lightheadedness, confusion, nausea, constipation, and dry mouth

Serious side effects may include: yellowing of the skin or whites of eyes (jaundice), unusually dark urine, loss of appetite that lasts for several days, severe nausea, rash or hives, convulsions, fainting, and long lasting erection. Contact your doctor immediately if you experience any of these serious symptoms.

Can I receive this medication if I am pregnant or breastfeeding?

The effects of nefazodone during pregnancy and breastfeeding are unknown. Tell your doctor if you are pregnant, planning to become pregnant or breastfeed, or become pregnant while taking nefazodone.

What should I do if I miss a dose of this medication?

If you miss a dose, skip it and return to your regular schedule. Never take two doses at the same time.

How should I store this medication?

Nefazodone should be stored at room temperature and protected from light.

NEMBUTAL

Generic name: Pentobarbital sodium

What is this medication?

Nembutal is a barbiturate, a central nervous system depressant used for the short-term treatment of insomnia. It is also used as an emergency antiseizure medication and as a pre-anesthetic.

What is the most important information I should know about this medication?

Barbiturates, including Nembutal, should not be used if you have a history of porphyria, a blood disorder.

Taking more than is recommended of this medication may result in tolerance and/or dependence, in which case you will need more of the drug to produce the same affect, which increases the risk of side effects.

Avoid performing activities that require alertness, such as operating an automobile, or any other machinery, until you know how this medication affects you.

To avoid serious side effects, avoid consumption of alcohol and other nervous system depressants, including narcotic pain killers, antihistamines, and sleep aids.

Who should not take this medication?

If you have a history of porphyria, you should not use Nembutal, or any other barbiturate.

What should I tell my doctor before I take the first dose of this medication?

Tell your doctor about all prescription, over-the-counter, and herbal medications you are taking before beginning treatment with Nembutal. Also, talk to your doctor about your complete medical history, especially if you have a history of drug abuse or dependence, depression, or any other condition.

What is the usual dosage?

The information below is based on the dosage guidelines your doctor uses. Depending on your condition and medical history, your doctor may prescribe a different regimen. Do not change the dosage or stop taking your medication without your doctor's approval.

Adults: The usual adult dose of Nembutal is 150 to 200 milligrams (mg) as a single intramuscular injection. Monitor vital signs carefully after injection.

If you are above the age of 65, or if you have liver or kidney disease, a lower dose of Nembutal may be used, since you might be more sensitive to this medication.

Children: The recommended pediatric dosage ranges from 2 to 6 mg/kg, as a single intramuscular injection, and is not to exceed 100 mg.

How should I take this medication?

Take this medication exactly as directed by your physician. Taking more or less of this medication than is prescribed might lead to serious side effects.

What should I avoid while taking this medication?

Avoid consumption of alcohol, or any other nervous system depressants, including narcotic pain killers, antihistamines, and sleep aids.

Avoid activities that require alertness, such as operating a vehicle, or any other machinery, until you know how this medication affects you.

What are possible food and drug interactions associated with this medication?

If Nembutal is used with certain other drugs, the effects of either could be increased, decreased, or altered. It is especially important to check with your doctor before combining Nembutal with the following: alcohol, anticoagulants/blood thinners (such as aspirin and warfarin), corticosteroids, doxycycline, estrogen, griseofulvin, phenytoin.

What are the possible side effects of this medication?

Side effects cannot be anticipated. If any develop or change in intensity, tell your doctor as soon as possible. Only your doctor can determine if it is safe for you to continue taking this drug.

Side effects may include: sleepiness, agitation, confusion, depression, nervousness, nightmares, breathing disorders, nausea, vomiting

Can I receive this medication if I am pregnant or breastfeeding?

Barbiturates, including Nembutal, can cause fetal damage when given during pregnancy. If you are pregnant, or plan to become pregnant, speak with your doctor about the possible harm to the fetus.

What should I do if I miss a dose of this medication?

Take the dose as soon as you remember, unless it is almost time for your next dose. Do not take more than one dose at a time.

How should I store this medication?

Store at controlled room temperature.

NIRAVAM

Generic name: Alprazolam

What is this medication?

Niravam is used to treat anxiety disorder, panic disorder, and to provide short-term relief of anxiety symptoms.

What is the most important information I should know about this medication?

Niravam may cause dependence. The risk of developing a dependency on Niravam is greater if you have a history of drug or alcohol abuse.

Until you experience how this medication affects you, do not drive a car or operate potentially dangerous machinery.

Do not increase the dose of this medication without consulting your physician.

Who should not take this medication?

You should not take Niravam if you have a known sensitivity to this drug or other benzodiazepines.

If you have acute narrow-angle glaucoma (increased eye pressure), or are taking a potent antifungal medication such as ketoconazole or itraconazole, you should not take Niravam.

What should I tell my doctor before I take the first dose of this medication?

Tell your doctor about all prescription, over-the-counter, and herbal medications you are taking before beginning treatment with Niravam. Also, talk to your doctor about your complete medical history, especially if you have kidney or liver problems, or if you are pregnant, plan to become pregnant, or are breastfeeding.

What is the usual dosage?

The information below is based on the dosage guidelines your doctor uses. Depending on your condition and medical history, your doctor may prescribe a different regimen. Do not change the dosage or stop taking your medication without your doctor's approval.

Anxiety Disorder

Adults: Initial dosage is 0.25 to 0.5 milligrams (mg) three times a day; dosage may increase every three to four days to a maximum of 4 mg/day.

Elderly: Initial dosage for the elderly is 0.25 mg, two to three times per day; dosage may increase as needed and tolerated.

Panic Disorder

Adults: Initial dosage is 0.5 mg, three times a day; dosage may increase every three to four days to a maximum of 10 mg/day. The average effective dose is approximately 5 to 6 mg daily.

How should I take this medication?

With clean, dry hands, place a Niravam tablet on your tongue. It will begin to dissolve within seconds with or without water.

What should I avoid while taking this medication?

Until you know how Niravam affects you, do not drive a car or operate heavy machinery.

Do not change or stop taking your prescribed dose of Niravam without talking to your doctor first.

Avoid alcohol and other medications that may have a depressant effect on your central nervous system.

What are possible food and drug interactions associated with this medication?

If Niravam is taken with certain other drugs, the effects of either could be increased, decreased, or altered. It is especially important to check with your doctor before combining Niravam with the following: alcohol, anticonvulsants, antifungals, antihistamines, cimetidine, desipramine, fluoxetine, fluvoxamine, imipramine, nefazodone, oral contraceptives, propoxyphene, psychotropic medications.

What are the possible side effects of this medication?
Side effects cannot be anticipated. If any develop or change in intensity, tell your doctor as soon as possible. Only your doctor can determine if it is safe for you to continue taking this drug.

Side effects may include: drowsiness, fatigue, headache, impaired coordination, insomnia, irritability, lightheadedness, memory impairment

Can I receive this medication if I am pregnant or breastfeeding?
It is not recommended to take Niravam while pregnant. If you are pregnant, planning to become pregnant, or are breastfeeding, talk to your doctor.

Where should I keep my supply of this medication?
Store at room temperature, away from moisture.

NORPRAMIN
Generic name: Desipramine hydrochloride

What is this medication?
Norpramin is used to treat the symptoms of depression.

What is the most important information I should know about this medication?
Norpramin is not approved for use in children.

Antidepressant medicines may increase suicidal thoughts or actions in some children, teenagers, and young adults when the medicine is first started. Depression and other serious mental illnesses are the most important causes of suicidal thoughts and actions. Some people may have a particularly high risk of having suicidal thoughts or actions. These include people who have (or have a family history of) bipolar disorder (also called manic-depressive illness) or suicidal thoughts or actions.

Pay close attention to any changes, especially sudden changes, in mood, behaviors, thoughts, or feelings. This is very important when an antidepressant medicine is first started or when the dose is changed.

Call the doctor right away to report new or sudden changes in mood, behavior, thoughts, or feelings. Signs to watch for include new or worsening depression, new or worsening anxiety, agitation, insomnia, hostility, panic attacks, restlessness, extreme hyperactivity, and suicidal thinking or behavior.

Keep all follow-up visits as scheduled, and call the doctor between visits as needed, especially if you have concerns about symptoms.

Who should not take this medication?
Do not take Norpramin if you are allergic to it or any of its components.
Do not take Norpramin if you have recently had a heart attack.

If you are taking or have taken antidepressant medications known as monoamine oxidase inhibitors (MAOIs) within the last 14 days, do not take Norpramin.

If you are planning to have elective surgery, make sure that your doctor is aware that you are taking Norpramin. It should be discontinued as soon as possible prior to surgery.

What should I tell my doctor before I take the first dose of this medication?

Tell your doctor about all prescription, over-the-counter, and herbal medications you are taking before beginning treatment with Norpramin. Also, talk to your doctor about your complete medical history, especially if you have heart disease, a history of heart attack, stroke, seizures, bipolar disorder (manic-depression), schizophrenia or other mental illness, liver disease, overactive thyroid, high blood sugar, increased pressure in the eyes (glaucoma), or problems with urination.

What is the usual dosage?

The information below is based on the dosage guidelines your doctor uses. Depending on your condition and medical history, your doctor may prescribe a different regimen. Do not change the dosage or stop taking your medication without your doctor's approval.

Adults: The usual dose ranges from 100 to 200 milligrams (mg) per day, taken in one dose or divided into smaller doses. If needed, dosages may gradually be increased to 300 mg a day. Dosages above 300 mg per day are not recommended.

Elderly and Adolescents: The usual dose ranges from 25 to 100 mg per day. If needed, dosages may gradually be increased to 150 mg a day. Doses above 150 mg per day are not recommended.

How should I take this medication?

Norpramin should be taken exactly as prescribed. Do not stop taking Norpramin if you feel no immediate effect. It can take up to 2 or 3 weeks for improvement to begin.

Norpramin can cause dry mouth. Sucking hard candy or chewing gum can help this problem.

What should I avoid while taking this medication?

Norpramin may increase your skin's sensitivity to sunlight. Overexposure could cause rash, itching, redness, or sunburn. Avoid direct sunlight or wear protective clothing.

This drug may impair your ability to drive a car or operate potentially dangerous machinery. Do not participate in any activities that require full alertness if you are unsure about your ability.

Avoid drinking alcohol. It can cause dangerous side effects when taken together with Norpramin.

What are possible food and drug interactions associated with this medication?

If Norpramin is taken with certain other drugs, the effects of either could be increased, decreased, or altered. It is especially important to check with your doctor before combining Norpramin with the following: alcohol, antidepressants (including MAOIs and SSRIs), cimetidine, drugs that improve breathing, muscle relaxants, guanethidine, sedatives/hypnotics, sertraline, thyroid medications.

What are the possible side effects of this medication?

Side effects cannot be anticipated. If any develop or change in intensity, tell your doctor as soon as possible. Only your doctor can determine if it is safe for you to continue taking this drug.

Side effects may include: anxiety, confusion, dizziness, dry mouth, frequent urination or problems urinating, high blood pressure, hallucinations, hives, impaired coordination, irregular heartbeat, low blood pressure, numbness, rapid heartbeat, sensitivity to sunlight, sex drive changes, tingling, and tremors

Can I receive this medication if I am pregnant or breastfeeding?

The effects of Norpramin during pregnancy and breastfeeding are unknown. Tell your doctor immediately if you are pregnant, plan to become pregnant, or are breastfeeding.

What should I do if I miss a dose of this medication?

If you do miss a dose, take it as soon as you remember. However, if it is almost time for your next dose, skip the missed dose and take only your next regularly scheduled dose. Do not take a double dose of this medication.

How should I store this medication?

Norpramin can be stored at room temperature. Protect it from excessive heat.

OXAZEPAM

What is this medication?

Oxazepam is used to treat anxiety disorders, including anxiety associated with depression. It is also prescribed to relieve symptoms of acute alcohol withdrawal.

What is the most important information I should know about this medication?

Oxazepam should be used for only a short time. Do not take this medication for longer than 4 months unless your doctor instructs you to.

Oxazepam may be habit-forming and should be used only by the person it was prescribed for. Oxazepam should never be shared with another person, especially someone who has a history of drug abuse or addiction.

Contact your doctor if this medicine seems to stop working as well in treating your symptoms. Do not stop using oxazepam suddenly without first talking to your doctor.

Your symptoms may return when you stop using oxazepam after using it over a long period of time. You may also have seizures or withdrawal symptoms when you stop using oxazepam. Withdrawal symptoms may include tremor, sweating, trouble sleeping, muscle cramps, stomach pain, vomiting, diarrhea, confusion, unusual thoughts or behavior, and seizures (convulsions).

Who should not take this medication?

If you are sensitive to or have ever had an allergic reaction to oxazepam or other tranquilizers such as Valium, you should not take oxazepam.

Oxazepam should not be prescribed if you are being treated for mental disorders more serious than anxiety.

What should I tell my doctor before I take the first dose of this medication?

Tell your doctor about all prescription, over-the-counter, and herbal medications you are taking before beginning treatment with oxazepam. Also, talk to your doctor about your complete medical history, especially if you have any breathing problems, glaucoma, porphyria, kidney or liver disease, or a history of depression, suicidal thoughts, or addiction to drugs or alcohol.

What is the usual dosage?

The information below is based on the dosage guidelines your doctor uses. Depending on your condition and medical history, your doctor may prescribe a different regimen. Do not change the dosage or stop taking your medication without your doctor's approval.

Mild to Moderate Anxiety with Tension, Irritability, Agitation

Adults: The usual dose is 10 to 15 milligrams (mg) 3 or 4 times per day.
Elderly: The usual starting dose is 10 mg, 3 times a day. Your doctor may increase the dose to 15 mg 3 or 4 times a day, if needed.
Children: Safety and effectiveness have not been established for children <6 years of age, nor have dosage guidelines been established for children 6 to 12 years. The doctor will adjust the dosage to fit your child's needs.

Severe Anxiety, Depression with Anxiety, or Alcohol Withdrawal

Adults: The usual dose is 15 to 30 mg, 3 or 4 times per day.

How should I take this medication?

Take oxazepam exactly as prescribed. Do not take the medication in larger amounts, or take it for longer than recommended by your doctor. Follow the directions on your prescription label.

What should I avoid while taking this medication?

Do not drink alcohol while taking oxazepam. This medication can increase the effects of alcohol. Oxazepam can cause side effects that may impair your thinking or reactions. Be careful if you drive or do anything that requires you to be awake and alert.

Avoid using other medicines that make you sleepy (such as cold medicine; pain medication; muscle relaxers; and medicine for seizures, depression or anxiety). They can increase some of the side effects of oxazepam.

What are possible food and drug interactions associated with this medication?

If oxazepam is taken with certain other drugs, the effects of either could be increased, decreased, or altered. It is especially important to check with your doctor before combining oxazepam with the following: alcohol, antihistamines, narcotic painkillers, sedatives, tranquilizers.

What are the possible side effects of this medication?

Side effects cannot be anticipated. If any develop or change in intensity, tell your doctor as soon as possible. Only your doctor can determine if it is safe for you to continue taking this drug.

Side effects may include: dizziness, drowsiness, headache, memory impairment, paradoxical excitement, transient amnesia, vertigo

Side effects due to rapid decrease in dose or abrupt withdrawal from oxazepam may include: abdominal and muscle cramps, convulsions, depression, inability to fall asleep or stay asleep, sweating, tremors, vomiting

Can I receive this medication if I am pregnant or breastfeeding?

Do not take oxazepam if you are pregnant or planning to become pregnant. There is an increased risk of birth defects. Oxazepam may appear in breast milk and could affect a nursing infant. If oxazepam is essential to your health, your doctor may advise you to stop breastfeeding until your treatment with oxazepam is finished.

What should I do if I miss a dose of this medication?

Take the missed dose as soon as you remember. However, if it is almost time for the next dose, skip the missed dose and take only the next regularly scheduled dose. Do not take a double dose of this medication.

Where should I keep my supply of this medication?

Store at room temperature in a tightly closed container.

PAMELOR

Generic name: Nortriptyline hydrochloride

What is this medication?

Pamelor is prescribed for the relief of symptoms of depression.

What is the most important information I should know about this medication?

Antidepressants can increase the risk of suicidal thinking and behavior in children and teenagers. Adult and pediatric patients taking antidepressants should be watched closely for changes in moods and actions, especially when their dose is increased or decreased. Patients and their families should contact the doctor immediately if new symptoms develop or seem to get worse. Signs to watch for include anxiety, hostility, insomnia, restlessness, impulsive or dangerous behavior, and thoughts about suicide or dying.

Who should not take this medication?

Do not use Pamelor Solution if you are allergic to any ingredient in Pamelor Solution or to similar medicines. Also, do not take Pamelor if you are recovering from a recent heart attack.

If you have taken furazolidone or a monoamine oxidase inhibitor (MAOI) like phenelzine within the last 14 days, or if you are taking astemizole, dofetilide, droperidol, terfenadine, or cisapride, you should not take Pamelor.

What should I tell my doctor before I take the first dose of this medication?

Tell your doctor about all prescription, over-the-counter, and herbal medications you are taking before beginning treatment with Pamelor. Also, talk to your doctor about your complete medical history, especially if you have: a history of suicidal thoughts or behavior; an overactive thyroid; bipolar disorder or any other mental disorder; diabetes; difficulty urinating; glaucoma; heart, kidney, or liver problems; seizures; porphyria (a blood disorder).

Be sure to let your doctor know if you are undergoing electroshock therapy, if you are scheduled to have any surgery, if you drink alcohol-containing beverages daily, or if you have a history of alcohol abuse.

What is the usual dosage?

The information below is based on the dosage guidelines your doctor uses. Depending on your condition and medical history, your doctor may prescribe a different regimen. Do not change the dosage or stop taking your medication without your doctor's approval.

This medication is available in tablet and liquid form. Only tablet dosages are listed. Consult your doctor if you cannot take the tablet form of Pamelor.

Adults: The usual starting dosage is 25 milligrams (mg) taken 3 or 4 times per day. Alternatively, your doctor may prescribe that the total daily dose be taken once a day. Doses above 150 mg per day are not recommended. Your doctor will monitor your response to Pamelor carefully and will gradually increase or decrease the dose to suit your needs.

Elderly: The usual dose is 30 to 50 mg taken in a single dose or divided into smaller doses, as determined by your doctor.

How should I take this medication?

Take Pamelor exactly as prescribed. Pamelor Solution may be taken with or without food. Pamelor may make your mouth dry. Sucking on hard candy, chewing gum, or melting ice chips in your mouth can provide relief.

What should I avoid while taking this medication?

Pamelor may cause you to become drowsy or less alert. Do not drive or operate dangerous machinery or participate in any hazardous activity that requires full mental alertness until you know how Pamelor affects you.

Pamelor may make your skin more sensitive to sunlight. Try to stay out of the sun, wear protective clothing, and apply sunblock.

Avoid drinking alcohol or taking other medications that cause drowsiness, such as sedatives.

What are possible food and drug interactions associated with this medication?

If Pamelor is taken with certain other drugs, the effects of either could be increased, decreased, or altered. It is especially important to check with your doctor before combining Pamelor with the following: albuterol, alcohol, antiarrhythmics, antidepressants, antihistamines, antispasmodics, blood pressure medication, cimetidine, chlorpropamide, levodopa, MAO inhibitors (combination with Pamelor can be fatal), quinidine, reserpine, stimulants such as dextroamphetamine, thyroid medication, tranquilizers, warfarin.

What are the possible side effects of this medication?

Side effects cannot be anticipated. If any develop or change in intensity, tell your doctor as soon as possible. Only your doctor can determine if it is safe for you to continue taking this drug.

Side effects may include: anxiety, blurred vision, confusion, dry mouth, hallucinations, heart attack or vascular heart blockage, heartbeat irregularities, high blood pressure, insomnia, loss of muscle coordination, low blood pressure, rapid heartbeat, sensitivity to sunlight, skin rash, stroke, tremors, weight loss

Side effects due to rapid decrease in dose or abrupt withdrawal from Pamelor after prolonged treatment include: headache, nausea, vague feeling of bodily discomfort

Can I receive this medication if I am pregnant or breastfeeding?

The effects of Pamelor during pregnancy and breastfeeding are unknown. Tell your doctor immediately if you are pregnant, plan to become pregnant, or are breastfeeding.

What should I do if I miss a dose of this medication?

Take it as soon as you remember. If it is almost time for the next dose, skip the dose you missed and go back to your regular schedule. If you take Pamelor once a day at bedtime and you miss a dose, do not take it in the morning, since disturbing side effects could occur. Never take two doses at once.

How should I store this medication?

Store Pamelor at room temperature in the container it came in, tightly closed and away from light.

PARNATE

Generic name: Tranylcypromine sulfate

What is this medication?

Parnate is prescribed for the treatment of major depression. This medication is usually given after other antidepressants have been tried without successful treatment of symptoms.

What is the most important information I should know about this medication?

Parnate is a potent antidepressant in the class of drugs called monoamine oxidase inhibitors (MAOIs). It works by increasing the concentration of chemicals in your brain such as epinephrine, norepinephrine, and serotonin. It can produce serious side effects. It is typically prescribed only if other antidepressants fail, and then only for adults who are under close medical supervision. It can interact with a long list of drugs and foods to produce life-threatening side effects (see "**What are possible food and drug interactions associated with this medication?**").

Antidepressants can increase the risk of suicidal thinking and behavior in children and teenagers. Adult and pediatric patients taking antidepressants should be watched closely for changes in moods or actions, especially when they first start therapy or when their dose is increased or decreased. Patients and their families should contact the doctor immediately if new symptoms develop or seem to get worse. Signs to watch for include anxiety, hostility, insomnia, restlessness, impulsive or dangerous behavior, and thoughts about suicide or dying.

Who should not take this medication?

Do not take Parnate if you have any of the following medical conditions: heart, kidney, or liver disease; high blood pressure; a history of headaches; a type of tumor known as pheochromocytoma; or if you will be undergoing elective surgery requiring general anesthesia.

What should I tell my doctor before I take the first dose of this medication?

Tell your doctor about all prescription, over-the-counter, and herbal medications you are taking before beginning treatment with Parnate. Also, talk to your doctor about your complete medical history (see "**Who should not take this medication?**").

What is the usual dosage?

The information below is based on the dosage guidelines your doctor uses. Depending on your condition and medical history, your doctor may prescribe a different regimen. Do not change the dosage or stop taking your medication without your doctor's approval.

Adults: The usual dosage is 30 milligrams (mg) per day, divided into smaller doses. If ineffective, the dosage may be slowly increased under your doctor's supervision to a maximum of 60 mg per day.

How should I take this medication?

Take this medication exactly as it was prescribed for you. Follow the instructions on your prescription label. Your doctor will adjust the dosage of Parnate according to your individual needs and response. It will usually take 48 hours to 3 weeks for you to see the benefits of Parnate.

What should I avoid while taking this medication?

While you are taking Parnate, avoid foods that are high in tyramine (see "**What are possible food and drug interactions associated with this medication?**").

Avoid alcohol and large amounts of caffeine while you are taking Parnate.

Avoid driving, operating machinery, or other dangerous tasks until you know how Parnate will affect you. Parnate may cause you to be very drowsy.

What are possible food and drug interactions associated with this medication?

Never take Parnate with the following drugs; the combination can trigger seizures or a dangerous spike in blood pressure: dibenzapine-related and other drugs classified as tricyclic antidepressants, such as amitriptyline, amoxapine, carbamazepine, clomipramine, cyclobenzaprine, desipramine, doxepin, imipramine, maprotiline, nortriptyline, perphenazine and amitriptyline, protriptyline, trimipramine maleate; other MAOIs such as furazolidone, isocarboxazid, pargyline, procarbazine, phenelzine.

When switching from one of these drugs to Parnate, or vice versa, allow an interval of at least 1 week between medications.

If Parnate is taken with certain other drugs, the effects of either could be increased, decreased, or altered. It is especially important to check with your doctor before combining Parnate with the following: alcohol, amphetamines, anesthetics, antidepressants classified as SSRIs, antihistamines, blood pressure medications, blood-vessel constricting medicines for colds, hay fever and weight loss, bupropion, buspirone, cocaine, cough remedies containing dextromethorphan, dexfenfluramine, disulfiram, diuretics (water pills), dopamine, guanethidine, meperidine and other narcotic painkillers, methyldopa, Parkinson's disease medications, reserpine, sedatives such as triazolam, pentobarbital, and secobarbital, tryptophan.

While taking Parnate, you should also avoid foods that contain a high amount of a substance called tyramine, including: anchovies, avocados, bananas, beer (including nonalcoholic beer), canned figs, caviar, cheese (especially strong and aged varieties), chianti wine, chocolate, dried fruits (including raisins, prunes), liqueurs, liver, meat extracts or meat prepared with tenderizers, overripe fruit, pickled herring, pods of broad beans like fava beans, raspberries, sauerkraut, sherry, sour cream, soy sauce, yeast extracts, yogurt.

What are the possible side effects of this medication?

Side effects cannot be anticipated. If any develop or change in intensity, tell your doctor as soon as possible. Only your doctor can determine if it is safe for you to continue taking this drug.

Side effects may include: abdominal pain, agitation, anxiety, blood disorders, blurred vision, chills, constipation, diarrhea, dizziness, drowsiness, dry mouth, headache, impotence, insomnia, muscle spasm, nausea, numbness, overstimulation, rapid or irregular heartbeat, restlessness, ringing in the ears, tremors, urinary retention, water retention, weakness, weight loss

Can I receive this medication if I am pregnant or breastfeeding?

If you are pregnant or plan to become pregnant, inform your doctor immediately. Parnate should be used during pregnancy only if its benefits outweigh potential risks.

Parnate is found in breast milk. If the drug is essential to your health, your doctor may advise you to stop nursing until your treatment is finished.

What should I do if I miss a dose of this medication?

Take the missed dose as soon as you remember. If it is almost time for your next dose, skip the missed dose and take the medicine at the next regularly scheduled time. Do not take extra medicine to make up for a missed dose.

How should I store this medication?

Store Parnate at room temperature.

PAXIL
Generic name: Paroxetine hydrochloride

What is this medication?
Paxil is used to treat depression, obsessive-compulsive disorder, panic disorder, social anxiety disorder, generalized anxiety disorder, and post-traumatic stress disorder.

What is the most important information I should know about this medication?
Paxil is not approved for use in pediatric patients.

Antidepressant medicines may increase suicidal thoughts or actions in some children, teenagers, and young adults when the medicine is first started. Depression and other serious mental illnesses are the most important causes of suicidal thoughts and actions. Some people may have a particularly high risk of having suicidal thoughts or actions. These include people who have (or have a family history of) bipolar disorder (also called manic-depressive illness) or suicidal thoughts or actions.

Pay close attention to any changes, especially sudden ones, in mood, behaviors, thoughts, or feelings. This is very important when an antidepressant medicine is first started or when the dose is changed.

Call the doctor right away to report new or sudden changes in mood, behavior, thoughts, or feelings. Signs to watch for include new or worsening depression, new or worsening anxiety, agitation, insomnia, hostility, panic attacks, restlessness, extreme hyperactivity, and suicidal thinking or behavior.

Keep all follow-up visits as scheduled, and call the doctor between visits as needed, especially if you have concerns about symptoms.

Who should not take this medication?
You should not take Paxil if you are allergic to it or any of its components. It should also be avoided if you are currently taking monoamine oxidase inhibitors (MAOIs), linezolid, thioridazine, or pimozide.

What should I tell my doctor before I take the first dose of this medication?
Tell your doctor about all prescription, over-the-counter, and herbal medications you are taking before beginning treatment with Paxil. Also, talk to your doctor about your complete medical history, especially if you intend on becoming pregnant or if you have a history of suicidal thoughts, panic attacks, insomnia, seizures, glaucoma, or severe kidney or liver impairment.

What is the usual dosage?
The information below is based on the dosage guidelines your doctor uses. Depending on your condition and medical history, your doctor may prescribe a different regimen. Do not change the dosage or stop taking your medication without your doctor's approval.

Depression

Adults: The recommended starting dose is 20 milligrams (mg) daily. Depending on how you respond to Paxil, your doses may be increased in 10 mg/day increments up to a maximum daily dose of 50 mg.

Obsessive-Compulsive Disorder

Adults: The recommended starting dose is 20 mg daily. Depending on how you respond to Paxil, your doses may be increased in 10 mg/day increments up to a maximum daily dose of 60 mg.

Panic Disorder

Adults: The recommended starting dose is 10 mg daily. Depending on how you respond to Paxil, your doses may be increased in 10 mg/day increments up to a maximum daily dose of 60 mg.

Social Anxiety Disorder

Adults: The recommended starting dose is 20 mg daily. Depending on how you respond to Paxil, your doses may be increased up to a maximum daily dose of 60 mg.

Generalized Anxiety Disorder

Adults: The recommended starting dose is 20 mg daily. Depending on how you respond to Paxil, your doses may be increased up to a maximum daily dose of 50 mg.

Post-traumatic Stress Disorder

Adults: The recommended starting dose is 20 mg daily. Depending on how you respond to Paxil, your dose may be increased up to a maximum daily dose to 50 mg.

How should I take this medication?

Paxil is taken once daily, usually in the morning, with or without food.

What should I avoid while taking this medication?

Avoid drinking alcohol during treatment with Paxil. Avoid driving or operating dangerous machinery or participating in any hazardous activity that requires full mental alertness until you know how this drug affects you.

What are possible food and drug interactions associated with this medication?

If Paxil is taken with certain other drugs, the effects of either could be increased, decreased, or altered. It is especially important to check with your doctor before combining Paxil with any of the following: alcohol, antidepressants such as amitriptyline, desipramine, fluoxetine, imipramine, and nortriptyline, aspirin, cimetidine, diazepam, digoxin, flecainide, linezolid, lithium, nonsteroidal anti-inflammatory drugs (NSAIDs) such as aspirin, ibuprofen, naproxen, and ketoprofen, phenobarbital, phenytoin, pimozide, procyclidine, propafenone, propranolol, quinidine, St. John's wort, sumatriptan, theophylline, thioridazine, tramadol, triptans (a class of medication used to treat migraines; examples include sumatriptan and zolmitriptan), tryptophan, warfarin.

What are the possible side effects of this medication?
Side effects cannot be anticipated. If any develop or change in intensity, tell your doctor as soon as possible. Only your doctor can determine if it is safe for you to continue taking this drug.

Side effects may include: abnormal ejaculation, abnormal orgasm, constipation, decreased appetite, decreased sex drive, diarrhea, dizziness, drowsiness, dry mouth, gas, impotence, male and female genital disorders, nausea, nervousness, sleeplessness, sweating, tremor, weakness, and vertigo

Can I receive this medication if I am pregnant or breastfeeding?
For women who intend to become pregnant or are in their first trimester of pregnancy, Paxil should only be initiated after consideration of the other available treatment options. The effects of Paxil during breastfeeding are unknown; discuss your options with your doctor.

What should I do if I miss a dose of this medication?
Skip the missed dose and go back to your regular schedule. Do not take a double dose to make up for the one you missed.

How should I store this medication?
Store at room temperature.

PAXIL CR
Generic name: Paroxetine hydrochloride

What is this medication?
Paxil CR is used to treat depression, panic disorder, social anxiety disorder, and premenstrual dysphoric disorder.

What is the most important information I should know about this medication?
Paxil CR is not approved for use in pediatric patients.

Antidepressant medicines may increase suicidal thoughts or actions in some children, teenagers, and young adults when the medicine is first started. Depression and other serious mental illnesses are the most important causes of suicidal thoughts and actions. Some people may have a particularly high risk of having suicidal thoughts or actions. These include people who have (or have a family history of) bipolar disorder (also called manic-depressive illness) or suicidal thoughts or actions.

Pay close attention to any changes, especially sudden ones, in mood, behaviors, thoughts, or feelings. This is very important when an antidepressant medicine is first started or when the dose is changed.

Call the doctor right away to report new or sudden changes in mood, behavior, thoughts, or feelings. Signs to watch for include new or worsening depression, new or worsening anxiety, agitation, insomnia, hostility, panic attacks, restlessness, extreme hyperactivity, and suicidal thinking or behavior.

Keep all follow-up visits as scheduled, and call the doctor between visits as needed, especially if you have concerns about symptoms.

Paxil CR is not approved for use in pediatric patients.

Who should not take this medication?

You should not take Paxil CR if you are allergic to it or any of its components. It should also be avoided if you are currently taking monoamine oxidase inhibitors (MAOIs), linezolid, thioridazine, or pimozide.

What should I tell my doctor before I take the first dose of this medication?

Tell your doctor about all prescription, over-the-counter, and herbal medications you are taking before beginning treatment with Paxil CR. Also, talk to your doctor about your complete medical history, especially if you intend on becoming pregnant or if you have a history of suicidal thoughts, panic attacks, insomnia, scizures, glaucoma, or severe kidney or liver impairment.

What is the usual dosage?

The information below is based on the dosage guidelines your doctor uses. Depending on your condition and medical history, your doctor may prescribe a different regimen. Do not change the dosage or stop taking your medication without your doctor's approval.

Depression

Adults: The recommended starting dose is 25 milligrams (mg) daily. Depending on how you respond to Paxil CR, your doses may be increased in 12.5 mg/day increments up to a maximum daily dose of 62.5 mg.

Panic Disorder

Adults: The recommended starting dose is 12.5 mg daily. Depending on how you respond to Paxil CR, your doses may be increased in 12.5 mg/day increments up to a maximum daily dose of 75 mg.

Social Anxiety Disorder

Adults: The recommended starting dose is 12.5 mg daily. Depending on how you respond to Paxil CR, your doses may be increased in 12.5 mg/day increments up to a maximum daily dose of 37.5 mg.

Premenstrual Dysphoric Disorder

Adults: The recommended starting dose is 12.5 mg daily. Depending on how you respond to Paxil CR, your dose may be increased 25 mg daily.

How should I take this medication?

Paxil CR is taken once daily, usually in the morning, with or without food. Swallow the tablets whole, and never chew or crush them.

What should I avoid while taking this medication?
Avoid drinking alcohol during treatment with Paxil CR. Avoid driving or operating dangerous machinery or participating in any hazardous activity that requires full mental alertness until you know how this drug affects you.

What are possible food and drug interactions associated with this medication?
If Paxil CR is taken with certain other drugs, the effects of either could be increased, decreased, or altered. It is especially important to check with your doctor before combining Paxil CR with the following: almotriptan, clorgyline, dexfenfluramine, dextromethorphan, droperidol, eletriptan, fenfluramine, frovatriptan, furazolidone, isoniazid, isocarboxazid, linezolid, moclobemide, naratriptan, nefazodone, nialamide, pargyline, phenelzine, pimozide, procarbazine, rasagiline, rizatriptan, selegiline, sibutramine, St. John's wort, sumatriptan, thioridazine, toloxatone, tramadol, tranylcypromine, trazodone, tryptophan, zolmitriptan.

What are the possible side effects of this medication?
Side effects cannot be anticipated. If any develop or change in intensity, tell your doctor as soon as possible. Only your doctor can determine if it is safe for you to continue taking this drug.

Side effects may include: somnolence, insomnia, nausea, asthenia, abnormal ejaculation, dry mouth, constipation, dizziness, diarrhea, decreased libido, sweating, female genital disorders, and tremor

Can I receive this medication if I am pregnant or breastfeeding?
For women who intend to become pregnant or are in their first trimester of pregnancy, Paxil CR should only be initiated after consideration of the other available treatment options. The effects of Paxil CR during breastfeeding are unknown; discuss your options with your doctor.

What should I do if I miss a dose of this medication?
Skip the missed dose and go back to your regular schedule. Do not take a double dose to make up for the one you missed.

How should I store this medication?
Store at room temperature.

PEMOLINE

What is this medication?
Pemoline is a nervous system stimulant used to treat attention-deficit/hyperactivity disorder (ADHD).

What is the most important information I should know about this medication?

Use of Pemoline has been linked with an increased risk of liver failure. Notify your doctor immediately if you notice a yellowish discoloration of your skin or eyes, have stomach discomfort, loss of appetite, darkened urine, or are constantly tired. Your physician should perform a liver function test before beginning treatment, and every two weeks while treatment is underway.

Your doctor will have you sign an informed consent form before beginning treatment, after he or she has explained the possible risks associated with Pemoline.

Who should not take this medication?

If you have liver disease, you should not use Pemoline, since this will increase your risk of liver failure.

Long-term therapy with Pemoline has been shown to stunt growth in children. Monitor your child's growth carefully if he or she is on Pemoline for a prolonged period of time.

What should I tell my doctor before I take the first dose of this medication?

Tell your doctor about all prescription, over-the-counter, and herbal medications you are taking before beginning treatment with Pemoline. Also, talk to your doctor about your complete medical history, especially if you have liver or kidney disease, or a history of depression or drug addiction.

What is the usual dosage?

The information below is based on the dosage guidelines your doctor uses. Depending on your condition and medical history, your doctor may prescribe a different regimen. Do not change the dosage or stop taking your medication without your doctor's approval.

Adults: The starting dose is 37.5 milligrams (mg) daily, taken in the morning. Your doctor may want to increase the dose in weekly intervals until the desired outcome is achieved. Let your doctor know if there is no improvement within three weeks of beginning therapy.

How should I take this medication?

You should take Pemoline in the morning, unless otherwise instructed by your physician.

What should I avoid while taking this medication?

Avoid taking anything that will cause hyperactivity, such as excessive caffeine.

What are possible food and drug interactions associated with this medication?

If Pemoline is used with certain other drugs, the effects of either could be increased, decreased, or altered. It is especially important to check with your doctor before combining Pemoline with the following: antiepileptic (antiseizure) drugs and other drugs that affect the nervous system (eg, sleep aids, anti-anxiety drugs, etc.).

What are the possible side effects of this medication?

Side effects cannot be anticipated. If any develop or change in intensity, tell your doctor as soon as possible. Only your doctor can determine if it is safe for you to continue taking this drug.

Side effects may include: sleeplessness, seizures, hallucinations, twitches, dizziness, drowsiness, headache

Can I receive this medication if I am pregnant or breastfeeding?

The effects of Pemoline during pregnancy and breastfeeding are unknown. Tell your doctor immediately if you are pregnant, plan to become pregnant, or are breastfeeding.

What should I do if I miss a dose of this medication?

Take the dose as soon as you remember. If your next dose is within 12 hours, skip the missed dose and continue with your normal dosing schedule, unless otherwise directed by your physician.

How should I store this medication?

Store at room temperature in a tightly sealed container.

PERPHENAZINE

What is this medication?

Perphenazine is indicated for use in the treatment of schizophrenia and for the control of severe nausea and vomiting in adults.

What is the most important information I should know about this medication?

Tardive dyskinesia, a syndrome consisting of potentially irreversible, involuntary movements, may develop in patients treated with antipsychotic drugs. Older patients are at an increased risk. There is no known treatment for established cases of tardive dyskinesia.

A potentially fatal symptom complex referred to as neuroleptic malignant syndrome (NMS) has been reported in association with antipsychotic drugs. Signs and symptoms of NMS include muscle rigidity, confusion, irregular pulse or blood pressure, etc. Contact your doctor immediately if you experience any of these symptoms.

Perphenazine may impair the mental and/or physical abilities required for the performance of hazardous tasks such as driving a car or operating machinery.

Perphenazine is not for use in children under 12 years of age.

Who should not take this medication?

Patients who have previously had a severe reaction to other phenothiazines should not take perphenazine.

Perphenazine should be used with caution in patients with depression.

Patients who have decreased kidney function should speak with their physician before taking perphenazine.

What should I tell my doctor before I take the first dose of this medication?

Tell your doctor about all prescription, over-the-counter, and herbal medications you are taking before beginning treatment with perphenazine. Also, talk to your doctor about your complete medical history, especially past or current kidney problems, respiratory problems, or a history of suicidality. Tell your doctor if you are pregnant, planning to become pregnant, or breastfeeding.

What is the usual dosage?

The information below is based on the dosage guidelines your doctor uses. Depending on your condition and medical history, your doctor may prescribe a different regimen. Do not change the dosage or stop taking your medication without your doctor's approval.

Dosage of perphenazine must be individualized and adjusted according to the severity of the condition and the response obtained. As with all drugs, the best dose is the lowest dose that will produce the desired effect.

Schizophrenia

Adults: 4 to 8 milligrams (mg) three times daily initially; dose wil be reduced as soon as possible to minimum effective dose.

Severe Nausea and Vomiting in Adults

Adults: 8 to 16 mg daily in divided doses; up to 24 mg may occasionally be necessary.

How should I take this medication?

Take perphenazine as directed by your physician.

What should I avoid while taking this medication?

Avoid alcohol since additive effects and decreased blood pressure may occur.

Use caution in extreme heat. Avoid excessive exposure to the sun.

Do not expose yourself to phosphorous insecticides.

What are possible food and drug interactions associated with this medication?
If perphenazine is taken with certain other drugs, the effects of either could be increased, decreased, or altered. It is especially important to check with your doctor before combining perphenazine with the following: antihistamines, analgesics, barbiturates, opiates, SSRIs (such as fluoxetine, sertraline, and paroxetine), tricyclic antidepressants.

What are the possible side effects of this medication?
Side effects cannot be anticipated. If any develop or change in intensity, tell your doctor as soon as possible. Only your doctor can determine if it is safe for you to continue taking this drug.

Side effects may include: drowsiness, yellowing of the skin and eyes (jaundice), movement disorders, aching and numbness of the limbs, slurred speech, seizures, headaches, insomnia, bizarre dreams, dry mouth, nasal congestion, fluctuations in blood pressure

Can I receive this medication if I am pregnant or breastfeeding?
Safe use of perphenazine during pregnancy and breastfeeding has not been established. Consult with your physician before becoming pregnant while taking perphenazine.

What should I do if I miss a dose of this medication?
If you miss a dose, take it as soon as you remember. If it is almost time for your next dose, skip the missed dose and resume your normal dosage schedule.

How should I store this medication?
Store perphenazine at room temperature, away from heat, light, and moisture.

PEXEVA
Generic name: Paroxetine mesylate

What is this medication?
Pexeva is used to treat depression, obsessive-compulsive disorder, panic disorder, and generalized anxiety disorder.

What is the most important information I should know about this medication?
Pexeva is not approved for use in pediatric patients.

Antidepressant medicines may increase suicidal thoughts or actions in some children, teenagers, and young adults when the medicine is first started. Depression and other serious mental illnesses are the most important causes of suicidal thoughts and actions. Some people may have a particularly high risk of having suicidal thoughts or actions. These include people who have (or have a family history of) bipolar disorder (also called manic-depressive illness) or suicidal thoughts or actions.

Pay close attention to any changes, especially sudden ones, in mood, behaviors, thoughts, or feelings. This is very important when an antidepressant medicine is first started or when the dose is changed.

Call the doctor right away to report new or sudden changes in mood, behavior, thoughts, or feelings. Signs to watch for include new or worsening depression, new or worsening anxiety, agitation, insomnia, hostility, panic attacks, restlessness, extreme hyperactivity, and suicidal thinking or behavior.

Keep all follow-up visits as scheduled, and call the doctor between visits as needed, especially if you have concerns about symptoms.

Who should not take this medication?
You should not take Pexeva if you are allergic to it or any of its components. It should also be avoided if you are currently taking monoamine oxidase inhibitors (MAOIs), linezolid, thioridazine, or pimozide.

What should I tell my doctor before I take the first dose of this medication?
Tell your doctor about all prescription, over-the-counter, and herbal medications you are taking before beginning treatment with Pexeva. Also, talk to your doctor about your complete medical history, especially if you intend on becoming pregnant or if you have a history of suicidal thoughts, panic attacks, insomnia, seizures, glaucoma, or severe kidney or liver impairment.

What is the usual dosage?
The information below is based on the dosage guidelines your doctor uses. Depending on your condition and medical history, your doctor may prescribe a different regimen. Do not change the dosage or stop taking your medication without your doctor's approval.

Depression
Adults: The recommended starting dose is 20 milligrams (mg) daily. Depending on you respond to Pexeva, your dose may be increased in 10 mg/day increments up to a maximum daily dose of 50 mg.

Obsessive-Compulsive Disorder
Adults: The recommended starting dose is 20 mg daily. Depending on how you respond to Pexeva, your dose may be increased in 10 mg/day increments up to a maximum daily dose of 60 mg.

Panic Disorder
Adults: The recommended starting dose is 10 mg daily. Depending on how you respond to Pexeva, your dose may be increased in 10 mg/day increments up to a maximum daily dose of 60 mg.

Generalized Anxiety Disorder
Adults: The recommended starting dose is 20 mg daily. Depending on how you respond to Pexeva, your dose may be increased up to a maximum daily dose of 50 mg.

How should I take this medication?

Pexeva is taken once daily, usually in the morning, with or without food. Pexeva should be swallowed whole, and never be chewed or crushed.

What should I avoid while taking this medication?

Avoid drinking alcohol during treatment with Pexeva. Avoid driving or operating dangerous machinery or participating in any hazardous activity that requires full mental alertness until you know how this drug affects you.

What are possible food and drug interactions associated with this medication?

If Pexeva is taken with certain other drugs, the effects of either could be increased, decreased, or altered. It is especially important to check with your doctor before combining Pexeva with any of the following: alcohol, antidepressants (such as amitriptyline, desipramine, fluoxetine, imipramine, and nortriptyline), aspirin, cimetidine, diazepam, digoxin, flecainide, linezolid, lithium, nonsteroidal anti-inflammatory drugs (NSAIDs, such as aspirin, ibuprofen, naproxen, and ketoprofen), pheno-barbital, phenytoin, pimozide, procyclidine, propafenone, propranolol, quinidine, St. John's wort, sumatriptan, theophylline, thioridazine, tra-madol, triptans (a class of medication used to treat migraines; examples include sumatriptan and zolmitriptan), tryptophan, warfarin.

What are the possible side effects of this medication?

Side effects cannot be anticipated. If any develop or change in intensity, tell your doctor as soon as possible. Only your doctor can determine if it is safe for you to continue taking this drug.

Side effects may include: abnormal ejaculation, abnormal orgasm, constipa-tion, decreased appetite, decreased sex drive, diarrhea, dizziness, drowsi-ness, dry mouth, gas, impotence, male and female genital disorders, nausea, nervousness, sleeplessness, sweating, tremor, weakness, vertigo

Can I receive this medication if I am pregnant or breastfeeding?

For women who intend to become pregnant or are in their first trimester of pregnancy, Pexeva should only be initiated after consideration of the other available treatment options. The effects of Pexeva during breast-feeding are unknown; discuss your options with your doctor.

What should I do if I miss a dose of this medication?

Skip the missed dose and go back to your regular schedule. Do not take a double dose to make up for the one you missed.

How should I store this medication?

Store at room temperature.

PHENOBARBITAL

What is this medication?

Phenobarbital, a barbiturate, is used in the treatment of certain types of epilepsy, including generalized or grand mal seizures and partial seizures. It is also used for short-term treatment of insomnia.

What is the most important information I should know about this medication?

Phenobarbital can be habit-forming. You may become tolerant and need more of the drug to achieve the same effect. You may become physically and psychologically dependent with continued use. Never increase the amount of phenobarbital you take without checking with your doctor.

Phenobarbital may cause excitement, depression, or confusion in elderly or weakened individuals, and excitement in children.

Barbiturates such as phenobarbital may cause you to become tired or less alert. Be careful driving, operating machinery, or doing any activity that requires full mental alertness until you know how this medication affects you.

Who should not take this medication?

Phenobarbital should not be used if you suffer from porphyria (a blood disorder), liver or lung disease, or if you have ever had an allergic reaction to or are sensitive to phenobarbital or other barbiturates.

Phenobarbital should be used with extreme caution, or not at all, by people who are depressed or who have a history of drug or alcohol dependence.

What should I tell my doctor before I take the first dose of this medication?

Tell your doctor about all prescription, over-the-counter, and herbal medications you are taking before beginning treatment with phenobarbital. Also, talk to your doctor about your complete medical history, especially if you have a history of depression, suicidal thoughts, drug or alcohol dependence, liver disease, adrenal gland problems, constant pain; or if you are pregnant, planning to become pregnant, or are breastfeeding.

What is the usual dosage?

The information below is based on the dosage guidelines your doctor uses. Depending on your condition and medical history, your doctor may prescribe a different regimen. Do not change the dosage or stop taking your medication without your doctor's approval.

Seizures

Adults: Phenobarbital dosage must be individualized on the basis of specific laboratory tests. Your doctor will determine the exact dose best for you. The typical doses are 50 to 100 milligrams (mg) taken two to three times daily.

Children: The phenobarbital dosage must be individualized on the basis of specific laboratory tests. Your doctor will determine the exact dose best for your child.

Sedation
Adults: The usual dose is 30 to 120 milligrams (mg) a day, divided into 2 to 3 doses.

Insomnia
Adults: The usual dose is 100 to 320 mg, taken at bedtime.

People who are elderly, debilitated, or who have liver or kidney disease may require a lower dose of phenobarbital.

How should I take this medication?
Take this medication exactly as indicated by your doctor. You should never stop taking this medication without consulting your doctor first, especially if you are using this medication for seizures.

What should I avoid while taking this medication?
Avoid driving, operating machinery, or doing any activity that requires full mental alertness until you know how this medication affects you.

What are possible food and drug interactions associated with this medication?
If phenobarbital is taken with certain other drugs, the effects of either could be increased, decreased, or altered. It is especially important to check with your doctor before combining this medication with any the following: Antidepressants known as MAOIs, antihistamines, blood-thinners, doxycycline, epilepsy drugs, griseofulvin, narcotic pain relievers, oral contraceptives, sedatives, steroids, tranquilizers.

What are the possible side effects of this medication?
Side effects cannot be anticipated. If any develop or change in intensity, inform your doctor as soon as possible. Only your doctor can determine if it is safe for you to continue taking this drug.

Side effects may include: allergic reactions, drowsiness, headache, lethargy, nausea, oversedation, sleepiness, slowed or delayed breathing, vertigo, and vomiting

Can I receive this medication if I am pregnant or breastfeeding?
Barbiturates such as phenobarbital may cause fetal damage. Withdrawal symptoms may occur in an infant whose mother took barbiturates during the last 3 months of pregnancy. If you are pregnant or plan to become pregnant, inform your doctor immediately.

Phenobarbital is secreted in breast milk. Talk to your doctor about whether you should stop breastfeeding while taking this medication.

What should I do if I miss a dose of this medication?
Take it as soon as you remember. If it is almost time for your next dose, skip the one you missed and go back to your regular schedule. Never take two doses at once.

How should I store this medication?
Store at room temperature in a tightly closed container protected from light.

PRISTIQ
Generic name: Desvenlafaxine succinate

What is this medication?
Pristiq is used to treat major depression.

What is the most important information I should know about this medication?
Antidepressants can increase the risk of suicidal thinking and behavior in children and teenagers. Adult and pediatric patients taking antidepressants should be watched closely for changes in moods or actions, especially when they first start therapy or when their dose is increased or decreased. Patients and their families should contact the doctor immediately if new symptoms develop or seem to get worse. Signs to watch for include anxiety, hostility, sleeplessness, restlessness, impulsive or dangerous behavior, and thoughts about suicide or dying.

Pristiq is not approved for use in pediatric patients.

Who should not take this medication?
Do not take Pristiq if you are allergic to any of its ingredients, or if you are allergic to venlafaxine hydrochloride, the active ingredient in Effexor.

Do not take monoamine oxidase inhibitors (MAOIs) within 2 weeks before or after treatment with this medication. In some cases, a serious, possibly fatal, reaction may occur. Examples of MAOIs include selegiline and the antidepressants phenelzine and tranylcypromine.

What should I tell my doctor before I take the first dose of this medication?
Tell your doctor about all prescription, over-the-counter, and herbal medications you are taking before beginning treatment with Pristiq. Also, talk to your doctor about your complete medical history, especially if you have high blood pressure, heart problems, high cholesterol or high triglycerides, history of stroke, glaucoma, kidney or liver problems, bleeding problems, seizures or convulsions, mania or bipolar disorder, or low sodium levels in your blood.

What is the usual dosage?
The information below is based on the dosage guidelines your doctor uses. Depending on your condition and medical history, your doctor may prescribe a different regimen. Do not change the dosage or stop taking your medication without your doctor's approval.

Adults: The recommended dose is 50 milligrams once daily with or without food. If you have poor kidney or liver function, your doctor may prescribe a different dose.

How should I take this medication?
Take Pristiq at the same time each day. You can take it with or without food. Tablets should be taken whole; do not crush, chew, dissolve, or divide them. When you take Pristiq, you may see something in your stool that looks like a tablet. This is the empty shell from the tablet after the medicine has been absorbed in your body.

What should I avoid while taking this medication?
Do not drive or operate dangerous machinery until you know how Pristiq affects you. You should also avoid alcohol.

What are possible food and drug interactions associated with this medication?
If Pristiq is taken with certain drugs, the effects of either could be increased, decreased, or altered. It is important to check with your doctor before combining Pristiq with the following: drugs that affect the central nervous system, lithium, migraine medications known as triptans, narcotic painkillers, sleep aids, weight-loss products such as phentermine, tranquilizers, antipsychotic medicines, antidepressants that affect serotonin such as fluoxetine and paroxetine, MAOIs, nonsteroidal anti-inflammatory drugs, blood thinners such as aspirin and warfarin, alcohol, ketoconazole, desimipramine.

What are the possible side effects of this medication?
Side effects cannot be anticipated. If any develop or change in intensity, tell your doctor as soon as possible. Only your doctor can determine if it is safe for you to continue taking this drug.

Side effects may include: abnormal bleeding or bruising, anxiety, constipation, decreased sex drive, delayed orgasm and ejaculation, dilated pupils, dizziness, dry mouth, glaucoma, headache, high blood pressure, increased cholesterol and triglyceride levels, low sodium levels, seizures, serotonin syndrome (including restlessness, increased blood pressure, diarrhea, nausea, vomiting, increased body temperature, fast heartbeat, hallucinations, and loss of coordination), sleepiness, tiredness, tremor

Can I receive this medication if I am pregnant or breastfeeding?
Tell your doctor immediately if you are pregnant, plan to become pregnant, or are breastfeeding. It is not known if Pristiq is safe to use during pregnancy.

Pristiq can pass into breast milk and may harm your baby. Talk with your doctor about the best way to feed your baby while taking this drug.

How should I store this medication?
Store at room temperature.

PROCHLORPERAZINE

What is this medication?
Prochlorperazine is used to treat symptoms of schizophrenia and is occasionally prescribed for anxiety. It is also used to control severe nausea and vomiting.

What is the most important information I should know about this medication?
Prochlorperazine may cause a potentially fatal condition called neuroleptic malignant syndrome (NMS). Symptoms include extremely high body temperature, rigid muscles, mental changes, irregular pulse or blood pressure, rapid heartbeat, excessive sweating, and changes in heart rhythm. Alert your doctor immediately if these symptoms develop.

Prochlorperazine may cause tardive dyskinesia, a potentially irreversible movement disorder. Elderly women appear to be at higher risk.

Because it prevents vomiting, prochlorperazine may mask symptoms of an overdose of other drugs. It may also mask symptoms of brain tumor, intestinal blockage, and the neurological condition known as Reye's syndrome.

Prochlorperazine should be used cautiously in children suffering from dehydration or an acute illness such as chickenpox, measles, or other infection. The drug should not be used in children and adolescents who have symptoms of Reye's syndrome, including persistent or recurrent vomiting, listlessness, irritability, combativeness, and disorientation.

Who should not take this medication?
Do not take prochlorperazine if you are sensitive to or have ever had an allergic reaction to prochlorperazine or other phenothiazine drugs.

Prochlorperazine should not be given to comatose patients or those who have taken large amounts of central nervous system depressants (eg, alcohol, barbiturates, narcotics, etc.).

Prochlorperazine should not be given to children who are undergoing surgery or children younger than 2 years old or under 20 pounds.

What should I tell my doctor before I take the first dose of this medication?
Tell your doctor about all prescription, over-the-counter, and herbal medications you are taking before beginning treatment with prochlorperazine. Also, talk to your doctor about your complete medical history, especially if you have kidney or liver disease, intestinal blockage, heart disease,

breast cancer, seizures, glaucoma, leukemia, or if you are being treated for a brain tumor.

What is the usual dosage?

The information below is based on the dosage guidelines your doctor uses. Depending on your condition and medical history, your doctor may prescribe a different regimen. Do not change the dosage or stop taking your medication without your doctor's approval.

Severe Nausea and Vomiting

Adults: Tablets: The usual dosage is one 5-milligram (mg) or 10-mg tablet 3 or 4 times a day.

"Spansule" Capsules: The usual starting dose is one 15-milligram capsule on getting out of bed or one 10-mg capsule every 12 hours.

Suppositories: The usual rectal dosage is 25 mg, taken 2 times a day.

Children: An oral or rectal dose of prochlorperazine is usually not needed for more than 1 day. The doctor will prescribe a dosage appropriate for the child's weight.

Nonpsychotic Anxiety

Adults: Tablets: The usual dose is 5 mg taken 3 or 4 times a day.

"Spansule" capsule: The usual starting dose is one 15-mg capsule on getting up or one 10-mg capsule every 12 hours.

Treatment should not continue for longer than 12 weeks, and daily doses should not exceed 20 mg.

Mild Schizophrenia

Adults: The usual dose is 5 or 10 mg, taken 3 or 4 times daily.

Children 2 to 12 years old: The starting oral or rectal dose is 2-1/2 mg 2 or 3 times daily. Do not exceed 10 mg the first day, then increase according to the patient's response.

Children 2 to 5 years old: The total daily dosage usually does not exceed 20 mg.

Moderate to Severe Schizophrenia

Adults: Dosages usually start at 10 mg, taken 3 or 4 times a day. If needed, the dose may be gradually increased to 50 to 75 mg daily.

Severe Schizophrenia

Adults: Dosages may range from 100 to 150 mg per day.

In general, older people will be prescribed lower dosages of prochlorperazine and will undergo regular blood pressure monitoring.

How should I take this medication?

Never take more prochlorperazine than prescribed.

If you are using the suppository form of prochlorperazine and find it is too soft to insert, chill it in the refrigerator for about 30 minutes or run cold water over it before removing the wrapper. To insert a suppository, first remove the wrapper and moisten the suppository with cold water. Then lie down on your side and use a finger to push the suppository well up into the rectum.

What should I avoid while taking this medication?
Avoid large amounts of alcohol, barbiturates, or narcotics when taking prochlorperazine.

This drug may impair your ability to drive a car or operate potentially dangerous machinery. Avoid activities that require full alertness until you are sure how this drug affects you.

While taking prochlorperazine, avoid or limit sun exposure. Use sunblock and wear protective clothing. Your eyes may become more sensitive to sunlight as well so wear sunglasses.

Prochlorperazine interferes with your ability to shed body heat. Be cautious in hot weather.

What are possible food and drug interactions associated with this medication?
If prochlorperazine is taken with certain other drugs, the effects of either could be increased, decreased, or altered. It is especially important to check with your doctor before combining prochlorperazine with the following: antiseizure drugs, anticoagulants such as warfarin, central nervous system depressants, guanethidine, lithium, narcotic painkillers, propranolol, thiazide diuretics.

What are the possible side effects of this medication?
Side effects cannot be anticipated. If any develop or change in intensity, tell your doctor as soon as possible. Only your doctor can determine if it is safe for you to continue taking this drug.

Side effects may include: blurred vision, dizziness, drowsiness, jaundice (yellowing of skin and eyes), jitteriness, insomnia, low blood pressure, menstrual irregularities, skin reactions, leukopenia (a decreased number of white blood cells)

Can I receive this medication if I am pregnant or breastfeeding?
Prochlorperazine is not usually recommended for pregnant women. However, your doctor may prescribe it for severe nausea and vomiting if the potential benefits of the drug outweigh the potential risks. Prochlorperazine is secreted in breast milk and may affect a nursing infant. If prochlorperazine is essential to your health, your doctor may recommend that you stop breastfeeding until your treatment is finished.

What should I do if I miss a dose of this medication?

If you miss a dose, take it as soon as possible. If it is almost time for your next dose, skip the missed dose and go back to your normal schedule. Do not take two doses at the same time.

How should I store this medication?

Store at room temperature. Protect from heat and light.

PROVIGIL

Generic name: Modafinil

What is this medication?

Provigil is used to treat narcolepsy, obstructive sleep apnea/hypopnea syndrome, and shift work sleep disorder.

What is the most important information I should know about this medication?

Provigil may cause a rash or a serious allergic reaction. Stop Provigil and call your doctor right away or get emergency treatment if you have any of the following: skin rash, hives, sores in your mouth, or if your skin blisters and peels; swelling of your face, eyes, lips, tongue, or throat; trouble swallowing or breathing; or hoarse voice.

Provigil is not approved for use in children.

Provigil is a controlled substance because it can be abused or lead to dependence. Keep Provigil in a safe place to prevent misuse and abuse.

Who should not take this medication?

Do not take Provigil if you are allergic to any of its ingredients.

It is not known if Provigil is safe for children under the age of 16. Reduced levels of white blood cells (cells that fight infections) have occurred in some children who have taken Provigil.

What should I tell my doctor before I take the first dose of this medication?

Tell your doctor about all prescription, over-the-counter, and herbal medications you are taking before beginning treatment with Provigil. Also, talk to your doctor about your complete medical history, especially if you have high blood pressure; or heart, liver, or kidney problems. Also tell your doctor if you have used stimulant medications or if you have or have had a mental disorder known as psychosis.

What is the usual dosage?

The information below is based on the dosage guidelines your doctor uses. Depending on your condition and medical history, your doctor may prescribe a different regimen. Do not change the dosage or stop taking your medication without your doctor's approval.

Adults: The usual dose of Provigil is 200 milligrams (mg) taken as a single dose in the morning. For patients with narcolepsy or obstructive sleep apnea/hypopnea syndrome, Provigil should be taken as a single dose in the morning. For patients with shift work sleep disorder, Provigil should be taken approximately 1 hour prior to the start of their work shift.

Adults ≥*65:* These patients may need a lower dose if they have liver or kidney disease, which reduce the body's ability to metabolize Provigil.

How should I take this medication?

Take Provigil exactly as prescribed by your doctor. Your doctor will tell you the right time of day to take Provigil. You can take Provigil with or without food.

If you take more than your prescribed dose, or take Provigil too late in your waking day, you may find it harder to go to sleep. Call your doctor if you have any concerns.

What should I avoid while taking this medication?

Avoid driving or operating hazardous machinery until you know how Provigil affects you.

Avoid drinking alcohol while taking Provigil.

What are possible food and drug interactions associated with this medication?

If Provigil is taken with certain other drugs, the effects of either could be increased, decreased, or altered. It is especially important to check with your doctor before combining Provigil with the following: antidepressants, carbamazepine, clomipramine, cyclosporine, diazepam, itraconazole, ketoconazole, MAOIs, methylphenidate, oral contraceptives and hormonal implants, phenobarbital, phenytoin, propranolol, rifampin, theophylline, warfarin.

What are the possible side effects of this medication?

Side effects cannot be anticipated. If any develop or change in intensity, tell your doctor as soon as possible. Only your doctor can determine if it is safe for you to continue taking this drug.

Side effects may include: headache, nausea, nervousness, stuffy nose, diarrhea, back pain, anxiety, trouble sleeping, dizziness, upset stomach

Serious side effects may include: chest pain; mental problems; allergic reactions, such as a rash or hives

Can I receive this medication if I am pregnant or breastfeeding?

The effects of Provigil during pregnancy and breastfeeding are unknown. Tell your doctor immediately if you are pregnant, plan to become pregnant, or are breastfeeding. It is not known whether Provigil may harm your unborn baby, or if Provigil is secreted in breast milk.

What should I do if I miss a dose of this medication?

Take it as soon as possible. If you don't remember until the next day, skip the dose you missed and go back to your regular schedule. Do not take two doses at the same time.

How should I store this medication?

Store at room temperature.

PROZAC

Generic name: Fluoxetine hydrochloride

What is this medication?

Prozac is prescribed for the treatment of major depressive disorder and for panic disorder. Prozac is also prescribed to treat obsessive-compulsive disorder, bulimia and other eating disorders, and obesity. In children and adolescents, Prozac is used to treat major depression and obsessive-compulsive disorder. Prozac Weekly is approved for treating major depression.

What is the most important information I should know about this medication?

Antidepressant medicines may increase suicidal thoughts or actions in some children, teenagers, and young adults when the medicine is first started. Depression and other serious mental illnesses are the most important causes of suicidal thoughts and actions. Some people may have a particularly high risk of having suicidal thoughts or actions. These include people who have (or have a family history of) bipolar disorder (also called manic-depressive illness) or suicidal thoughts or actions.

Pay close attention to any changes, especially sudden changes, in mood, behaviors, thoughts, or feelings. This is very important when an antidepressant medicine is first started or when the dose is changed.

Call the doctor right away to report new or sudden changes in mood, behavior, thoughts, or feelings. Signs to watch for include new or worsening depression, new or worsening anxiety, agitation, insomnia, hostility, panic attacks, restlessness, extreme hyperactivity, and suicidal thinking or behavior.

Keep all follow-up visits as scheduled, and call the doctor between visits as needed, especially if you have concerns about symptoms.

If you get a rash or hives while taking Prozac, call your doctor right away because this can be a sign of a serious medical condition.

Who should not take this medication?

Do not take Prozac while using an MAOI, or within 14 days of stopping treatment with an MAOI. You should also not use Prozac if you are taking pimozide or thioridazine. Do not start thioridazine within 5 weeks of stopping Prozac.

If you are sensitive to or have ever had an allergic reaction to Prozac or similar drugs, you should not take Prozac. Make sure that your doctor is aware of any drug reactions that you have experienced.

What should I tell my doctor before I take the first dose of this medication?

Tell your doctor about all prescription, over-the-counter, and herbal medications you are taking before beginning treatment with Prozac. Also, talk to your doctor about your complete medical history, especially if you have liver or kidney disease, diabetes, seizures or epilepsy, bipolar disorder (manic depression) or a history of drug abuse or suicidal thoughts.

What is the usual dosage?

The information below is based on the dosage guidelines your doctor uses. Depending on your condition and medical history, your doctor may prescribe a different regimen. Do not change the dosage or stop taking your medication without your doctor's approval.

Depression

Adults: The recommended starting dose is 20 milligrams (mg) a day, usually taken in the morning. If needed, your doctor may gradually increase the dose to a maximum of 80 mg a day. The usual daily dose ranges from 20 to 60 mg. Daily doses above 20 mg should be taken in the morning or in two smaller doses taken in the morning and at noon.

It may take 4 weeks before the full antidepressant effect of Prozac is seen.

Prozac Weekly: You need to wait at least 7 days after stopping your daily dose of Prozac before switching to the once-weekly formulation. One Prozac Weekly capsule contains 90 mg of medication.

Children ≥8 years: The usual starting dose is 10 or 20 mg a day. Children starting at 10 mg will have their dose increased to 20 mg a day after 1 week. Underweight children may need to remain at the 10-mg dose.

Obsessive-Compulsive Disorder

Adults: The recommended starting dose is 20 mg a day, usually taken in the morning. If needed, your doctor may gradually increase the dose up to a maximum of 80 mg a day. The usual daily dose ranges from 20 to 60 mg. Daily doses above 20 mg should be taken in the morning or in two smaller doses taken in the morning and at noon.

It may take 5 weeks before the full effects of Prozac are seen.

Children ≥7 years: The recommended starting dose is 10 mg a day. After 2 weeks, the doctor will increase the dose to 20 mg. If needed, the doctor may further increase the dose up to a maximum of 60 mg a day. The recommended dosage range for underweight children is 10 to 30 mg a day.

Bulimia

Adults: The recommended dose is 60 mg day taken in the morning. The doctor may start you at a lower dose and gradually increase it over a period of several days.

Panic Disorder

Adults: The recommended starting dose is 10 mg a day. After 1 week, the doctor will increase the dose to 20 mg. If no improvement is seen after several weeks, the doctor may increase the dose to a maximum of 60 mg a day.

How should I take this medication?

Prozac should be taken exactly as prescribed by your doctor. Do not stop taking Prozac without first talking to your doctor.

Prozac usually is taken once or twice a day, at the same time each day. To be effective, it should be taken regularly.

What should I avoid while taking this medication?

Avoid driving or operating dangerous machinery or participating in any hazardous activity that requires full mental alertness until you know how this medication affects you.

Avoid alcohol while taking Prozac.

What are possible food and drug interactions associated with this medication?

If Prozac is taken with certain other drugs, the effects of either could be increased, decreased, or altered. It is especially important to check with your doctor before combining Prozac with the following: alcohol, alprazolam, antidepressants, antipsychotics, carbamazepine, central nervous system drugs, clozapine, desipramine, diazepam, digitoxin, flecainide, haloperidol, imipramine, linezolid, lithium, MAOIs, narcotic painkillers, nonsteroidal anti-inflammatory drugs (NSAIDs) such as aspirin, ibuprofen, naproxen, and ketoprofen, phenytoin, pimozide, propafenone, sleep aids, St. John's wort, sumatriptan, terfenadine, tryptophan, tramadol, vinblastine, warfarin.

Never take Prozac with MAOIs or thioridazine.

What are the possible side effects of this medication?

Side effects cannot be anticipated. If any develop or change in intensity, tell your doctor as soon as possible. Only your doctor can determine if it is safe for you to continue taking this drug.

Side effects may include: abnormal dreams, abnormal ejaculation, abnormal vision, anxiety, chest pain, chills, confusion, diarrhea, diminished sex drive, dizziness, dry mouth, flu-like symptoms, flushing, gas, headache, hives, impotence, impaired thinking, insomnia, itching, loss of appetite, nausea, nervousness, rash, seizures, sinusitis, sleepiness, sore throat, sweating, tremors, upset stomach, vomiting, weakness, yawning

Can I receive this medication if I am pregnant or breastfeeding?

The effects of Prozac during pregnancy are unknown. Tell your doctor immediately if you are pregnant, or plan to become pregnant.

Prozac is secreted in breast milk, and breastfeeding is not recommended while you are taking Prozac.

What should I do if I miss a dose of this medication?

Take it as soon as possible. If you don't remember until the next day, skip the dose you missed and go back to your regular schedule. Do not take a double dose.

How should I store this medication?

Store Prozac at room temperature.

REMERON

Generic name: Mirtazapine

What is this medication?

Remeron is a tetracyclic antidepressant used for the treatment of major depressive disorder.

What is the most important information I should know about this medication?

Antidepressant medicines may increase suicidal thoughts or actions in some children, teenagers, and young adults when the medicine is first started. Depression and other serious mental illnesses are the most important causes of suicidal thoughts and actions. Some people may have a particularly high risk of having suicidal thoughts or actions. These include people who have (or have a family history of) bipolar disorder (also called manic-depressive illness) or suicidal thoughts or actions.

Pay close attention to any changes, especially sudden changes, in mood, behaviors, thoughts, or feelings. This is very important when an antidepressant medicine is first started or when the dose is changed.

Call the doctor right away to report new or sudden changes in mood, behavior, thoughts, or feelings. Signs to watch for include new or worsening depression, new or worsening anxiety, agitation, insomnia, hostility, panic attacks, restlessness, extreme hyperactivity, and suicidal thinking or behavior.

Keep all follow-up visits as scheduled, and call the doctor between visits as needed, especially if you have concerns about symptoms.

Do not use this medication if you have used an MAO inhibitor (such as isocarboxazid, phenelzine, rasagiline, selegiline, or tranylcypromine) within the past 14 days.

If you of your family member develop signs and symptoms of fever, sore throat, stomatitis, or other signs of infection contact your doctor because this may be a sign of a serious side effect.

While you may notice improvements with Remeron therapy in 1 to 4 weeks, you should continue therapy as directed.

Never stop an antidepressant, such as Remeron, without first talking to a healthcare provider. Stopping an antidepressant medicine suddenly can cause other symptoms.

This drug may impair the mental and/or physical abilities required for performing potentially hazardous tasks such as driving or operating machinery. These effects may become worse if you combine Remeron with alcohol or certain medicines.

Who should not take this medication?

Remeron should not be used if you are known to be hypersensitive to this medication or any of its ingredients.

Do not use Remeron if you have used an MAO inhibitor within the past 14 days.

What should I tell my doctor before I take the first dose of this medication?

Tell your doctor about all prescription, over-the-counter, and herbal medications you are taking before beginning treatment with Remeron. Also, talk to your doctor about your complete medical history, especially if you have liver disease of kidney disease, a low white blood cell count, if you are have taken a MAO inhibitor (such as isocarboxazid, phenelzine, rasagiline, selegiline, or tranylcypromine) within the past 14 days, or if you have attempted or thought about suicide in the past.

What is the usual dosage?

The information below is based on the dosage guidelines your doctor uses. Depending on your condition and medical history, your doctor may prescribe a different regimen. Do not change the dosage or stop taking your medication without your doctor's approval.

Adults: The recommended starting dose of Remeron is 15 milligrams (mg) daily taken as a single dose. Preferably, this dose is to be taken in the evening, prior to sleep. The effective dose range is 15 mg to 45 mg daily. If dose changes are needed, they should not be made at intervals of less than one to two weeks in order to allow sufficient time for evaluation of the drug's effect.

Elderly or patients with serious liver of kidney problems: These patients may require a lower dose of this medication.

How should I take this medication?

Remeron should be taken exactly as prescribed. Follow the directions on your prescription label.

Take Remeron by mouth with or without food daily. Take Remeron in the evening before bedtime unless your doctor tells you otherwise.

Improvements should be noticed within 1 to 4 weeks of taking this medication. Continue to take Remeron even if you feel well, do not miss a dose.

What should I avoid while taking this medication?

Avoid driving or operating potentially dangerous machinery. Do not participate in any activities that require full alertness until you know how this drug affects you.

Avoid drinking alcohol. It can cause dangerous side effects when taken with Remeron.

Do not use Remeron if you have used an MAO inhibitor (such as isocarboxazid, phenelzine, rasagiline, selegiline, or tranylcypromine) within the past 14 days.

What are possible food and drug interactions associated with this medication?

If Remeron is taken with certain other drugs, the effects of either could be increased, decreased, or altered. It is especially important to check with your doctor before combining Remeron with the following: alcohol, clonidine, fluvoxamine, furazolidone, MAO inhibitors (including Nardil and Parnate), hydantoins such as phenytoin.

What are the possible side effects of this medication?

Side effects cannot be anticipated. If any develop or change in intensity, tell your doctor as soon as possible. Only your doctor can determine if it is safe for you to continue taking this drug.

Side effects may include: abnormal dreams, abnormal thinking, constipation, dizziness, drowsiness, dry mouth, flu symptoms, increased appetite, weakness, weight gain, decreased ability to fight infection (fever, chill, sore throat), mental or mood changes, mouth sores, thoughts or hurting yourself, tremors, worsening of depression

Can I receive this medication if I am pregnant or breastfeeding?

The effects of Remeron during pregnancy and breastfeeding are unknown. Tell your doctor immediately if you are pregnant, plan to become pregnant, or are breastfeeding.

What should I do if I miss a dose of this medication?

If you do miss a dose, take it as soon as you remember. However, if it is almost time for your next dose, skip the missed dose and take only your next regularly scheduled dose. Do not double the dose.

How should I store this medication?

Store Remeron at room temperature away from heat, moisture, and light. Do not store in the bathroom.

RESERPINE

What is this medication?

Reserpine is used to treat mild hypertension (high blood pressure) and to relieve symptoms of agitated patients with mental disorders such as schizophrenia. It is also used as a combination therapy with other blood pressure medication to treat severe cases of hypertension.

What is the most important information I should know about this medication?

Do not stop taking this medication without consulting your doctor first.

If you develop symptoms such as depression, nightmares, fainting, slow heartbeat, chest pain, swollen ankles or feet, call your doctor immediately.

Reserpine is not approved for use in children.

Who should not take this medication?

You should not take reserpine if you are allergic to it or any of its components. You should avoid taking this medication if you have mental depression, especially with suicidal tendencies, ulcers, or are receiving electroconvulsive (ECT) therapy.

What should I tell my doctor before I take the first dose of this medication?

Tell your doctor about all prescription, over-the-counter, and herbal medications you are taking before beginning treatment with reserpine. Also, talk to your doctor about your complete medical history, especially if you have a history of depression, suicidal thoughts, seizures, or gallstones.

What is the usual dosage?

The information below is based on the dosage guidelines your doctor uses. Depending on your condition and medical history, your doctor may prescribe a different regimen. Do not change the dosage or stop taking your medication without your doctor's approval.

High Blood Pressure

Adults: The usual starting dose is 0.5 milligrams (mg) daily for 1 to 2 weeks. If used long term, your dose may be reduced to 0.1 to 0.25 mg daily.

Mental Disorders

Adults: The usual starting dose is 0.5 mg daily, but it can range from 0.1 to 1 mg. Your dose may be changed based on how you respond to this drug.

How should I take this medication?

Take this medication exactly as indicated by your doctor.

What should I avoid while taking this medication?

Do not stop taking reserpine without talking to your doctor first. Abruptly stopping reserpine may increase blood pressure and cause unwanted side effects.

What are possible food and drug interactions associated with this medication?

If reserpine is taken with certain other drugs, the effects of either could be increased, decreased, or altered. It is especially important to check with your doctor before combining reserpine with any of the following: antidepressants, digoxin, isoproterenol, MAOIs, metaraminol, norepinephrine, phenylephrine, quinidine.

What are the possible side effects of this medication?

Side effects cannot be anticipated. If any develop or change in intensity, tell your doctor as soon as possible. Only your doctor can determine if it is safe for you to continue taking this drug.

Side effects may include: dizziness, loss of appetite, diarrhea, upset stomach, vomiting, stuffy nose, headache, dry mouth, and decreased sexual ability

Can I receive this medication if I am pregnant or breastfeeding?

The effects of reserpine in pregnant women are not well known. Reserpine is secreted in breast milk. Tell your doctor know if you are pregnant, planning to become pregnant, or are breastfeeding.

What should I do if I miss a dose of this medication?

Skip the missed dose and go back to your regular schedule. Do not double the dose to make up for the one you missed.

How should I store this medication?

Store at room temperature and in a dry place.

RESTORIL

Generic name: Temazepam

What is this medication?

Restoril is used for the relief of insomnia.

What is the most important information I should know about this medication?

Sleep problems are usually temporary, requiring treatment for only a short time, usually 1 or 2 days and no more than 2 to 3 weeks. Insomnia that lasts longer than this may be a sign of another medical problem. If you find you need this medicine for more than 7 to 10 days, be sure to check with your doctor.

After you stop taking Restoril, you may have more trouble sleeping than you did before you started taking it. This is called "rebound insomnia" and should clear up after one or two nights.

When you first start taking Restoril, until you know how this medicine affects you, try to avoid activities that require alertness, such as driving a car, or operating heavy machinery.

While taking Restoril, you may get up out of bed while not being fully awake and perform an activity that you do not know you are doing—nor remember the next morning. You have a greater chance of this if you drink alcohol or take other medicines that make you sleepy.

If you take Restoril every night for more than a few weeks, it loses its effectiveness to help you sleep. You can also develop physical dependence on this drug, especially if you take it regularly for more than a few weeks, or if you take more than is prescribed.

Who should not take this medication?
If you are pregnant or plan to become pregnant, you should not take this medicine. It poses a potential risk to the developing baby.

What should I tell my doctor before I take the first dose of this medication?
Tell your doctor about all prescription, over-the-counter, and herbal medications you are taking before beginning treatment with Restoril. Also, talk to your doctor about your complete medical history, especially if you are, or have been diagnosed with depression in the past, have kidney or liver problems, or if you have chronic lung disease. Let your doctor know if you have a history of alcohol or drug abuse.

What is the usual dosage?
The information below is based on the dosage guidelines your doctor uses. Depending on your condition and medical history, your doctor may prescribe a different regimen. Do not change the dosage or stop taking your medication without your doctor's approval.

Adults: The usual recommended dose is 15 milligrams (mg) at bedtime; however, 7.5 mg may be adequate. Your doctor will tailor your dose depending on your needs.

How should I take this medication?
Take Restoril exactly as prescribed; do not take more than is prescribed by your doctor.

Take Restoril right before you get into bed, not sooner.

Do not take Restoril unless you are able to get a full night's sleep (7 to 8 hours) before you must be active again.

What should I avoid while taking this medication?
Avoid drinking alcohol, or taking other medicines that can make you sleepy.

What are possible food and drug interactions associated with this medication?
If Restoril is used with certain other drugs, the effects of either could be increased, decreased, or altered. It is especially important to check with your doctor before combining Restoril with the following: alcohol, antidepressants, antihistamines, benzodiazepines, narcotic pain killers.

What are the possible side effects of this medication?

Side effects cannot be anticipated. If any develop or change in intensity, tell your doctor as soon as possible. Only your doctor can determine if it is safe for you to continue taking this drug.

Side effects may include: drowsiness, headache, fatigue, nervousness, dizziness, nausea, "hangover" feeling the next morning

Side effects due to rapid decrease in dose or abrupt withdrawal from Restoril: abdominal and muscle cramps, convulsions, feeling of discomfort, inability to fall asleep or stay asleep, sweating, tremors, vomiting

Side effects due to overdose: coma, confusion, diminished reflexes, low blood pressure, difficulty breathing

Can I receive this medication if I am pregnant or breastfeeding?

Do not take Restoril if you are pregnant or planning to become pregnant. There is an increased risk of birth defects. This drug may appear in breast milk and could affect a nursing infant. If this medication is essential to your health, your doctor may advise you to stop breastfeeding until your treatment with this medication is finished.

What should I do if I miss a dose of this medication?

Take this medicine only when you need it.

How should I store this medication?

Store at room temperature in a tightly sealed container. Do not share this medicine with anyone.

REVIA

Generic Name: Naltrexone hydrochloride

What is this medication?

Revia is indicated in the treatment of alcohol dependence and for blocking the effects of certain opioids.

What is the most important information I should know about this medication?

You should carry identification to alert medical personnel to the fact that you are taking Revia. A Revia medication card may be obtained from your physician and can be used for this purpose. Carrying the card should help to ensure that you can obtain adequate treatment in an emergency.

If you attempt to self-administer large doses of heroin or any other opioid, including methadone, while on Revia you may fall into a coma, sustain serious injury, or die.

Revia is well-tolerated in the recommended doses, but may cause liver injury when taken in excess or in people who develop liver disease from other causes. If you develop abdominal pain lasting more than a few days, pale bowel movements, dark urine, or yellowing of the eyes, you should stop taking Revia immediately and see you doctor as soon as possible.

Who should not take this medication?

You should not take Revia if you: are receiving opioid analgesics; are currently dependent on opioids; are in acute opioid withdrawal; have failed the naloxone challenge test or have a positive urine screen for opioids; have a sensitivity to Revia or any other components of the product; or have acute hepatitis or liver failure.

What should I tell my doctor before I take the first dose of this medication?

Tell your doctor about all prescription, over-the-counter, and herbal medications you are taking before beginning treatment with Revia. Talk to your doctor about your complete medical history. Tell your doctor if you are pregnant, planning to become pregnant, or are breastfeeding.

What is the usual dosage?

The information below is based on the dosage guidelines your doctor uses. Depending on your condition and medical history, your doctor may prescribe a different regimen. Do not change the dosage or stop taking your medication without your doctor's approval.

Adults: The recommended dosages are 50 milligrams (mg) every weekday with a 100 mg dose on Saturday; or 100 mg every other day; or 150 mg every third day.

Administration and single doses of Revia higher than 50 mg may be associated with an increased risk of liver injury even though three-times-a-week dosing has been well tolerated.

How should I take this medication?

Take Revia as directed by your physician.

What should I avoid while taking this medication?

Avoid taking opioid-containing preparations.

What are possible food and drug interactions associated with this medication?

If Revia is taken with certain other drugs, the effects of either could be increased, decreased, or altered. It is especially important to check with your doctor before combining Revia with the following: disulfiram; opioid-containing medicines, such as cough and cold preparations, antidiarrheal preparations, and opioid analgesics; opioids; thioridazine.

What are the possible side effects of this medication?

Side effects cannot be anticipated. If any develop or change in intensity, tell your doctor as soon as possible. Only your doctor can determine if it is safe for you to continue taking this drug.

Side effects may include: abdominal cramps, anxiety, bone or joint pain, chills, cough, decreased energy, difficulty sleeping, dizziness, headache, irritability, itching, mild nausea, muscle pain, nasal symptoms, nervousness, restlessness, runny nose, shortness of breath, skin rash, sneezing, tearfulness, vomiting

Can I receive this medication if I am pregnant or breastfeeding?
There are no adequate and well-controlled studies in pregnant women. In animal studies, Revia as well as its metabolite were found to be secreted in lactating rats. It is not known whether or not Revia is secreted in human breast milk.

What should I do if I miss a dose of this medication?
If you miss a dose, take it as soon as you remember. If it is almost time for your next dose, skip the missed dose, and resume your normal dosage schedule.

How should I store this medication?
Store Revia at room temperature, away from heat, light, and moisture.

RISPERDAL
Generic name: Risperidone

What is this medication?
Risperdal is an antipsychotic medication prescribed for the treatment of schizophrenia and for the short-term treatment of mania associated with bipolar disorder. It is also used in the treatment of irritability associated with autistic disorder in children.

What is the most important information I should know about this medication?
Risperdal may increase the risk of death when used to treat mental problems caused by dementia in elderly patients. Risperdal is not approved to treat mental problems caused by dementia.

Risperdal may cause tardive dyskinesia, a potentially irreversible condition that causes involuntary muscle spasms and twitches in the face and body. Elderly women appear to be at a higher risk for this condition. Tell your doctor immediately if you begin to have any involuntary movements. You may need to discontinue Risperdal therapy.

Risperdal may mask signs and symptoms of drug overdose and of conditions such as intestinal obstruction, brain tumor, and Reye's syndrome (a dangerous neurological condition that may follow viral infections, usually occurring in children). Risperdal may also cause difficulty when swallowing, which in turn can cause a type of pneumonia.

Risperdal may cause neuroleptic malignant syndrome (NMS), a potentially fatal condition marked by muscle stiffness or rigidity, fast heartbeat or irregular pulse, increased sweating, high fever, and blood pressure irregularities. Call your doctor immediately if you notice any of these symptoms.

Certain antipsychotic drugs, including Risperdal, are associated with an increased risk of developing high blood sugar, which on rare occasions has led to coma or death. See your doctor right away if you develop signs of high blood sugar, including dry mouth, unusual thirst, increased urination, and fatigue. If you have diabetes or have a high risk of developing it, see your doctor regularly for blood sugar testing.

Risperdal may cause dizziness, lightheadedness, or fainting; alcohol, hot weather, exercise, or fever may increase these effects. To prevent them, sit up or stand slowly, especially in the morning. Sit or lie down at the first sign of any of these effects. This effect may be more prominent when you first start taking Risperdal.

Do not drive or perform other possibly unsafe tasks until you know how you react to Risperdal.

Do not drink alcohol while you are using Risperdal.

Check with your doctor before taking medicines that may cause drowsiness (eg, sleep aids, muscle relaxers) while you are using Risperdal, because the drug may add to their effects.

Risperdal may increase the amount of a certain hormone (prolactin) in your blood. Symptoms may include enlarged breasts, missed menstrual period, decreased sexual ability, or nipple discharge. Contact your doctor right away if you experience any of these symptoms.

Risperdal may rarely cause a prolonged, painful erection. This could happen even when you are not having sex. If this is not treated right away, it could lead to permanent sexual problems such as impotence. Contact your doctor right away if this happens.

Who should not take this medication?
If you are sensitive to or have ever had an allergic reaction to Risperdal or other major tranquilizers, you should not take Risperdal.

Risperdal should not be used to treat elderly patients who have dementia because the drug could increase the risk of stroke.

What should I tell my doctor before I take the first dose of this medication?
Tell your doctor about all prescription, over-the-counter, and herbal medications you are taking before beginning treatment with Risperdal. Also, talk to your doctor about your complete medical history, especially if you have breast cancer, liver, kidney or heart disease, high or low blood pressure, heart rhythm problems, a history of heart attack or stroke, seizures, epilepsy, alcohol or substance abuse or dependence, diabetes, Alzheimer's disease, stomach or bowel problems, history of neuroleptic malignant syndrome, a history of suicidal thoughts, phenylketonuria, Parkinson's disease, or trouble swallowing. In addition, tell your doctor if you are pregnant, plan to become pregnant, or are breastfeeding.

What is the usual dosage?

The information below is based on the dosage guidelines your doctor uses. Depending on your condition and medical history, your doctor may prescribe a different regimen. Do not change the dosage or stop taking your medication without your doctor's approval.

Schizophrenia

Adults: Doses of Risperdal can be taken once a day, or divided in half and taken twice daily. The usual dose on the first day is 1 milligram (mg) taken twice a day. Incremental increases in dose are recommended. On the second day, the dose increases to 2 mg taken twice a day (for a second-day total of 4 mg). On the third day, the dose rises to 3 mg taken twice a day (for a third-day total of 6 mg). Further dosage adjustments can be made at intervals of 1 week. Over the long term, typical daily doses range from 2 to 8 mg. When dosage adjustments are necessary, small increases/decreases of 1 to 2 mg are recommended.

Bipolar Mania (Short-term Treatment of Acute Episodes)

Adults: The recommended starting dose is 2 to 3 mg per day, given as a single dose. If needed, the doctor will adjust the dose by 1 mg at intervals of at least 24 hours. The effective dosage range is 1 to 6 mg a day.

Debilitated, elderly, liver or kidney disease, or high risk for low blood pressure: The usual starting dose is 0.5 mg (or 0.5 milliliter of oral solution) twice a day. The doctor may switch you to a once-a-day dosing schedule after the first 2 to 3 days of treatment. You may also need your Risperdal dose adjusted if you're taking certain medications. Dosage increases in these patients should be in increments of no more than 0.5 mg twice a day. Increases to dosages above 1.5 mg twice a day should generally occur at intervals of at least 1 week.

Irritability Associated with Autistic Disorder

Children ≥5 years: The recommended starting dose is 0.25 mg once a day for patients <44 pounds and 0.5 mg once a day for patients ≥44 pounds. The patient should continue on the starting dose for a minimum of 4 days. The dose can then be increased to the recommended dose of 0.5 mg per day for patients <44 pounds and 1 mg per day for patients ≥44 pounds. This dose should be maintained for a minimum of 14 days. If sufficient clinical response is not achieved, dose increases of 0.25 mg per day for patients <44 pounds and 0.5 mg per day for patients ≥44 pounds can be made at no less than 2-week intervals.

No dosing data are available for children under 33 pounds. Patients who experience persistent drowsiness may benefit from once-a-day dosing given at bedtime.

The safety and effectiveness of Risperdal in pediatric patients with autistic disorder <5 years of age have not been established.

How should I take this medication?

Do not take more or less of Risperdal than prescribed. Higher doses are more likely to cause unwanted side effects.

Risperdal may be taken with or without food. Risperdal oral solution comes with a calibrated pipette to use for measuring. The oral solution can be taken with water, coffee, orange juice, and low-fat milk, but not with cola drinks or tea.

Take Risperdal on a regular schedule to get the most benefit from it. Taking Risperdal at the same time each day will help you remember to take it.

Continue to take Risperdal even if you feel well. Do not miss any doses.

What should I avoid while taking this medication?

Avoid driving or operating potentially dangerous machinery. Do not participate in any activities that require full alertness if you are not sure of how this medication affects you.

Do not drink alcohol with Risperdal.

Check with your doctor before taking medicines that may cause drowsiness (eg, sleep aids, muscle relaxers) while you are using Risperdal; it may add to their effects.

What are possible food and drug interactions associated with this medication?

If Risperdal is taken with certain other drugs, the effects of either could be increased, decreased, or altered. It is especially important to check with your doctor before combining Risperdal with the following: blood pressure medicines, bromocriptine mesylate, carbamazepine, clozapine, fluoxetine, levodopa, paroxetine, phenobarbital, phenytoin, quinidine, rifampin, valproic acid.

You may experience drowsiness and other potentially serious effects if Risperdal is combined with alcohol and other drugs that slow the central nervous system.

What are the possible side effects of this medication?

Side effects cannot be anticipated. If any develop or change in intensity, tell your doctor as soon as possible. Only your doctor can determine if it is safe for you to continue taking this drug.

Side effects may include: agitation, anxiety, constipation, dizziness, hallucinations, headache, indigestion, insomnia, rapid or irregular heartbeat, restlessness, runny nose, sleepiness, vomiting, weight change

Can I receive this medication if I am pregnant or breastfeeding?

The effects of Risperdal during pregnancy are unknown. Tell your doctor immediately if you are pregnant or plan to become pregnant.

Risperdal is secreted in breast milk. Do not breastfeed.

What should I do if I miss a dose of this medication?
Take it as soon as you remember. If it is almost time for your next dose, skip the one you missed and go back to your regular schedule. Do not take two doses at once.

How should I store this medication?
Store Risperdal at room temperature. Protect tablets from light and moisture; protect oral solution from light and freezing.

RISPERDAL CONSTA
Generic name: Risperidone

What is this medication?
Risperdal Consta is an antipsychotic medication used to treat schizophrenia.

What is the most important information I should know about this medication?
Risperdal Consta may increase the risk of death when used to treat mental problems caused by dementia in elderly patients. Risperdal Consta is not approved to treat mental problems caused by dementia.

Risperdal Consta is usually given as an injection at your doctor's office, hospital, or clinic. Be sure to keep all doctor appointments while using Risperdal Consta.

Risperdal Consta may cause tardive dyskinesia, a potentially irreversible condition that causes involuntary muscle spasms and twitches in the face and body. Elderly women appear to be at a higher risk for this condition. Tell your doctor immediately if you begin to have any involuntary movements. You may need to discontinue Risperdal Consta therapy.

Risperdal Consta may mask signs and symptoms of drug overdose and of conditions such as intestinal obstruction, brain tumor, and Reye's syndrome (a dangerous neurological condition that may follow viral infections, usually occurring in children). Risperdal Consta may also cause difficulty when swallowing, which in turn can cause a type of pneumonia.

Risperdal Consta may cause neuroleptic malignant syndrome (NMS), a potentially fatal condition marked by muscle stiffness or rigidity, fast heartbeat or irregular pulse, increased sweating, high fever, and blood pressure irregularities. Call your doctor immediately if you notice any of these symptoms.

Certain antipsychotic drugs, including Risperdal Consta, are associated with an increased risk of developing high blood sugar, which on rare occasions has led to coma or death. See your doctor right away if you develop signs of high blood sugar, including dry mouth, unusual thirst, increased urination, and tiredness. If you have diabetes or have a high risk of developing it, see your doctor regularly for blood sugar testing.

Risperdal Consta may cause dizziness, lightheadedness, or fainting; alcohol, hot weather, exercise, or fever may increase these effects. To prevent them, sit up or stand slowly, especially in the morning. Sit or lie down at the first sign of any of these effects. This effect may be more prominent when you first start taking Risperdal Consta.

Do not drive or perform other possibly unsafe tasks until you know how you react to Risperdal Consta.

Do not drink alcohol while you are using Risperdal Consta.

Check with your doctor before taking medicines that may cause drowsiness (eg, sleep aids, muscle relaxers) while you are using Risperdal Consta because the drug may add to their effects.

Risperdal Consta may increase the amount of a certain hormone (prolactin) in your blood. Symptoms may include enlarged breasts, missed menstrual period, decreased sexual ability, or nipple discharge. Contact your doctor right away if you experience any of these symptoms.

Risperdal Consta may rarely cause a prolonged, painful erection. This could happen even when you are not having sex. If this is not treated right away, it could lead to permanent sexual problems such as impotence. Contact your doctor right away if this happens.

Who should not take this medication?

If you are sensitive to or have ever had an allergic reaction to Risperdal Consta or other major tranquilizers, you should not take Risperdal Consta.

Risperdal Consta should not be used to treat elderly patients who have dementia because the drug could increase the risk of stroke.

What should I tell my doctor before I take the first dose of this medication?

Tell your doctor about all prescription, over-the-counter, and herbal medications you are taking before beginning treatment with Risperdal Consta. Also, talk to your doctor about your complete medical history, especially if you have breast cancer, liver, kidney or heart disease, high or low blood pressure, heart rhythm problems, a history of heart attack or stroke, seizures, epilepsy, alcohol or substance abuse or dependence, diabetes, Alzheimer's disease, stomach or bowel problems, history of neuroleptic malignant syndrome, a history of suicidal thoughts, phenylketonuria, Parkinson's disease, or trouble swallowing. In addition, tell your doctor if you are pregnant, plan to become pregnant, or are breastfeeding.

What is the usual dosage?

The information below is based on the dosage guidelines your doctor uses. Depending on your condition and medical history, your doctor may prescribe a different regimen. Do not change the dosage or stop taking your medication without your doctor's approval.

Schizophrenia

Adults: For patients who have never taken Risperdal, it is recommended to establish tolerability with oral Risperdal prior to initiating treatment with Risperdal Consta.

Risperdal Consta should be administered every 2 weeks by deep intramuscular (IM) gluteal injection. Each injection should be administered by a healthcare professional using the safety needle that is included with the medication. Injections should alternate between the two buttocks. Risperdal Consta should not be administered intravenously.

The recommended dose is 25 milligrams (mg) IM every 2 weeks. Those patients who do not respond to 25 mg may benefit from a higher dose of 37.5 mg or 50 mg. The maximum dose of Risperdal Consta should not exceed 50 mg every 2 weeks. No additional benefit was observed with dosages greater than 50 mg; however, a higher incidence of adverse effects was observed.

Oral Risperdal (or another antipsychotic medication) should be given with the first injection of Risperdal Consta and continued for 3 weeks to ensure adequate amounts of the drug in the blood. (The oral Risperdal/other antipsychotic medication should be discontinued after 3 weeks.)

Upward dosage adjustment should not be made more frequently than every 4 weeks. The clinical effects of this dose adjustment should not be anticipated earlier than 3 weeks after the first injection with the higher dose. Risperdal Consta has not been studied in children younger than 18 years old.

Elderly: For elderly patients treated with Risperdal Consta, the recommended dosage is 25 mg IM every 2 weeks. Oral Risperdal, or another antipsychotic medication, should be given with the first injection of Risperdal Consta and should be continued for 3 weeks to ensure adequate amounts of the drug in the blood.

Kidney or liver problems: Patients with kidney or liver dysfunction should be treated with titrated doses of oral Risperdal prior to initiating treatment with Risperdal Consta. The recommended starting dose is 0.5 mg oral Risperdal two times a day during the first week, which can be increased to 1 mg twice daily or 2 mg once daily during the second week. If a total daily dose of at least 2 mg oral Risperdal is well tolerated, an injection of 25 mg Risperdal Consta can be administered every 2 weeks.

Alternatively, a starting dose of Risperdal Consta of 12.5 mg may be appropriate for patients with kidney or liver dysfunction, for certain drug interactions that increase Risperdal concentrations in the blood, or in patients who have a history of poor tolerability to psychotropic medications. The efficacy of the 12.5 mg dose has not been investigated in clinical trials.

How should I take this medication?

Risperdal Consta is usually given as an injection at your doctor's office, hospital, or clinic. Be sure to keep all doctor appointments while using Risperdal Consta to maintain a regular schedule and gain the most benefit from the drug. Continue to take Risperdal Consta even if you feel well.

What should I avoid while taking this medication?

This drug may impair your ability to drive a car or operate potentially dangerous machinery. Do not participate in any activities that require full alertness if you are unsure of your ability.

Do not drink alcohol with Risperdal Consta.

When you first start treatment, avoid sitting up or standing up too quickly, especially in the morning. Risperdal Consta may cause dizziness, lightheadedness, or fainting due to a decrease in blood pressure. Alcohol, hot weather, exercise, or fever may increase these effects. Sit or lie down at the first sign of any of these effects.

Check with your doctor before taking medicines that may cause drowsiness (eg, sleep aids, muscle relaxers) while you are using Risperdal Consta; it may add to their effects.

What are possible food and drug interactions associated with this medication?

If Risperdal Consta is taken with certain other drugs, the effects of either could be increased, decreased, or altered. It is especially important to check with your doctor before combining Risperdal Consta with the following: blood pressure medicines, bromocriptine mesylate, carbamazepine, clozapine, fluoxetine, levodopa, paroxetine, phenobarbital, phenytoin, quinidine, rifampin, valproic acid.

You may experience drowsiness and other potentially serious effects if Risperdal Consta is combined with alcohol and other drugs that slow the central nervous system.

What are the possible side effects of this medication?

Side effects cannot be anticipated. If any develop or change in intensity, tell your doctor as soon as possible. Only your doctor can determine if it is safe for you to continue taking this drug.

Side effects may include: agitation, anxiety, constipation, dizziness, hallucinations, headache, indigestion, insomnia, rapid or irregular heartbeat, restlessness, runny nose, sleepiness, vomiting, weight change

Can I receive this medication if I am pregnant or breastfeeding?

The effects of Risperdal Consta during pregnancy are unknown. Tell your doctor immediately if you are pregnant, or plan to become pregnant.

Risperdal Consta is secreted in breast milk. Do not breastfeed.

What should I do if I miss a dose of this medication?

Take it as soon as you remember. If it is almost time for your next dose, skip the one you missed and go back to your regular schedule. Do not take two doses at once.

How should I store this medication?

The entire dose pack should be stored in the refrigerator and protected from light. If refrigeration is unavailable, Risperdal Consta can be stored at temperatures of <77°F (25°C) for < 7 days prior to administration. Do not expose unrefrigerated product to temperatures above 77°F.

RISPERDAL M-TAB ORALLY DISINTEGRATING TABLETS
Generic name: Risperidone

What is this medication?
Risperdal M-Tab is an antipsychotic medication prescribed for the treatment of schizophrenia and for the short-term treatment of mania associated with bipolar disorder. It is also used in the treatment of irritability associated with autistic disorder in children.

What is the most important information I should know about this medication?
Risperdal M-Tab may increase the risk of death when used to treat mental problems caused by dementia in elderly patients. Risperdal is not approved to treat mental problems caused by dementia.

Risperdal may cause tardive dyskinesia, a potentially irreversible condition that causes involuntary muscle spasms and twitches in the face and body. Elderly women appear to be at a higher risk for this condition. Tell your doctor immediately if you begin to have any involuntary movements. You may need to discontinue Risperdal M-Tab therapy.

Risperdal M-Tab may mask signs and symptoms of drug overdose and of conditions such as intestinal obstruction, brain tumor, and Reye's syndrome (a dangerous neurological condition that may follow viral infections, usually occurring in children). Risperdal M-Tab may also cause difficulty when swallowing, which in turn can cause a type of pneumonia.

Risperdal M-Tab may cause neuroleptic malignant syndrome (NMS), a potentially fatal condition marked by muscle stiffness or rigidity, fast heartbeat or irregular pulse, increased sweating, high fever, and blood pressure irregularities. Call your doctor immediately if you notice any of these symptoms.

Certain antipsychotic drugs, including Risperdal M-Tab, are associated with an increased risk of developing high blood sugar, which on rare occasions has led to coma or death. See your doctor right away if you develop signs of high blood sugar, including dry mouth, unusual thirst, increased urination, and fatigue. If you have diabetes or have a high risk of developing it, see your doctor regularly for blood sugar testing.

Risperdal M-Tab may cause dizziness, lightheadedness, or fainting; alcohol, hot weather, exercise, or fever may increase these effects. To prevent them, sit up or stand slowly, especially in the morning. Sit or lie down at the first sign of any of these effects. This effect may be more prominent when you first start taking Risperdal M-Tab.

Do not drive or perform other possibly unsafe tasks until you know how you react to Risperdal M-Tab.

Do not drink alcohol while you are using Risperdal M-Tab.

Check with your doctor before taking medicines that may cause drowsiness (eg, sleep aids, muscle relaxers) while you are using Risperdal M-Tab because the drug may add to their effects.

Risperdal M-Tab may increase the amount of a certain hormone (prolactin) in your blood. Symptoms may include enlarged breasts, missed menstrual period, decreased sexual ability, or nipple discharge. Contact your doctor right away if you experience any of these symptoms.

Risperdal may rarely cause a prolonged, painful erection. This could happen even when you are not having sex. If this is not treated right away, it could lead to permanent sexual problems such as impotence. Contact your doctor right away if this happens.

Who should not take this medication?

If you are sensitive to or have ever had an allergic reaction to Risperdal M-Tab or other major tranquilizers, you should not take Risperdal M-Tab.

Risperdal M-Tab should not be used to treat elderly patients who have dementia because the drug could increase the risk of stroke.

What should I tell my doctor before I take the first dose of this medication?

Tell your doctor about all prescription, over-the-counter, and herbal medication you are taking before beginning treatment with Risperdal M-Tab. Also, talk to your doctor about your complete medical history, especially if you have breast cancer, liver, kidney or heart disease, high or low blood pressure, heart rhythm problems, a history of heart attack or stroke, seizures, epilepsy, alcohol or substance abuse or dependence, diabetes, Alzheimer's disease, stomach or bowel problems, history of neuroleptic malignant syndrome, a history of suicidal thoughts, phenylketonuria, Parkinson's disease, or trouble swallowing. In addition, tell your doctor if you are pregnant, plan to become pregnant, or are breastfeeding.

What is the usual dosage?

The information below is based on the dosage guidelines your doctor uses. Depending on your condition and medical history, your doctor may prescribe a different regimen. Do not change the dosage or stop taking your medication without your doctor's approval.

Schizophrenia

Adults: Doses of Risperdal M-Tab can be taken once a day, or divided in half and taken twice daily. The usual dose on the first day is 1 milligram (mg) taken twice a day. Incremental increases in dose are recommended. On the second day, the dose increases to 2 mg taken twice a day (for a second-day total of 4 mg). On the third day, the dose rises to 3 mg taken twice a day (for a third-day total of 6 mg). Further dosage adjustments can be made at intervals of 1 week. Over the long term, typical daily doses range from 2 to 8 mg. When dosage adjustments are necessary, small increases/decreases of 1 to 2 mg are recommended.

Bipolar Mania (Short-term Treatment of Acute Episodes)

Adults: The recommended starting dose is 2 to 3 mg per day, given as a single dose. If needed, the doctor will adjust the dose by 1 mg at intervals of at least 24 hours. The effective dosage range is 1 to 6 mg a day.

Debilitated, elderly, liver or kidney disease, or high risk for low blood pressure: The usual starting dose is 0.5 milligram (or 0.5 milliliter of oral solution) twice a day. The doctor may switch you to a once-a-day dosing schedule after the first 2 to 3 days of treatment. You may also need your Risperdal dose adjusted if you're taking certain medications. Dosage increases in these patients should be in increments of no more than 0.5 mg twice a day. Increases to dosages above 1.5 mg twice a day should generally occur at intervals of at least 1 week.

Irritability Associated with Autistic Disorder

Children ≥5 years: The recommended starting dose is 0.25 mg once a day for patients <44 pounds and 0.5 mg once a day for patients >44 pounds. The patient should continue on the starting dose for a minimum of 4 days. The dose can then be increased to the recommended dose of 0.5 mg per day for patients <44 pounds and 1 mg per day for patients ≥44 pounds. This dose should be maintained for a minimum of 14 days. If sufficient clinical response is not achieved, dose increases of 0.25 mg per day for patients <44 pounds and 0.5 mg per day for patients ≥44 pounds can be made at no less than 2-week intervals.

No dosing data is available with children under 33 pounds. Patients who experience persistent drowsiness may benefit from once-a-day dosing given at bedtime.

The safety and effectiveness of Risperdal M-Tab in pediatric patients with autistic disorder <5 years of age have not been established.

How should I take this medication?

Do not take more or less of Risperdal M-Tab than prescribed. Higher doses are more likely to cause unwanted side effects.

Risperdal M-Tab orally disintegrating tablets come in blister packs and should not be removed from the package until you are ready to take them. When it's time for your dose, use dry fingers to separate one of the four blister units by tearing apart at the perforation. Bend the corner where indicated and peel back the foil of the blister pack to remove the tablet; do not push the tablet through the foil because this could damage the tablet. Immediately place the tablet on your tongue. The medication dissolves in the mouth quickly and can be swallowed with or without liquid.

You should not split, chew, or swallow the orally disintegrating tablets. Risperdal M-Tab may be taken with or without food.

Take Risperdal M-Tab on a regular schedule to get the most benefit from it. Taking Risperdal M-Tab at the same time each day will help you remember to take it.

Continue to take Risperdal M-Tab even if you feel well. Do not miss any doses.

What should I avoid while taking this medication?

Avoid driving or operating potentially dangerous machinery. Do not participate in any activities that require full alertness if you are not sure of how this medication affects you.

Do not drink alcohol with Risperdal M-Tab.

When you first start treatment, avoid sitting up or standing up too quickly, especially in the morning. Risperdal M-Tab may cause dizziness, lightheadedness, or fainting due to a decrease in blood pressure. Alcohol, hot weather, exercise, or fever may increase these effects. Sit or lie down at the first sign of any of these effects.

Check with your doctor before taking medicines that may cause drowsiness (eg, sleep aids, muscle relaxers) while you are using Risperdal M-Tab; it may add to their effects.

What are possible food and drug interactions associated with this medication?

If Risperdal M-Tab is taken with certain other drugs, the effects of either could be increased, decreased, or altered. It is especially important to check with your doctor before combining Risperdal M-Tab with the following: blood pressure medicines, bromocriptine mesylate, carbamazepine, clozapine, fluoxetine, levodopa, paroxetine, phenobarbital, phenytoin, quinidine, rifampin, valproic acid.

You may experience drowsiness and other potentially serious effects if Risperdal M-Tab is combined with alcohol and other drugs that slow the central nervous system.

What are the possible side effects of this medication?

Side effects cannot be anticipated. If any develop or change in intensity, tell your doctor as soon as possible. Only your doctor can determine if it is safe for you to continue taking this drug.

Side effects may include: agitation, anxiety, constipation, dizziness, hallucinations, headache, indigestion, insomnia, rapid or irregular heartbeat, restlessness, runny nose, sleepiness, vomiting, weight change

Can I receive this medication if I am pregnant or breastfeeding?

The effects of Risperdal M-Tab during pregnancy are unknown. Tell your doctor immediately if you are pregnant, or plan to become pregnant.

Risperdal is secreted in breast milk. Do not breastfeed.

What should I do if I miss a dose of this medication?

Take it as soon as you remember. If it is almost time for your next dose, skip the one you missed and go back to your regular schedule. Do not take two doses at once.

How should I store this medication?

Store Risperdal M-Tab at room temperature and protect from light and moisture.

RITALIN/RITALIN SR/RITALIN LA

Generic name: Methylphenidate hydrochloride

What is this medication?

Ritalin and other brands of methylphenidate are mild central nervous system stimulants used in the treatment of attention-deficit/hyperactivity disorder (ADHD) in children.

Ritalin is also used in adults to treat narcolepsy (an uncontrollable desire to sleep).

What is the most important information I should know about this medication?

When given for ADHD, Ritalin should be an integral part of a total treatment program that includes psychological, educational, and social measures.

There are reports of heart and mental problems in patients taking Ritalin or other related stimulants. Some of the problems are sudden death in patients with previous heart problems, heart attacks in adults, increased blood pressure and heart rate, new or worsening symptoms of behavior problems, bipolar disorder, and aggressive or hostile behavior. Call your doctor right away if you or your child develop signs of heart problems such as chest pain, shortness of breath, or fainting while taking Ritalin.

Excessive doses of Ritalin over a long period of time may cause addiction. It is also possible to develop tolerance to the drug, so that larger doses are needed to produce the original effect. Be sure to check with your doctor before making any change in dosage; and stop the drug only under your doctor's supervision.

There is no information regarding the safety and effectiveness of long-term treatment in children. However, slowing of growth has been seen with the long-term use of stimulants, so your doctor will monitor your child carefully while he or she is taking Ritalin.

The use of Ritalin in children less than 6 years old is not recommended.

Who should not take this medication?

This drug should not be prescribed for anyone experiencing anxiety, tension, and agitation, since the drug may aggravate these symptoms. Individuals sensitive or allergic to Ritalin should not take it.

This medication should not be taken by individuals with glaucoma, those who suffer from tics (repeated, involuntary twitches) or with a family history of Tourette's syndrome (severe and multiple tics).

This drug is not intended for use in children whose symptoms may be caused by stress or a psychiatric disorder.

This medication should not be used for the prevention or treatment of normal fatigue, nor should it be used for the treatment of severe depression.

Do not take Ritalin if you or your child are taking or have taken antidepressants known as monoamine oxidase inhibitors (MAOIs) in the last 14 days.

What should I tell my doctor before I take the first dose of this medication?

Tell your doctor about all prescription, over-the-counter, and herbal medications you are taking before beginning treatment with Ritalin, especially if you are currently taking or have recently taken MAOIs. Also, talk to your doctor about your complete medical history, especially if you have a heart problems such as a congenital heart defect, heart failure, heart rhythm disorder or recent heart attack, high blood pressure, a personal or family history of mental illness, psychotic disorder, bipolar disorder, depression, suicide attempt, epilepsy or other seizure disorder, a history of drug or alcohol addiction, glaucoma, a personal or family history of tics or Tourette's syndrome, severe anxiety, tension, or agitation.

What is the usual dosage?

The information below is based on the dosage guidelines your doctor uses. Depending on your condition and medical history, your doctor may prescribe a different regimen. Do not change the dosage or stop taking your medication without your doctor's approval.

Ritalin Tablets

Adults: The average dosage is 20 to 30 milligrams (mg) a day, divided into 2 or 3 doses, preferably taken 30 to 45 minutes before meals. Some people may need 40 to 60 mg daily, others only 10 to 15 mg. Your doctor will determine the best dose.

Children ≥6 years: The usual starting dose is 5 mg taken twice a day, before breakfast and lunch; your doctor may increase the dose by 5 to 10 mg a week. Your child should not take more than 60 mg in a day. If you do not see any improvement over a period of one month, check with your doctor.

Ritalin-SR Tablets

Adults: These are suspended-release tablets that keep working for 8 hours. They may be used in place of Ritalin tablets if they deliver a comparable dose over an 8-hour period.

Children ≥6 years: These tablets continue working for 8 hours. Your doctor will decide if they should be used in place of the regular tablets.

This drug should not be given to children under 6 years of age.

Ritalin LA Capsules

Children ≥6 years: The recommended starting dose is 20 mg once daily in the morning. At weekly intervals, your doctor may increase the dose by 10 mg, up to a maximum of 60 mg once a day.

How should I take this medication?

Follow your doctor's directions carefully. Ritalin should be taken 30 to 45 minutes before meals. If the drug interferes with sleep, give the child the last dose before 6 p.m.

Ritalin-SR and Ritalin LA are long-acting forms of the drug and are taken less frequently. They should be swallowed whole, never crushed or chewed. Ritalin LA may also be given by sprinkling the contents of the capsule on a tablespoon of cool applesauce and administering immediately, followed by a drink of water.

What should I avoid while taking this medication?

Some people have had visual disturbances such as blurred vision while being treated with Ritalin. Be careful if you drive or do anything that requires you to be awake and alert until you know how this drug affects you.

What are possible food and drug interactions associated with this medication?

If Ritalin is taken with certain other drugs, the effects of either could be increased, decreased, or altered. It is especially important to check with your doctor before combining Ritalin with the following: antidepressants, antiseizure drugs, blood pressure drugs, blood thinners such as warfarin, clonidine, guanethidine, MAO inhibitors, phenylbutazone.

What are the possible side effects of this medication?

Side effects cannot be anticipated. If any develop or change in intensity, tell your doctor as soon as possible. Only your doctor can determine if it is safe for you to continue taking this drug.

Side effects may include: inability to fall or stay asleep, nervousness

These side effects can usually be controlled by reducing the dosage and omitting the drug in the afternoon or evening.

More common side effects in children may include: loss of appetite, abdominal pain, weight loss during long-term therapy, inability to fall or stay asleep, abnormally fast heartbeat

Can I receive this medication if I am pregnant or breastfeeding?

The effects of Ritalin during pregnancy and breastfeeding are unknown. Tell your doctor immediately if you are pregnant, plan to become pregnant, or are breastfeeding.

What should I do if I miss a dose of this medication?

Give it to the child as soon as you remember. Give the remaining doses for the day at regularly spaced intervals. Do not give two doses at once.

How should I store this medication?

Store at room temperature in a tightly closed, light-resistant container protected from moisture.

ROZEREM

Generic name: Ramelteon

What is this medication?

Rozerem is used for the treatment of insomnia characterized by difficulty with sleep onset.

What is the most important information I should know about this medication?

If you experience worsening of insomnia or any new behavioral signs or symptoms of concern, consult your healthcare provider.

Rozerem is not approved for use in children.

Who should not take this medication?

Do not take Rozerem if you are allergic to the medication or any of its ingredients.

Rozerem should not be used in combination with fluvoxamine or if you have severe liver disease.

What should I tell my doctor before I take the first dose of this medication?

Tell your doctor about all prescription, over-the-counter, and herbal medications you are taking before beginning treatment with Rozerem. Also, talk to your doctor about your complete medical history, especially if you have liver disease, sleep apnea (pauses in breathing during sleep), depression, or if you have suicidal thoughts.

What is the usual dosage?

The information below is based on the dosage guidelines your doctor uses. Depending on your condition and medical history, your doctor may prescribe a different regimen. Do not change the dosage or stop taking your medication without your doctor's approval.

Adults: The recommended dose is 8 milligrams (mg) taken within 30 minutes of going to bed. Do not take this medicine with, or immediately after a high-fat meal.

How should I take this medication?

Take Rozerem exactly as directed by your doctor. Take Rozerem within 30 minutes prior to going to bed and limit your activities to those necessary to prepare for bed.

You can take Rozerem with or without food, but for Rozerem to work best, do not take it with or immediately after a high-fat, heavy meal.

Do not crush or chew the tablets. Take each tablet whole.

What should I avoid while taking this medication?
Avoid using alcoholic beverages.

Use caution when driving, operating machinery, or performing other hazardous activities. Rozerem will cause drowsiness and may cause dizziness. If you experience drowsiness or dizziness, avoid these activities.

What are possible food and drug interactions associated with this medication?
If Rozerem is taken with certain other drugs, the effects of either could be increased, decreased, or altered. It is especially important to check with your doctor before combining Rozerem with the following: fluconazole, fluvoxamine, ketoconazole, rifampin.

What are the possible side effects of this medication?
Side effects cannot be anticipated. If any develop or change in intensity, tell your doctor as soon as possible. Only your doctor can determine if it is safe for you to continue taking this drug.

Side effects may include: dizziness, fatigue, headache, nausea, drowsiness, upper respiratory tract infection

Can I receive this medication if I am pregnant or breastfeeding?
The effects of Rozerem during pregnancy and breastfeeding are unknown. Tell your doctor immediately if you are pregnant, plan to become pregnant, or are breastfeeding.

What should I do if I miss a dose of this medication?
Rozerem is usually taken only if you need it to help you sleep; missing a dose will not cause problems.

How should I store this medication?
Store Rozerem at room temperature, away from moisture and heat.

SARAFEM
Generic Name: Fluoxetine hydrochloride

What is this medication?
Sarafem is indicated for the treatment of premenstrual dysphoric disorder (PMDD).

What is the most important information I should know about this medication?
Antidepressant medicines may increase suicidal thoughts or actions in some children, teenagers, and young adults when the medicine is first started. Depression and other serious mental illnesses are the most important causes of suicidal thoughts and actions. Some people may have a particularly high risk of having suicidal thoughts or actions. These include people who have (or have a family history of) bipolar disorder (also called manic-depressive illness) or suicidal thoughts or actions.

Pay close attention to any changes, especially sudden changes, in mood, behaviors, thoughts, or feelings. This is very important when an antidepressant medicine is first started or when the dose is changed.

Call the doctor right away to report new or sudden changes in mood, behavior, thoughts, or feelings. Signs to watch for include new or worsening depression, new or worsening anxiety, agitation, insomnia, hostility, panic attacks, restlessness, extreme hyperactivity, and suicidal thinking or behavior.

Keep all follow-up visits as scheduled, and call the doctor between visits as needed, especially if you have concerns about symptoms.

Who should not take this medication?
You should not take Sarafem if you have a known hypersensitivity to any of its ingredients.

Do not take Sarafem if you are taking a monoamine oxidase inhibitor (MAOI) or have stopped taking an MAOI less than 14 days ago.

If you are taking pimozide you should not take Sarafem.

If you are taking thioridazine, you should not take Sarafem or wait a minimum of 5 weeks after Sarafem has been discontinued.

What should I tell my doctor before I take the first dose of this medication?
Tell your doctor about all prescription, over-the-counter, and herbal medications you are taking before beginning treatment with Sarafem. Talk to your doctor about your complete medical history, especially past or current liver or kidney disease. Tell your doctor if you are pregnant, planning to become pregnant, or are breastfeeding.

What is the usual dosage?
The information below is based on the dosage guidelines your doctor uses. Depending on your condition and medical history, your doctor may prescribe a different regimen. Do not change the dosage or stop taking your medication without your doctor's approval.

Adults: The recommended starting dose of Sarafem for the treatment of PMDD is 20 milligrams (mg) a day given continuously (every day of the menstrual cycle) or intermittently for up to 3 months at a dose of 20 mg a day (defined as starting a daily dose 14 days prior to the anticipated onset of menstruation through the first full day of menses and repeating with each new cycle).

The maximum dose of Sarafem should not exceed 80 mg a day.

How should I take this medication?
Take Sarafem as directed by your physician.

What should I avoid while taking this medication?
Avoid taking Sarafem with other medications that affect serotonin; see the next page for more on drug interactions.

What are possible food and drug interactions associated with this medication?

If Sarafem is taken with certain other drugs, the effects of either could be increased, decreased, or altered. It is especially important to check with your doctor before combining Sarafem with the following: anticonvulsants, antipsychotics, benzodiazepines, digoxin, electroconvulsive therapy, lithium, MAOIs, nonsteroidal anti-inflammatory drugs (NSAIDs), pimozide, selective norepinephrine reuptake inhibitors, selective serotonin reuptake inhibitors (eg, Prozac, Zoloft), thioridazine, triptans (eg, Imitrex, Maxalt, Frova), tryptophan, warfarin.

What are the possible side effects of this medication?

Side effects cannot be anticipated. If any develop or change in intensity, tell your doctor as soon as possible. Only your doctor can determine if it is safe for you to continue taking this drug.

Side effects may include: headache, body pain, nausea, diarrhea, insomnia, dizziness, nervousness, abnormalities in thinking, decreased libido, runny nose, sore throat

Can I receive this medication if I am pregnant or breastfeeding?

Sarafem should be used during pregnancy only if the potential benefit justifies the potential risk to the fetus. Sarafem is secreted in breast milk, hence nursing while on Sarafem is not recommended.

What should I do if I miss a dose of this medication?

If you miss a dose, take it as soon as you remember. If it is almost time for your next dose, skip the missed dose, and resume your normal dosage schedule.

How should I store this medication?

Store Sarafem at room temperature, away from heat, light, and moisture.

SECONAL

Generic Name: Secobarbital

What is this medication?

Seconal is used for the short-term treatment of insomnia. It is also used as a pre-anesthetic in certain medical procedures.

What is the most important information I should know about this medication?

Complex behaviors such as "sleep driving" (ie, driving while not fully awake after taking this medication, or other similar medications, with amnesia of the event) have been reported. Although behaviors such as sleep-driving may occur with this medication alone, the use of alcohol and other depressants, such as narcotics, tranquilizers, and antihistamines increase the risk of such behavior. If any such acts occur, notify your doctor immediately.

Seconal may be habit-forming; tolerance and physical dependence may occur with continued use. Do not increase the dose of the drug without consulting with your physician. If you have a history of drug abuse, consult with your physician before taking Seconal.

Seconal may impair your mental and/or physical abilities required for potentially hazardous tasks, such as driving a car or operating machinery.

Who should not take this medication?
You should not take Seconal if you are hypersensitive to barbiturates.

Seconal should not be taken if you have marked impairment of liver function or certain respiratory diseases.

What should I tell my doctor before I take the first dose of this medication?
Tell your doctor about all prescription, over-the-counter, and herbal medications you are taking before beginning treatment with Seconal. Also, talk to your doctor about your complete medical history, especially past or current liver problems, drug abuse, and acute or chronic pain. Tell your doctor if you are pregnant, planning to become pregnant, or are breastfeeding.

What is the usual dosage?
The information below is based on the dosage guidelines your doctor uses. Depending on your condition and medical history, your doctor may prescribe a different regimen. Do not change the dosage or stop taking your medication without your doctor's approval.

Dosages of barbiturates vary on a patient to patient basis. Your doctor will prescribe you an appropriate dose based on your age, weight, and condition.

Insomnia
Adults: 100 milligrams (mg) at bedtime.
Elderly: Dosage will be reduced for elderly patients because they are more sensitive to barbiturates.

Presurgical Anesthesia
Adults: 200 to 300 mg 1 to 2 hours before surgery.

How should I take this medication?
Take Seconal as directed by your physician. It is usually taken once at bedtime.

What should I avoid while taking this medication?
Avoid drinking alcohol while taking Seconal; also avoid taking any other medications that may cause drowsiness or decrease your alertness.

Do not drive or operate machinery until you know how this medication affects you.

What are possible food and drug interactions associated with this medication?

If Seconal is taken with certain other drugs, the effects of either could be increased, decreased, or altered. It is especially important to check with your doctor before combining Seconal with the following: antihistamines, blood thinners such as warfarin, corticosteroids, doxycycline, griseofulvin, phenytoin, steroid hormones, tranquilizers, valproic acid.

What are the possible side effects of this medication?

Side effects cannot be anticipated. If any develop or change in intensity, tell your doctor as soon as possible. Only your doctor can determine if it is safe for you to continue taking this drug.

Side effects may include: agitation, confusion, nightmares, anxiety, dizziness, hallucinations, decreased blood pressure and heart rate, nausea, vomiting

Can I receive this medication if I am pregnant or breastfeeding?

Barbiturates such as Seconal can cause fetal harm when administered to a pregnant woman. Barbiturates cross the placenta and high concentrations are found in the fetal liver and brain. Consult with your physician before breastfeeding while taking Seconal.

What should I do if I miss a dose of this medication?

If you miss a dose, take it as soon as you remember. If it is almost time for your next dose, skip the missed dose, and resume your normal dosage schedule.

How should I store this medication?

Store at room temperature, away from heat, light, and moisture.

SEROQUEL

Generic name: Quetiapine fumarate

What is this medication?

Seroquel is an antipsychotic medication prescribed for the treatment of schizophrenia. It is also used for the short-term treatment of mania associated with bipolar disorder as well as for the treatment of depressive episodes associated with bipolar disorder.

What is the most important information I should know about this medication?

Safety and effectiveness of Seroquel in children has not been established.

Antidepressants have increased the risk of suicidal thoughts and actions in children and teenagers. All patients starting treatment should be watched closely for worsening of depression, suicidal thoughts or actions, unusual changes in behavior, agitation, and irritability. Families and caregivers should watch patients daily and report these symptoms immediately to their physician.

Seroquel may increase the risk of death when used to treat mental problems caused by dementia in elderly patients and therefore should not be used in these patients. Most of the deaths were linked to heart problems or infection.

Seroquel may cause tardive dyskinesia, a potentially irreversible condition characterized by uncontrollable muscle spasms and twitches in the face and body. Older adults, especially women, appear to be at greater risk.

Seroquel may cause neuroleptic malignant syndrome (NMS), a serious, and potentially fatal, reaction to the drug. Call your doctor immediately if you develop muscle stiffness, confusion, irregular or rapid heartbeat, excessive sweating, and high fever. Be especially wary if you have a history of heart attack, heart disease, heart failure, circulation problems, or irregular heartbeat.

Certain antipsychotic drugs, including Seroquel, are associated with an increased risk of developing high blood sugar, which on rare occasions has led to coma or death. See your doctor right away if you develop signs of high blood sugar, including dry mouth, unusual thirst, increased urination, and tiredness. If you have diabetes or have a high risk of developing it, see your doctor regularly for blood sugar testing

When you first start treatment, avoid sitting up or standing up too quickly, especially in the morning. Seroquel may cause dizziness, lightheadedness, or fainting due to a decrease in blood pressure. Alcohol, hot weather, exercise, or fever may increase these effects. Sit or lie down at the first sign of any of these effects.

Seroquel may rarely cause a prolonged, painful erection. This could happen even when you are not having sex. If this is not treated right away, it could lead to permanent sexual problems, such as impotence. Contact your doctor right away if this happens.

Do not drink alcohol while you are using Seroquel.

Do not become overheated or dehydrated in hot weather or while you are being active; heatstroke, dizziness, or fainting may occur.

Several weeks may pass before your symptoms improve. Do NOT take more than the recommended dose or use for longer than prescribed without checking with your doctor.

Seroquel may cause drowsiness, dizziness, or decreased vision. These effects may be worse if you take it with alcohol or certain medicines. Use Seroquel with caution. Do not drive or perform other possibly unsafe tasks until you know how you react to it.

Seroquel should be used with particular caution in patients with known cardiovascular disease (history of heart attack or ischemic heart disease, heart failure or conduction abnormalities), cerebrovascular disease or conditions that would predispose patients to decreased blood pressure (dehydration, hypovolemia, and treatment with antihypertensive medications).

An eye exam for cataracts is recommended at the beginning of treatment and every six months.

Do not suddenly stop taking Seroquel without first talking with your doctor. You may have an increased risk of side effects. If you need to stop Seroquel or add a new medicine, your doctor will gradually lower your dose.

Rarely, Seroquel may lower the ability of your body to fight infection. Avoid contact with people who have colds or infections. Tell your doctor if you notice signs of infection like fever, sore throat, rash, or chills.

Who should not take this medication?

Do not take Seroquel if you are allergic to the medication or any of its ingredients.

What should I tell my doctor before I take the first dose of this medication?

Tell your doctor about all prescription, over-the-counter, and herbal medications you are taking before beginning treatment with Seroquel. Also, talk to your doctor about your complete medical history, especially if you have liver, kidney, or heart disease, high or low blood pressure, high cholesterol, heart rhythm problems, a history of heart attack or stroke, a thyroid disorder, seizures, epilepsy, Alzheimer's disease, obesity, breast cancer, thyroid problems, cataracts, narrow-angle glaucoma, high blood prolactin levels, neuroleptic malignant syndrome, a personal or family history of diabetes, or trouble swallowing.

What is the usual dosage?

The information below is based on the dosage guidelines your doctor uses. Depending on your condition and medical history, your doctor may prescribe a different regimen. Do not change the dosage or stop taking your medication without your doctor's approval.

Bipolar Mania (Short-term Treatment of Acute Episodes)

Adults: The usual dosage range is 400 to 800 milligrams (mg) a day. Doses above 800 mg a day have not been tested for safety. The dosage will be gradually increased over 4 to 6 days until the most effective dose is reached.

Schizophrenia

Adults: The usual dosage range is 300 to 400 mg a day, divided into two or three smaller doses. Doses as low as 150 mg a day sometimes prove effective; the dose rarely exceeds 750 mg per day. Doses above 800 mg per day have not been tested for safety. The dose is gradually increased over 4 days until the most effective dose is reached.

Liver problems: If you have liver problems, you may be started at 25 mg a day. The doctor will increase the dose as needed.

Debilitated, elderly, or prone to low blood pressure: You may also need your dose adjusted.

How should I take this medication?
Your doctor will increase your dose gradually until the drug takes effect. If you stop Seroquel for more than one week, you'll need to build up to your ideal dosage once again.

What should I avoid while taking this medication?
Seroquel tends to cause drowsiness, especially at the start of therapy, and can impair your judgment, thinking, and motor skills. Avoid driving or operating machinery until you know how the medication affects you.

Avoid exposure to extreme heat, strenuous exercise, and dehydration.

Avoid drinking alcohol while taking Seroquel. The drug increases the effects of alcohol.

When you first start treatment, avoid sitting up or standing up too quickly, especially in the morning. Seroquel may cause dizziness, lightheadedness, or fainting due to a decrease in blood pressure. Alcohol, hot weather, exercise, or fever may increase these effects. Sit or lie down at the first sign of any of these effects.

Rarely, Seroquel may lower the ability of your body to fight infection. Avoid contact with people who have colds or infections. Tell your doctor if you notice signs of infection like fever, sore throat, rash, or chills.

What are possible food and drug interactions associated with this medication?
If Seroquel is taken with certain other drugs, the effects of either could be increased, decreased, or altered. It is especially important to check with your doctor before combining Seroquel with the following: alcohol, barbiturates such as phenobarbital, carbamazepine, cimetidine, divalproex, erythromycin, fluconazole, itraconazole, ketoconazole, levodopa, lorazepam, phenytoin, rifampin, steroids such as hydrocortisone and prednisone, thioridazine.

What are the possible side effects of this medication?
Side effects cannot be anticipated. If any develop or change in intensity, tell your doctor as soon as possible. Only your doctor can determine if it is safe for you to continue taking this drug.

Side effects may include: abdominal pain, constipation, diminished movement, dizziness, drowsiness, dry mouth, excessive muscle tone, fatigue, headache, indigestion, low blood pressure (especially upon standing), nasal inflammation, neck rigidity, rapid or irregular heartbeat, rash, sleepiness, tremor, uncontrollable movements, vomiting, weakness, weight gain

Can I receive this medication if I am pregnant or breastfeeding?

The effects of Seroquel during pregnancy and breastfeeding are unknown. Tell your doctor immediately if you are pregnant, plan to become pregnant, or are breastfeeding. Seroquel should only be used during pregnancy if the potential benefit justifies the potential risk to the fetus.

What should I do if I miss a dose of this medication?

Take it as soon as you remember. If it is almost time for the next dose, skip the one you missed and go back to your regular schedule. Do not take two doses at once.

How should I store this medication?

Store at room temperature. Store away from heat, moisture, and light. Do not store in the bathroom.

SEROQUEL XR

Generic name: Quetiapine fumarate

What is this medication?

Seroquel XR is an antipsychotic medication prescribed for the treatment of schizophrenia.

What is the most important information I should know about this medication?

Seroquel XR is not approved for use in children.

Antidepressants have increased the risk of suicidal thoughts and actions in children and teenagers. All patients starting treatment should be watched closely for worsening of depression, suicidal thoughts or actions, unusual changes in behavior, agitation, and irritability. Families and caregivers should watch patients daily and report these symptoms immediately to their physician.

Seroquel XR may increase the risk of death when used to treat mental problems caused by dementia in elderly patients and therefore should not be used in these patients. Most of the deaths were linked to heart problems or infection.

Seroquel XR may cause tardive dyskinesia, a potentially irreversible condition characterized by uncontrollable muscle spasms and twitches in the face and body. Older adults, especially women, appear to be at greater risk.

Seroquel XR may cause neuroleptic malignant syndrome (NMS), a serious, and potentially fatal, reaction to the drug. Call your doctor immediately if you develop muscle stiffness, confusion, irregular or rapid heartbeat, excessive sweating, and high fever. Be especially wary if you have a history of heart attack, heart disease, heart failure, circulation problems, or irregular heartbeat.

Certain antipsychotic drugs, including Seroquel XR, are associated with an increased risk of developing high blood sugar, which on rare occasions has led to coma or death. See your doctor right away if you develop signs of high blood sugar, including dry mouth, unusual thirst, increased urination, and tiredness. If you have diabetes or have a high risk of developing it, see your doctor regularly for blood sugar testing.

When you first start treatment, avoid sitting up or standing up too quickly, especially in the morning. Seroquel XR may cause dizziness, lightheadedness, or fainting due to a decrease in blood pressure. Alcohol, hot weather, exercise, or fever may increase these effects. Sit or lie down at the first sign of any of these effects.

Seroquel XR may rarely cause a prolonged, painful erection. This could happen even when you are not having sex. If this is not treated right away, it could lead to permanent sexual problems, such as impotence. Contact your doctor right away if this happens.

Do not drink alcohol while you are using Seroquel XR.

Do not become overheated or dehydrated in hot weather or while you are being active; heatstroke, dizziness, or fainting may occur.

Seroquel XR should be used with particular caution in patients with known cardiovascular disease (history of heart attack or ischemic heart disease, heart failure or conduction abnormalities), cerebrovascular disease or conditions that would predispose patients to decreased blood pressure (dehydration, hypovolemia, and treatment with antihypertensive medications).

Do not suddenly stop taking Seroquel XR without first talking with your doctor. You may have an increased risk of side effects. If you need to stop Seroquel XR or add a new medicine, your doctor will gradually lower your dose.

Rarely, Seroquel XR may lower the ability of your body to fight infection. Avoid contact with people who have colds or infections. Tell your doctor if you notice signs of infection like fever, sore throat, rash, or chills.

Who should not take this medication?
Do not take Seroquel XR if you are allergic to the medication or any of its ingredients.

What should I tell my doctor before I take the first dose of this medication?
Tell your doctor about all prescription, over-the-counter, and herbal medications you are taking before beginning treatment with Seroquel XR. Also, talk to your doctor about your complete medical history, especially if you have liver, kidney or heart disease, high or low blood pressure, heart rhythm problems, high cholesterol, a history of heart attack or stroke, breast cancer, a thyroid disorder, seizures, epilepsy, Alzheimer's disease, dementia or mood problems, suicidal thoughts, obesity, history of alcohol or substance abuse, thyroid problems, cataracts, narrow-angle

glaucoma, blood problems, a history of neuroleptic malignant syndrome, a personal or family history of diabetes, or trouble swallowing.

What is the usual dosage?
The information below is based on the dosage guidelines your doctor uses. Depending on your condition and medical history, your doctor may prescribe a different regimen. Do not change the dosage or stop taking your medication without your doctor's approval.

Schizophrenia
Adults: The recommended starting dose of Seroquel XR is 300 milligrams (mg) a day, preferably taken in the evening. The effective dose range is 400 mg to 800 mg daily depending on the response and tolerance of the individual patient. Dose increases can be made at 1-day intervals at increments of up to 300 mg per day. Individual dosage adjustments may be necessary. The safety of doses higher than 800 mg daily have not been studied in clinical trials.

How should I take this medication?
Seroquel XR sustained-release tablets are best taken in the evening. Take Seroquel XR by mouth on an empty stomach or with a light meal (approximately 300 calories).

Continue with the medication even if you start to feel better; do not skip any doses.

Do not suddenly stop taking Seroquel XR without first contacting your doctor. You may have an increased risk of experiencing side effects.

What should I avoid while taking this medication?
Seroquel XR tends to cause drowsiness, especially at the start of therapy, and can impair your judgment, thinking, and motor skills. Until you are certain how the drug affects you, use caution when operating machinery or driving a car.

Avoid exposure to extreme heat, strenuous exercise, and dehydration.

Avoid drinking alcohol while taking Seroquel XR. The drug increases the effects of alcohol.

Rarely, Seroquel XR may lower the ability of your body to fight infection. Avoid contact with people who have colds or infections. Tell your doctor if you notice signs of infection like fever, sore throat, rash, or chills.

What are possible food and drug interactions associated with this medication?
If Seroquel XR is taken with certain other drugs, the effects of either could be increased, decreased, or altered. It is especially important to check with your doctor before combining Seroquel XR with the following: alcohol, barbiturates such as phenobarbital, carbamazepine, cimetidine, divalproex, erythromycin, fluconazole, itraconazole, ketoconazole, levodopa, lorazepam, phenytoin, rifampin, steroids such as hydrocortisone and prednisone, thioridazine.

What are the possible side effects of this medication?

Side effects cannot be anticipated. If any develop or change in intensity, tell your doctor as soon as possible. Only your doctor can determine if it is safe for you to continue taking this drug.

Side effects may include: constipation, dizziness, drowsiness, dry mouth, stomach upset, lightheadedness, weight gain, confusion, fainting, fever, chills, sore throat, increased saliva production or drooling, increased sweating, memory loss, menstrual changes, muscle pain, and allergic reactions (eg, rash, hives, itching, difficulty breathing, swelling of the mouth, face, lips, or tongue)

Can I receive this medication if I am pregnant or breastfeeding?

The effects of Seroquel XR during pregnancy and breastfeeding are unknown. Tell your doctor immediately if you are pregnant, plan to become pregnant, or are breastfeeding.

Seroquel XR should only be used during pregnancy if the potential benefit justifies the potential risk to the fetus.

What should I do if I miss a dose of this medication?

Take it as soon as you remember. If it is almost time for the next dose, skip the one you missed and go back to your regular schedule. Do not take 2 doses at once. If you miss taking Seroquel XR for longer than 1 week, contact your doctor.

How should I store this medication?

Store Seroquel XR at room temperature. Store away from heat, moisture, and light. Do not store in the bathroom.

SINEQUAN

Generic name: Doxepine hydrochloride

What is this medication?

Sinequan is a tricyclic antidepressant used to treat depression and anxiety.

What is the most important information I should know about this medication?

Sinequan is not approved for use in children under 12.

Antidepressant medicines may increase suicidal thoughts or actions in some children, teenagers, and young adults when the medicine is first started. Depression and other serious mental illnesses are the most important causes of suicidal thoughts and actions. Some people may have a particularly high risk of having suicidal thoughts or actions. These include people who have (or have a family history of) bipolar disorder (also called manic-depressive illness) or suicidal thoughts or actions.

Pay close attention to any changes, especially sudden changes, in mood, behaviors, thoughts, or feelings. This is very important when an antidepressant medicine is first started or when the dose is changed.

Call the doctor right away to report new or sudden changes in mood, behavior, thoughts, or feelings. Signs to watch for include new or worsening depression, new or worsening anxiety, agitation, insomnia, hostility, panic attacks, restlessness, extreme hyperactivity, and suicidal thinking or behavior.

Keep all follow-up visits as scheduled, and call the doctor between visits as needed, especially if you have concerns about symptoms.

Who should not take this medication?

If you are sensitive to or have ever had an allergic reaction to Sinequan or similar antidepressants, you should not take Sinequan. Make sure that your doctor is aware of any drug reactions that you have experienced.

Unless you are directed to do so by your doctor, do not take Sinequan if you have difficulty urinating or the eye condition known as glaucoma.

What should I tell my doctor before I take the first dose of this medication?

Tell your doctor about all prescription, over-the-counter, and herbal medications you are taking before beginning treatment with Sinequan. Also, talk to your doctor about your complete medical history, especially if you have glaucoma, or difficulty urinating.

What is the usual dosage?

The information below is based on the dosage guidelines your doctor uses. Depending on your condition and medical history, your doctor may prescribe a different regimen. Do not change the dosage or stop taking your medication without your doctor's approval.

Adults: The starting dose for mild to moderate illness is usually 75 milligrams (mg) per day. This dose can be increased or decreased by your doctor according to individual need. The total daily dose can be given once a day or divided into smaller doses. If you are taking Sinequan once a day, the recommended dose is 150 mg at bedtime.

The 150-mg capsule strength is intended for long-term therapy only and is not recommended as a starting dose.

For more severe illness, gradually increased doses of up to 300 mg may be required as determined by your doctor.

Elderly: Due to a greater risk of drowsiness and confusion, older people are usually started on a low dose.

How should I take this medication?

Take Sinequan exactly as prescribed. It may take several weeks for you to feel better.

What should I avoid while taking this medication?

Sinequan may cause you to become drowsy or less alert; do not drive, operate dangerous machinery, or participate in any hazardous activity that requires full mental alertness until you know how this medication affects you.

Do not drink alcohol while taking Sinequan. Alcohol increases the danger of a Sinequan overdose.

What are possible food and drug interactions associated with this medication?

If Sinequan is taken with certain other drugs, the effects of either could be increased, decreased, or altered. It is especially important to check with your doctor before combining Sinequan with the following: alcohol, antidepressants, carbamazepine, cimetidine, clonidine, flecainide, guanethidine, MAOIs, major tranquilizers, propafenone, quinidine, tolazamide.

What are the possible side effects of this medication?

Side effects cannot be anticipated. If any develop or change in intensity, tell your doctor as soon as possible. Only your doctor can determine if it is safe for you to continue taking this drug.

Side effects may include: blurred vision, constipation, diarrhea, dizziness, drowsiness, dry mouth, itchy or scaly skin (pruritus), light sensitivity, loss of appetite, low blood pressure, nausea, rapid or irregular heartbeat, rash, trouble urinating, vomiting, water retention, weight changes

Can I receive this medication if I am pregnant or breastfeeding?

The effects of Sinequan during pregnancy are unknown. Tell your doctor immediately if you are pregnant, or plan to become pregnant. Sinequan may appear in breast milk and could affect a nursing infant. If Sinequan is essential to your health, your doctor may advise you to stop breastfeeding your baby until your treatment is finished.

What should I do if I miss a dose of this medication?

Take it as soon as you remember. If it is almost time for the next dose, skip the one you missed and go back to your regular schedule. Do not take two doses at once.

How should I store this medication?

Store at room temperature.

SONATA
Generic name: Zaleplon

What is this medication?

Sonata is prescribed for people who have trouble falling asleep at bedtime. Because it has a short duration of action, it doesn't help those who suffer from frequent awakenings during the night or those who wake too early in the morning. It is intended only for short-term use.

What is the most important information I should know about this medication?

Sonata is not approved for use in children.

Do not take Sonata unless you plan to be in bed for at least 4 hours after taking it. If you need to be alert and active in less than 4 hours, your performance could be impaired. Never attempt to drive a car or operate other dangerous machinery right after taking Sonata.

Problems with sleep are usually temporary and require only short-term treatment with medication. Call your doctor immediately if it seems the medication is making the problem worse, or if you notice any unusual changes in your thinking or behavior, such as hallucinations, amnesia, agitation, or a lack of inhibition.

Use Sonata only for temporary relief of insomnia; sleep medicines tend to lose their effect when taken for more than a few weeks. Taking sleeping pills for extended periods or in high doses can lead to physical dependence and the danger of a withdrawal reaction when the drug is abruptly stopped.

If you have worsening insomnia or the emergence of new thinking or behavior abnormalities, see your doctor, this may be due to an unrecognized disorder.

Complex behaviors, such as "sleep-driving" have been reported. These events can occur if you have not taken a sedative in the past as well as if you have.

Who should not take this medication?

Sonata is not recommended for people with severe liver disease.

Do not take it if you are allergic to any of its ingredients. It contains the coloring agent FD&C Yellow No. 5, which causes a reaction in some individuals. This allergic reaction is more likely in people who are sensitive to aspirin.

What should I tell my doctor before I take the first dose of this medication?

Tell your doctor about all prescription, over-the-counter, and herbal medications you are taking before beginning treatment with Sonata. Also, talk to your doctor about your complete medical history, especially if you have depression, liver disease, sleep apnea (stopping breathing for short periods while asleep), asthma, bronchitis, emphysema, or another respiratory disease, myasthenia gravis (a muscle weakness), or a history of drug or alcohol addiction.

What is the usual dosage?

The information below is based on the dosage guidelines your doctor uses. Depending on your condition and medical history, your doctor may prescribe a different regimen. Do not change the dosage or stop taking your medication without your doctor's approval.

Adults: The usual dose is 10 milligrams (mg) taken once daily at bedtime. Your doctor may adjust the dose to your individual need, especially if you are in a weakened condition or have a low body weight. A dose of 5 mg is recommended if you have liver disease or use the drug cimetidine. Doses above 20 mg have not been adequately evaluated and are not recommended.

Elderly: This population is more sensitive to the effects of Sonata and respond to 5 mg. Doses over 10 mg in the elderly are not recommended.

How should I take this medication?

Sonata is very fast-acting and should be taken only at bedtime. Sonata should be taken immediately before bedtime or if you have difficulty falling asleep after you have gone to bed. Taking Sonata while still up and about may result in short-term memory impairment, hallucinations, impaired coordination, dizziness, and lightheadedness.

What should I avoid while taking this medication?

Avoid alcoholic beverages when taking Sonata.

Never attempt to drive a car or operate other dangerous machinery right after taking Sonata.

What are possible food and drug interactions associated with this medication?

If Sonata is taken with certain other drugs, the effects of either could be increased, decreased, or altered. It is especially important to check with your doctor before combining Sonata with the following: alcohol, carbamazepine, cimetidine, diphenhydramine, erythromycin, imipramine, ketoconazole, phenobarbital, promethazine, rifampin, thioridazine.

Avoid high-fat meals immediately before taking Sonata; they tend to slow or reduce the drug's effect.

What are the possible side effects of this medication?

Side effects cannot be anticipated. If any develop or change in intensity, tell your doctor as soon as possible. Only your doctor can determine if it is safe for you to continue taking this drug.

Side effects may include: abdominal pain, amnesia, back pain, chest pain, constipation, dizziness, drowsiness, dry mouth, eye pain, headache, memory loss, menstrual pain, migraine, muscle pain, nausea, sleepiness, tingling, weakness

Can I receive this medication if I am pregnant or breastfeeding?

The effects of Sonata during pregnancy are unknown. Tell your doctor immediately if you are pregnant, or plan to become pregnant. Sonata is secreted in breast milk and may affect a nursing baby. Do not take this medication without first talking to your doctor if you are breastfeeding.

What should I do if I miss a dose of this medication?

Take Sonata only when you're ready to sleep. Never double your dose.

How should I store this medication?

Store at room temperature in a light-resistant container.

STRATTERA

Generic name: Atomoxetine hydrochloride

What is this medication?

Strattera is used to treat attention-deficit/hyperactivity disorder (ADHD). Strattera may help increase attention and decrease impulsiveness and hyperactivity. It should be used as part of a total treatment program for ADHD that may include counseling or other therapies.

What is the most important information I should know about this medication?

In some children and teenagers, Strattera may increase the risk of suicidal thoughts. Call your doctor right away if your child has thoughts of suicide or sudden changes in mood or behavior, especially at the beginning of treatment or after a change in dose. New mental problems in children and teenagers may also occur. Call your doctor right away if your child has new psychotic symptoms (such as hearing voices, believing things that are not true, being suspicious), or new manic symptoms.

Strattera can cause liver damage. Call your doctor right away if you or your child has itching, right upper belly pain, dark urine, yellow skin or eyes, or unexplained flu-like symptoms.

Strattera use has been associated with heart-related problems, including sudden death in people who have heart problems or heart defects, stroke or heart attack in adults, and increased blood pressure and heart rate. Call your doctor right away if you or your child has any signs of heart problems such as chest pain, shortness of breath, or fainting.

Strattera has not been studied in children less than 6 years of age.

Who should not take this medication?

Do not take Strattera within 14 days of taking antidepressants called monoamine oxidase inhibitors (MAOIs), including phenelzine, tranylcypromine, and selegiline. The combination of Strattera and an MAOI can cause severe, even fatal, reactions. If you experience high fever, rigid muscles, rapid changes in heart rate, delirium, and coma, call your doctor immediately.

You should not take Strattera if you have narrow-angle glaucoma (high pressure in the eye) or if you are allergic to anything in Strattera.

What should I tell my doctor before I take the first dose of this medication?

Tell your doctor about all prescription, over-the-counter, and herbal medications you are taking before beginning treatment with Strattera. Also, talk to your doctor about your complete medical history, especially if there is a history of bipolar disorder or depression, heart problems, high or low blood pressure, irregular heart beat, liver disease, mental problems, psychosis, or suicidal thoughts or actions.

What is the usual dosage?

The information below is based on the dosage guidelines your doctor uses. Depending on your condition and medical history, your doctor may prescribe a different regimen. Do not change the dosage or stop taking your medication without your doctor's approval.

The daily dose of Strattera can be taken as a single dose in the morning, or divided into 2 equal doses taken in the morning and late afternoon or early evening.

Adults and teenagers >154 pounds: The usual starting dosage is 40 milligrams (mg) per day. After at least 3 days, your doctor may increase the daily total to a recommended level of 80 mg. After another 2-4 weeks, dosage may be increased to a maximum of 100 mg daily. If you have liver problems, your dosage will be reduced.

Children and teenagers ≤154 pounds: The usual starting dosage is 0.5 mg per 2.2 pounds of body weight per day. After at least 3 days, the doctor may increase the daily total to a recommended level of 1.2 mg per 2.2 pounds. Daily doses should never exceed 1.4 mg per 2.2 pounds, or a total of 100 mg, whichever is less.

Strattera has not been tested in children less than 6 years of age.

How should I take this medication?

Take Strattera exactly as prescribed by your doctor. Do not chew, crush, or open the capsules. Swallow the capsules whole with water or other liquids. Strattera can be taken with or without food. Take your dose at the same time each day to help you remember.

What should I avoid while taking this medication?

Avoid touching a broken Strattera capsule. Wash hands and surfaces that touched an open capsule. If any powder gets in your eyes or your child's eyes, rinse them with water right away and call your doctor.

Use caution when driving, operating machinery, or performing other hazardous activities.

What are possible food and drug interactions associated with this medication?

If Strattera is taken with certain other drugs, the effects of either could be increased, decreased, or altered. It is especially important to check with your doctor before combining Strattera with the following: albuterol and similar asthma medications, dopamine, dobutamine, fluoxetine, paroxetine, quinidine.

What are the possible side effects of this medication?

Side effects cannot be anticipated. If any develop or change in intensity, tell your doctor as soon as possible. Only your doctor can determine if it is safe for you to continue taking this drug.

Side effects in adults may include: constipation, decreased appetite, dizziness, dry mouth, menstrual cramps, nausea, problems urinating, sexual side effects, trouble sleeping

Side effects in children and teenagers may include: decreased appetite, dizziness, nausea or vomiting, mood swings, tiredness, upset stomach

Erections that won't go away (priapism) have occurred rarely during treatment with Strattera. If you have an erection that lasts more than 4 hours, seek medical help right away because of the potential for lasting damage, including the potential inability to have erections.

Can I receive this medication if I am pregnant or breastfeeding?

The effects of Strattera during pregnancy and breastfeeding are unknown. Tell your doctor immediately if you are pregnant, plan to become pregnant, or are breastfeeding.

What should I do if I miss a dose of this medication?

Take it as soon as remember on that day. If you miss a day of Strattera, do not double your dose. Just skip the day you missed.

How should I store this medication?

Store at room temperature.

SUBOXONE

Generic name: Buprenorphine hydrochloride and naloxone hydrochloride

What is this medication?

Suboxone is a sublingual tablet used to treat opioid addiction.

What is the most important information I should know about this medication?

If you use drugs like narcotic pain killers, anti-anxiety medicines, or sleep aids while taking Suboxone, you may experience difficulty breathing and other nervous system side effects.

Do not take more than is recommended, nor should you abruptly stop taking this medicine, since this can cause withdrawal symptoms.

If you are admitted to an emergency room, be sure to notify the staff that you are being treated with Suboxone. Have a family member notify the staff if you are unable to do so.

When you first start treatment with Suboxone, avoid performing activities that require alertness, such as driving a car, until you know how this medicine affects you.

Suboxone is a controlled substance; taking this medicine in a way that is not prescribed may lead to tolerance, dependence, and serious nervous system side effects.

Who should not take this medication?

If you have kidney, liver, or chronic lung disease, take Suboxone under close supervision.

Do not take this medicine if you have allergies to any of its components.

What should I tell my doctor before I take the first dose of this medication?

Tell your doctor about all prescription, over-the-counter, and herbal medications you are taking before beginning treatment with Suboxone. Also, talk to your doctor about your complete medical history, especially if you have liver or kidney disease, chronic lung disease, or any stomach or intestinal conditions.

What is the usual dosage?

The information below is based on the dosage guidelines your doctor uses. Depending on your condition and medical history, your doctor may prescribe a different regimen. Do not change the dosage or stop taking your medication without your doctor's approval.

Adults: Suboxone is administered sublingually (under the tongue) as a single daily dose in the range of 12 to 16 milligrams (mg) per day.

How should I take this medication?

Before taking Suboxone, drink some water to moisten your mouth. This will help the tablets dissolve more easily.

Place the Suboxone tablets under your tongue, lean your head slightly forward, and let the tablets completely dissolve, which might take 5 to 10 minutes. Try not to talk while the tablet is dissolving, since this can affect the absorption of the medicine.

Do not chew or swallow the tablet(s), allow them to dissolve completely under your tongue.

What should I avoid while taking this medication?

While taking Suboxone, do not take other nervous system depressants, such as sleep aids, or anti-anxiety medications, since this can cause serious, life-threatening side effects.

Do not take more than is prescribed, and do not stop taking this medicine unless told to do so by your doctor.

What are possible food and drug interactions associated with this medication?
If Suboxone is used with certain other drugs, the effects of either could be increased, decreased, or altered. It is especially important to check with your doctor before combining Suboxone with the following: antianxiety medications such as benzodiazepines, antibiotics, antifungals, HIV medications such as ritonavir, indinavir, and saquinavir.

What are the possible side effects of this medication?
Side effects cannot be anticipated. If any develop or change in intensity, tell your doctor as soon as possible. Only your doctor can determine if it is safe for you to continue taking this drug.

Side effects may include: chills, headache, abdominal pain, constipation, nausea, sleeplessness, sweating

Can I receive this medication if I am pregnant or breastfeeding?
The effects of Suboxone during pregnancy and breastfeeding are unknown. Tell your doctor immediately if you are pregnant, plan to become pregnant, or are breastfeeding.

What should I do if I miss a dose of this medication?
Take the dose as soon as you remember. If you are within 12 hours of your next dose, skip the missed dose and continue with your normal dosing schedule, unless your doctor tells you otherwise. Never take two doses at once.

How should I store this medication?
Store at room temperature.

SURMONTIL
Generic name: Trimipramine maleate

What is this medication?
Surmontil is a tricyclic antidepressant used to treat depression.

What is the most important information I should know about this medication?
Never take Surmontil if you are taking an antidepressant drug called a monoamine oxidase inhibitor (MAOI) or if you have stopped taking an MAOI in the last 14 days. MAOI drugs include phenelzine, tranylcypromine, and isocarboxazid. Taking Surmontil close in time to an MAOI can result in serious—sometimes fatal—reactions, including high body temperature, coma, and seizures.

Antidepressants can increase the risk of suicidal thinking and behavior in children and teenagers. Adult and pediatric patients taking antidepressants should be watched closely for changes in moods or actions, especially when they first start therapy or when their dose is increased or decreased. Patients and their families should contact the doctor immediately if new symptoms develop or seem to get worse. Signs to watch for include anxiety, hostility, insomnia, restlessness, impulsive or dangerous behavior, and thoughts about suicide or dying.

Never stop an antidepressant medication without first talking to your healthcare provider. Abruptly stopping Surmontil can cause other symptoms.

Antidepressant medications have other side effects. Talk to your healthcare provider about the side effects of the medicine prescribed for you or your family member.

Who should not take this medication?

Surmontil should not be used if you are recovering from a recent heart attack or if you are sensitive to the drug.

What should I tell my doctor before I take the first dose of this medication?

Tell your doctor about all prescription, over-the-counter, and herbal medications you are taking before beginning treatment with Surmontil. Also, talk to your doctor about your complete medical history, especially if you have a family history of suicide, bipolar disorder, or depression. Also let your doctor know if you have a history of diabetes, glaucoma (increased pressure in the eye), heart, kidney, or liver disease, overactive thyroid, seizure disorder, or urinary retention.

What is the usual dosage?

The information below is based on the dosage guidelines your doctor uses. Depending on your condition and medical history, your doctor may prescribe a different regimen. Do not change the dosage or stop taking your medication without your doctor's approval.

Adults: The usual starting dose is 75 milligrams (mg) per day, divided into equal, smaller doses. Your doctor may gradually increase your dose to 150 mg per day, again, divided into smaller doses. Doses over 200 mg a day are not recommended. Doses for long-term therapy may range from 50 to 150 mg daily. You can take this total daily dosage at bedtime or spread it throughout the day.

Elderly or Adolescents: Dosages usually start at 50 mg per day. Your doctor may increase the dose to 100 mg a day, if needed.

Surmontil is not approved for use in children.

How should I take this medication?

Surmontil is taken by mouth. Many people take one dose at bedtime. Others may find it works better to take Surmontil more than once a day.

It is important to take Surmontil exactly as prescribed, even if the drug seems to have no effect. It may take up to 4 weeks for its benefits to appear.

Surmontil can make your mouth dry. Sucking hard candy or chewing gum can help this problem.

What should I avoid while taking this medication?
Avoid driving a car, operating machinery, or participating in any activities that require full alertness if you are sure of the drug's effect on you.

Avoid using alcohol, which may increase drowsiness and dizziness while taking Surmontil.

What are possible food and drug interactions associated with this medication?
If Surmontil is taken with certain other drugs, the effects of either could be increased, decreased, or altered. It is especially important to check with your doctor before combining Surmontil with the following: antidepressants, antispasmodic drugs such as benztropine, atropine, cimetidine, decongestants, drugs for heart irregularities such as flecainide and propafenone, epinephrine, guanethidine, quinidine, tranquilizers, thyroid medications.

What are the possible side effects of this medication?
Side effects cannot be anticipated. If any develop or change in intensity, tell your doctor as soon as possible. Only your doctor can determine if it is safe for you to continue taking this drug.

Side effects may include: allergic reactions, black tongue, blood disorders, blurred vision, breast development in men, confusion, dizziness, drowsiness, dry mouth, fluctuations in blood pressure, heartbeat irregularities, high or low blood pressure, insomnia, lack of coordination, stomach and intestinal problems, urination problems, vomiting

Can I receive this medication if I am pregnant or breastfeeding?
The effects of Surmontil during pregnancy and breastfeeding are unknown. Tell your doctor immediately if you are pregnant, plan to become pregnant, or are breastfeeding. There is no information on whether Surmontil appears in breast milk. The doctor may tell you to stop breastfeeding until your treatment is finished.

What should I do if I miss a dose of this medication?
Take it as soon as you remember. If it is almost time for the next dose, skip the missed dose and go back to your regular schedule. Do not take two doses at once. If you take Surmontil once a day at bedtime and you miss a dose, do not take it in the morning; it could cause disturbing side effects during the day.

How should I store this medication?
Store at room temperature in a tightly closed container, away from moisture.

SYMBYAX

Generic name: Olanzapine and fluoxetine hydrochloride

What is this medication?

Symbyax contains two medicines, olanzapine and fluoxetine. Symbyax is used to treat adults who have depressive episodes associated with bipolar disorder.

What is the most important information I should know about this medication?

Symbyax is not for use in dementia-related psychosis (decreased mental functioning complicated by seeing or hearing things or having irrational thoughts or fears). There is an increased risk of death in elderly patients with dementia-related psychosis who are treated with Symbyax.

A life-threatening condition called serotonin syndrome (serious changes in how your brain, muscles, and digestive system work) can happen when you take Symbyax with medicines known as triptans, which are used to treat migraine headaches. Signs and symptoms of serotonin syndrome include restlessness, diarrhea, hallucinations, coma, loss of coordination, nausea, fast heartbeat, vomiting, increased body temperature, rapid changes in blood pressure, and overactive reflexes. Serotonin syndrome may be more likely to occur when starting or increasing the dose of Symbyax or a triptan.

Antidepressants can increase the risk of suicidal thinking and behavior in children and teenagers. Adult and pediatric patients taking antidepressants should be watched closely for changes in moods or actions, especially when they first start therapy or when their dose is increased or decreased. Patients and their families should contact the doctor immediately if new symptoms develop or seem to get worse. Signs to watch for include anxiety, hostility, insomnia, restlessness, impulsive or dangerous behavior, and thoughts about suicide or dying.

Symbyax may cause drowsiness or dizziness. These effects may be worse if you take it with alcohol or certain medicines. Take Symbyax with caution. Do not drive or perform other possibly unsafe tasks until you know how you react to it.

Do not drink alcohol or use medicines that may cause drowsiness (eg, sleep aids, muscle relaxers) while you are using Symbyax; it may add to their effects.

Symbyax may cause dizziness, lightheadedness, or fainting; alcohol, hot weather, exercise, or fever may increase these effects. To prevent them, sit up or stand slowly, especially in the morning. Sit or lie down at the first sign of any of these effects.

Do not become overheated in hot weather or while you are being active; heatstroke may occur.

Several weeks may pass before your symptoms improve. Do NOT take more than the recommended dose, change your dose, or take Symbyax for longer than prescribed without checking with your doctor.

Symbyax may rarely cause a prolonged, painful erection. This could happen even when you are not having sex. If this is not treated right away, it could lead to permanent sexual problems such as impotence. Contact your doctor right away if this happens.

Symbyax may raise your blood sugar. High blood sugar may make you feel confused, drowsy, or thirsty. It can also make you flush, breathe faster, or have a fruit-like breath odor. If these symptoms occur, tell your doctor right away.

Neuroleptic malignant syndrome (NMS) is a potentially fatal syndrome that can be caused by Symbyax. Symptoms may include fever, stiff muscles, confusion, abnormal thinking, fast or irregular heartbeat, and sweating. Contact your doctor at once if you have any of these symptoms.

Some patients who take Symbyax may develop tardive dyskinesia, a potentially irreversible disorder characterized by involuntary muscle movements and twitches. Older people, especially women, appear to be at greater risk. The chance that this will happen or that it will become permanent is greater in those who take Symbyax in higher doses or for a long time. Tell your doctor at once if you have muscle problems with your arms, legs, tongue, face, mouth, or jaw (eg, tongue sticking out, puffing of cheeks, mouth puckering, chewing movements) while taking Symbyax.

Who should not take this medication?

Never take Symbyax if you are taking antidepressant drugs called monoamine oxidase inhibitors (MAOIs), or if you have stopped taking an MAOI in the last 14 days. Taking Symbyax close in time to an MAOI can result in serious—sometimes fatal—reactions, including high body temperature, coma, or seizures. Do not take an MAOI within 5 weeks of stopping Symbyax. MAOI drugs include isocarboxazid, phenelzine, and tranylcypromine.

Never take Symbyax while you are taking thioridazine and do not take thioridazine within 5 weeks of stopping Symbyax. Simultaneously taking these drugs can result in serious heart rhythm problems.

Do not take Symbyax if you are taking pimozide or if you are sensitive to any component of the drug.

What should I tell my doctor before I take the first dose of this medication?

Tell your doctor about all prescription, over-the-counter, and herbal medications you are taking before beginning treatment with Symbyax. Also, talk to your doctor about your complete medical history, especially if you are older than 65 and have dementia, Alzheimer's disease, a history of certain types of cancer (breast, pancrease, pituitary) or if you are at risk for breast cancer, have a history of high blood sugar or diabetes, a family history of diabetes, or if you currently smoke, drink alcohol, exercise often, or are often in hot places. Be sure to also let your doctor know if you have any of the following conditions: a stomach problem called paralytic ileus; an enlarged prostate; narrow-angle glaucoma; history of heart attack; high or low blood pressure; liver, kidney, or heart problems; seizures, strokes, or mini-strokes.

You should especially tell your doctor if you are taking or plan to take Prozac, Prozac Weekly, Sarafem, olanzapine, Zyprexa, or Zyprexa Zydis. These medicines each contain an ingredient that is also found in Symbyax.

What is the usual dosage?

The information below is based on the dosage guidelines your doctor uses. Depending on your condition and medical history, your doctor may prescribe a different regimen. Do not change the dosage or stop taking your medication without your doctor's approval.

Adults: The usual starting dose is 1 capsule containing 6 milligrams (mg) of olanzapine and 25 mg of fluoxetine, taken once a day in the evening. If needed, your doctor may gradually increase the dose. The usual dose range is 6 to 12 mg of olanzapine and 25-50 mg of fluoxetine. The efficacy of Symbyax was demonstrated in a dose range of 6 mg to 12 mg of olanzapine and 25 mg to 50 mg of fluoxetine. The safety of doses above 18 mg olanzapine and 75 mg fluoxetine has not been evaluated in clinical studies.

Your doctor may adjust your dose if you have liver problems, a high risk of low blood pressure, or a combination of factors that may slow your body's processing of Symbyax (female, older age, nonsmoker).

How should I take this medication?

Take Symbyax exactly as instructed by your doctor. Your doctor will usually start you on a low dose of Symbyax. Your dose may be adjusted depending on your body's response to Symbyax. Do not stop taking Symbyax or change your dose even if you feel better. Do not suddenly stop taking Symbyax without checking with your doctor.

Symbyax is usually taken once a day in the evening. Take Symbyax at the same time each day.

You can take Symbyax with or without food.

What should I avoid while taking this medication?

Avoid driving, operating machinery, or performing other hazardous activities until you know how this medication affects you. If you experience dizziness or drowsiness, avoid these activities. Dizziness may be more likely to occur when you rise from a sitting or lying position. Rise slowly to prevent dizziness and a possible fall.

Do not drink alcohol while taking Symbyax. The combination can cause a sudden drop in blood pressure.

Avoid becoming overheated while taking Symbyax. Drink plenty of fluid and use caution in hot weather and during exercise.

What are possible food and drug interactions associated with this medication?

If Symbyax is taken with certain other drugs, the effects of either could be increased, decreased, or altered. It is especially important to check with your doctor before combining Symbyax with the following: alprazolam, antidepressants known as MAOIs or tricyclics, blood pressure drugs, carbamazepine, clozapine, diazepam, dopamine, fluvoxamine, haloperidol, levodopa, lithium, omeprazole, phenytoin, pimozide, rifampin, St. John's wort, thioridazine, tramadol, triptans such as sumatriptan or eletriptan, tryptophan, warfarin.

Be careful about combining Symbyax with aspirin or nonsteroidal anti-inflammatory drugs (NSAIDs) such as ibuprofen, or with other drugs that affect blood clotting. The combination may increase the risk of bleeding.

What are the possible side effects of this medication?

Side effects cannot be anticipated. If any develop or change in intensity, tell your doctor as soon as possible. Only your doctor can determine if it is safe for you to continue taking this drug.

Side effects may include: diarrhea, constipation, decreased sexual desire or ability, dizziness, dry mouth, feeling weak, increased appetite, problems keeping your body temperature regulated, sleepiness, black or tarry stools, confusion, anxiety, memory problems, irritability, sore throat, swelling of your hands and feet, tremors, trouble concentrating, weight gain, or allergic reactions (such as hives, rash, itching, difficulty breathing, swelling of lips, face, mouth, or tongue)

Can I receive this medication if I am pregnant or breastfeeding?

The effects of Symbyax during pregnancy and breastfeeding are unknown. Tell your doctor immediately if you are pregnant, plan to become pregnant, or are breastfeeding. Do not breastfeed while you are taking Symbyax.

Neonates exposed to fluoxetine, a component of Symbyax, late in the third trimester have developed complications requiring prolonged hospitalizations, respiratory support, and tube feeding. The risks and benefits of treatment should be carefully considered when using Symbyax during pregnancy.

What should I do if I miss a dose of this medication?

Take it as soon as you remember. However, if it is almost time for your next dose, skip the missed dose and take only your regularly scheduled dose. Do not take two doses at once.

How should I store this medication?

Store at room temperature, away from heat, moisture, and light. Do not store in the bathroom.

THIORIDAZINE HYDROCHLORIDE

What is this medication?

Thioridazine hydrochloride is used to treat schizophrenia.

What is the most important information I should know about this medication?

Thioridazine hydrochloride has been associated with arrhythmias (life-threatening irregular heartbeats) and sudden death. This medication should be reserved for people in whom other medication therapies did not work.

If you experience symptoms such as fast, irregular, or pounding heartbeat, dizziness, lightheadedness, fainting or seizures, call your doctor right away.

Who should not take this medication?

Do not take this medication if you are allergic to thioridazine hydrochloride or any of its components.

What should I tell my doctor before I take the first dose of this medication?

Tell your doctor about all prescription, over-the-counter, and herbal medications you are taking before beginning treatment with thioridazine hydrochloride. Also, talk to your doctor about your complete medical history, especially if you have a history of heart problems, and if you are pregnant, planning to become pregnant, or are breastfeeding.

What is the usual dosage?

The information below is based on the dosage guidelines your doctor uses. Depending on your condition and medical history, your doctor may prescribe a different regimen. Do not change the dosage or stop taking your medication without your doctor's approval.

Adults: The usual starting dose is 50 to 100 milligrams (mg), taken 3 times daily. If necessary, your doctor may increase your dose up to a maximum daily dose of 800 mg, divided into 2 or 4 doses.

Children: Your child's doctor will determine the exact dose based on your child's weight.

How should I take this medication?

Take this medication exactly as indicated by your doctor.

What should I avoid while taking this medication?

You should never stop taking this medication without consulting your doctor first.

Avoid driving or operating dangerous machinery or participating in any hazardous activity that requires full mental alertness until you know how this medication affects you.

Avoid drinking alcohol while on this medication.

What are possible food and drug interactions associated with this medication?

If thioridazine hydrochloride is taken with certain other drugs, the effects of either could be increased, decreased, or altered. It is especially important to check with your doctor before combining this medication with any of the following: fluvoxamine, fluoxetine, paroxetine, pindolol, propranolol.

What are the possible side effects of this medication?

Side effects cannot be anticipated. If any develop or change in intensity, inform your doctor as soon as possible. Only your doctor can determine if it is safe for you to continue taking this drug.

Side effects may include: drowsiness, dizziness, restlessness, blurred vision, dry mouth, constipation, and weight gain

Can I receive this medication if I am pregnant or breastfeeding?

The effects of thioridazine hydrochloride during pregnancy and breast-feeding are unknown. Tell your doctor immediately if you are pregnant, plan to become pregnant, or are breastfeeding.

What should I do if I miss a dose of this medication?

Take the missed dose as soon as you remember. However, if you remember a missed dose when it is almost time for your next scheduled dose, skip the missed dose. Do not take two doses to make up for a missed one.

How should I store this medication?

Thioridazine hydrochloride should be stored at room temperature, protected from light.

TOFRANIL/TOFRANIL-PM

Generic name: Imipramine

What is this medication?

Tofranil and Tofranil-PM are used to treat depression. Tofranil is also used on a short-term basis, along with behavioral therapies, to treat bed-wetting in children ages 6 and older.

What is the most important information I should know about this medication?

Antidepressants can increase the risk of suicidal thinking and behavior in children and teenagers. Adult and pediatric patients taking antidepressants should be watched closely for changes in moods or actions, especially when they first start therapy or when their dose is increased or decreased. Patients and their families should contact the doctor immediately if new symptoms develop or seem to get worse. Signs to watch for include anxiety, hostility, insomnia, restlessness, impulsive or dangerous behavior, and thoughts about suicide or dying.

Never take Tofranil if you are taking another antidepressant drug called a monoamine oxidase inhibitor (MAOI) or if you have stopped taking an MAOI in the last 14 days. MAOI drugs include phenelzine, tranylcypromine, and isocarboxazid. Taking Tofranil close in time to an MAOI can result in serious—sometimes fatal—reactions, including high body temperature, coma, and seizures.

You should not take this medicine if you are recovering from a heart attack.

Who should not take this medication?

Do not take Tofranil if you are recovering from a heart attack, if you are sensitive to the drug, or if you are using MAOI drugs or have used an MAOI in the last 14 days.

What should I tell my doctor before I take the first dose of this medication?

Tell your doctor about all prescription, over-the-counter, and herbal medications you are taking before beginning treatment with Tofranil. Also, talk to your doctor about your complete medical history, especially if you have a history of heart disease, congestive heart failure, abnormal heart rhythm, have had a heart attack, stroke, rapid heartbeat, glaucoma (increased pressure in the eye), urinary retention, an enlarged prostate, overactive thyroid, seizure disorder, schizophrenia, bipolar disorder, kidney or liver disease, diabetes, if you will be undergoing surgery, or if you will be undergoing electroconvulsive therapy (ECT).

What is the usual dosage?

The information below is based on the dosage guidelines your doctor uses. Depending on your condition and medical history, your doctor may prescribe a different regimen. Do not change the dosage or stop taking your medication without your doctor's approval.

Depression

Adults: The usual dose is 75 milligrams (mg) a day. Your doctor may increase this to 150 mg a day. The maximum daily dose is 200 mg. People who need to take 75 mg or more a day may use Tofranil-PM capsules instead of the regular tablets.

Elderly and Adolescents: The usual dose is 30 to 40 mg daily. Effective dosages usually do not exceed 100 mg a day.

Bedwetting

Children ≥6 years: The starting dose is 25 mg daily taken 1 hour before bedtime. If needed, this dose may be increased after 1 week to 50 mg (ages 6 to 11) or 75 mg (ages 12 and up), taken in one dose at bedtime or divided into 2 doses, 1 taken in the mid-afternoon and 1 at bedtime.

Safety and effectiveness in children under the age of 6 have not been established. Tofranil-PM should not be used in children for any reason.

How should I take this medication?

Take Tofranil exactly as prescribed by your doctor. Do not stop taking Tofranil if you feel no immediate effect. It can take anywhere from 1-3 weeks before you feel better. An abrupt decrease in dose could result in general feelings of illness, headache, and nausea.

Tofranil may be taken with or without food. It may be taken several times a day or in one daily dose at bedtime.

Tofranil can cause dry mouth. Sucking hard candy or chewing gum can help this problem.

What should I avoid while taking this medication?

Do not drive or operate machinery, or participate in any activities that require full alertness until you know how this drug affects you.

Use alcohol cautiously. Alcohol may increase drowsiness and dizziness while taking Tofranil.

Tofranil can make you sensitive to light. Try to stay out of the sun as much as possible while you are taking it.

What are possible food and drug interactions associated with this medication?

If Tofranil is taken with certain other drugs, the effects of either could be increased, decreased, or altered. It is especially important to check with your doctor before combining Tofranil with the following: albuterol, antidepressants, antipsychotic drugs, barbiturates, such as phenobarbital, benztropine, blood pressure medications, carbamazepine, cimetidine, epinephrine, flecainide, guanethidine, methylphenidate, narcotic painkillers, such as codeine and oxycodone, norepinephrine, phenytoin, propafenone, pseudoephedrine, quinidine, thyroid medications, tranquilizers.

If you are switching from fluoxetine, wait at least 5 weeks after your last dose of fluoxetine before starting Tofranil.

What are the possible side effects of this medication?

Side effects cannot be anticipated. If any develop or change in intensity, tell your doctor as soon as possible. Only your doctor can determine if it is safe for you to continue taking this drug.

Side effects may include: breast development in males, breast enlargement in females, breast milk production, confusion, diarrhea, dry mouth, hallucinations, hives, high blood pressure, low blood pressure upon standing, nausea, numbness, tremors, vomiting

Side effects in children being treated for bedwetting include: anxiety, collapse, constipation, convulsions, emotional instability, fainting, fatigue, nervousness, sleep disorders, stomach and intestinal problems

Can I receive this medication if I am pregnant or breastfeeding?
The effects of Tofranil during pregnancy and breastfeeding are unknown. Tell your doctor immediately if you are pregnant, plan to become pregnant, or are breastfeeding.

What should I do if I miss a dose of this medication?
If you take one dose a day at bedtime, contact your doctor. Do not take the dose in the morning because of possible side effects.

If you take two or more doses a day, take the forgotten dose as soon as you remember. If it is almost time for your next dose, skip the one you missed and go back to your regular schedule. Do not take two doses at once.

How should I store this medication?
Store Tofranil at room temperature in a tightly closed container.

TRANXENE
Generic name: Clorazepate dipotassium

What is this medication?
Tranxene T-Tab and Tranxene SD tablets belong to a class of drugs known as benzodiazepines. Tranxene is used to treat anxiety disorders and for the short-term relief of anxiety symptoms. The drug is also used to relieve the symptoms of acute alcohol withdrawal and to help in treating certain convulsive disorders such as epilepsy.

What is the most important information I should know about this medication?
Tranxene may be habit-forming if taken regularly over a long period. You may experience withdrawal symptoms if you stop using this drug abruptly. Consult your doctor before discontinuing Tranxene or making any change in your dose.

This drug has not been studied in children less than 9 years old.

Who should not take this medication?
Do not use Tranxene if you have a known hypersensitivity to the drug or if you have an eye condition known as acute narrow-angle glaucoma.

What should I tell my doctor before I take the first dose of this medication?
Tell your doctor about all prescription, over-the-counter, and herbal medications you are taking before beginning treatment with Tranxene. Also, talk to your doctor about your complete medical history, especially if you are being treated for depression or anxiety or if you have a history of drug abuse or dependence.

What is the usual dosage?

The information below is based on the dosage guidelines your doctor uses. Depending on your condition and medical history, your doctor may prescribe a different regimen. Do not change the dosage or stop taking your medication without your doctor's approval.

Anxiety

Adults: Tranxene T-Tab is administered orally in divided doses. The usual daily dose is 30 milligrams (mg). The dose should be adjusted gradually within the range of 15-60 mg daily depending on your response. In elderly or debilitated patients, treatment may start at a daily dose of 7.5-15 mg. It can be given as a single dose at bedtime starting at 15 mg. Tranxene SD tablets may be given as a single dose every 24 hours after you are stable on a fixed dose divided throughout the day and can be switched to a once daily dose for convenience.

Alcohol Withdrawal Symptoms

Adults: The doctor will provide a schedule of reducing daily doses until your condition is stable.

Add-on Therapy with Antiepileptic Drugs

Adults and Children over 12 years old: The starting dose is 7.5 mg 3 times a day. Your doctor may increase the dosage by 7.5 mg per week to a maximum of 90 mg a day.

Children 9-12 years old: The starting dose is 7.5 mg 2 times a day. Your doctor may increase the dosage by 7.5 mg per week to a maximum of 60 mg a day.

How should I take this medication?

Take Tranxene exactly as prescribed. Do not increase the amount you take or the number of doses per day without your doctor's approval.

What should I avoid while taking this medication?

Avoid driving a car or operating machinery until you know how Tranxene affects you. Also avoid alcohol and other central nervous system depressants while taking this drug.

What are possible food and drug interactions associated with this medication?

If Tranxene is taken with certain other drugs, the effects of either could be increased, decreased, or altered. Always check with your doctor before combining Tranxene T-Tabs with the following: antidepressants including monoamine oxidase inhibitors or tricyclics, antipsychotics, barbiturates, narcotic pain relievers, central nervous system depressants including alcohol.

What are the possible side effects of this medication?

Side effects cannot be anticipated. If any develop or change in intensity, tell your doctor as soon as possible. Only your doctor can determine if it is safe for you to continue taking this drug.

Side effects may include: drowsiness, dizziness, stomach complaints, nervousness, blurred vision, dry mouth, headache, mental confusion

Can I receive this medication if I am pregnant or breastfeeding?
Tell your doctor if you are pregnant, plan to become pregnant, or are breastfeeding before taking this drug. Several studies have suggested an increased risk of birth defects associated with using minor tranquilizers during the first trimester of pregnancy. Because treatment with minor tranquilizers is rarely a matter of urgency, their use during this period should almost always be avoided. Tranxene should not be given to nursing mothers.

What should I do if I miss a dose of this medication?
Take it as soon as you remember. If it is almost time for your next dose, skip the one you missed and go back to your regular schedule. Never take 2 doses at the same time.

How should I store this medication?
Store at room temperature in a tightly closed, light-resistant container. Protect from moisture and excessive heat.

TRAZODONE HYDROCHLORIDE
What is this medication?
Trazodone is an antidepressant chemically unrelated to other known antidepressants.

What is the most important information I should know about this medication?
Antidepressant medicines may increase suicidal thoughts or actions in some children, teenagers, and young adults when the medicine is first started. Depression and other serious mental illnesses are the most important causes of suicidal thoughts and actions. Some people may have a particularly high risk of having suicidal thoughts or actions. These include people who have (or have a family history of) bipolar disorder (also called manic-depressive illness) or suicidal thoughts or actions.

Pay close attention to any changes, especially sudden changes, in mood, behaviors, thoughts, or feelings. This is very important when an antidepressant medicine is first started or when the dose is changed.

Call the doctor right away to report new or sudden changes in mood, behavior, thoughts, or feelings. Signs to watch for include new or worsening depression, new or worsening anxiety, agitation, insomnia, hostility, panic attacks, restlessness, extreme hyperactivity, and suicidal thinking or behavior.

Keep all follow-up visits as scheduled, and call the doctor between visits as needed, especially if you have concerns about symptoms.

Who should not take this medication?

Trazodone is not recommended for use during the initial recovery phase of myocardial infarction (heart attack).

The safety and efficacy of trazodone has not been established in children.

Caution should be used when administering trazodone to patients with cardiac disease, since antidepressants have been associated with the occurrence of cardiac arrhythmias.

What should I tell my doctor before I take the first dose of this medication?

Tell your doctor about all prescription, over-the-counter, and herbal medications you are taking before beginning treatment with trazodone. Also, talk to your doctor about your complete medical history, especially if you have been diagnosed with bipolar disorder in the past, have or had any heart problems, are currently taking other antidepressants, or have liver or kidney problems.

What is the usual dosage?

The information below is based on the dosage guidelines your doctor uses. Depending on your condition and medical history, your doctor may prescribe a different regimen. Do not change the dosage or stop taking your medication without your doctor's approval.

Adults: The usual starting dose is 150 milligrams (mg) daily in divided doses. The dose may be increased by 50 mg per day every three to four days if needed. The maximum daily dose should not exceed 400 mg. Although symptomatic relief may be seen during the first week of therapy, it is generally recommended that a course of antidepressant drug treatment should continue for several months.

How should I take this medication?

Take a major portion of the total daily dose at bedtime, preferably after a meal or light snack.

What should I avoid while taking this medication?

Since trazodone may cause drowsiness, avoid performing activities that require alertness, such as driving or operating machinery, until you learn how this medication affects you. Also avoid alcohol while on trazodone, since this may cause excessive sedation.

What are possible food and drug interactions associated with this medication?

If trazodone is used with certain other drugs, the effects of either could be increased, decreased, or altered. It is especially important to check with your doctor before combining trazodone with the following: aspirin and aspirin products, carbamazepine, digoxin, indinavir, itraconazole, ketoconazole, MAOIs, nefazodone, phenytoin, ritonavir, and warfarin.

What are the possible side effects of this medication?
Side effects cannot be anticipated. If any develop or change in intensity, tell your doctor as soon as possible. Only your doctor can determine if it is safe for you to continue taking this drug.

Side effects may include: changes in mood or behavior, dizziness, drowsiness, nausea, blurred vision, dry mouth, muscle aches, decreased libido, weight gain or loss, priapism (prolonged or inappropriate erections)

Can I receive this medication if I am pregnant or breastfeeding?
The effects of trazodone during pregnancy and breastfeeding are unknown. Tell your doctor immediately if you are pregnant, plan to become pregnant, or are breastfeeding.

What should I do if I miss a dose of this medication?
Skip the dose and continue with your normal dosing schedule, never double the dose.

How should I store this medication?
Store at room temperature.

TRIFLUOPERAZINE HYDROCHLORIDE

What is this medication?
Trifluoperazine is used to treat schizophrenia. It is also prescribed for generalized anxiety that has not responded to other treatments.

What is the most important information I should know about this medication?
Trifluoperazine may cause tardive dyskinesia, a condition that causes involuntary muscle spasms and twitches in the face and body. This condition can become permanent and is most common among older people, especially women. Tell your doctor immediately if you begin to experience any involuntary movements.

Trifluoperazine may hide the signs of overdose of other drugs and may make it more difficult for your doctor to diagnose an intestinal obstruction, brain tumor, or Reye's syndrome.

Tell your doctor if you have ever had an allergic reaction to any major tranquilizer similar to trifluoperazine. The liquid concentrate form of trifluoperazine contains a sulfite that may cause allergic reactions, especially in those with asthma.

Tell your doctor immediately if you experience symptoms such as a fever or sore throat, mouth, or gums. These signs of infection may signal the need to stop trifluoperazine treatment. Notify your doctor, too, if you develop flu-like symptoms with fever.

Trifluoperazine can cause neuroleptic malignant syndrome (NMS), a dangerous and possibly life-threatening condition marked by high body temperature, rigid muscles, irregular pulse or blood pressure, rapid or abnormal heartbeat, excessive sweating, and high fever. Seek medical attention immediately if you develop any of these symptoms.

If you have any trouble with your vision, tell your doctor. Trifluoperazine has been known to cause vision problems.

Who should not take this medication?

You should not use trifluoperazine if you have liver damage, bone marrow abnormalities, a blood disorder, or if you allergic to phenothiazines.

This drug should also not be used in people who are comatose or in a greatly depressed state due to central nervous system depressants such as alcohol, barbiturates, or narcotic pain relievers.

What should I tell my doctor before I take the first dose of this medication?

Tell your doctor about all prescription, over-the-counter, and herbal medications you are taking before beginning treatment with trifluoperazine. Also, talk to your doctor about your complete medical history, especially if you have ever had a brain tumor, breast cancer, intestinal blockage, glaucoma, heart or liver disease, or seizures. In addition, tell your doctor if you are exposed to certain pesticides or extreme heat on a regular basis.

What is the usual dosage?

The information below is based on the dosage guidelines your doctor uses. Depending on your condition and medical history, your doctor may prescribe a different regimen. Do not change the dosage or stop taking your medication without your doctor's approval.

Nonpsychotic Anxiety

Adults: Usual dosage is 1 or 2 milligrams (mg) twice daily. Do not administer at doses of more than 6 mg per day or for longer than 12 weeks.

Psychotic Disorders

Adults: The usual starting dose is 2 to 5 mg two times a day. The usual effective dose is 15-20 mg daily, although some people may require 40 mg a day or more.

Children: The dosage will be adjusted based on your child's weight and the severity of the symptoms.

How should I take this medication?

Take it exactly as prescribed. Do not change the dose without talking to your doctor first.

If you are taking trifluoperazine in a liquid concentrate form, you will need to dilute it with another liquid such as a carbonated beverage, coffee, fruit juice, milk, tea, tomato juice, or water. You can also use pud-

dings, soups, and other semi-solid foods. Trifluoperazine should be diluted just before you take it. Do not take trifluoperazine with alcohol.

If dry mouth occurs, take sips of water, suck on ice chips or sugarless
hard candy, or chew sugarless gum.

What should I avoid while taking this medication?
Do not drink alcohol while taking trifluoperazine.

Follow your doctor's instructions when discontinuing trifluoperazine.
Dizziness, nausea, vomiting, and tremors can result if you suddenly stop
taking it.

This drug may impair your ability to drive a car or operate potentially
dangerous machinery, especially during the first few days of treatment.
Do not participate in any potentially hazardous activities until you know
how this drug affects you.

Avoid strenuous activity during periods of high temperature or humidity.

Trifluoperazine may cause sensitivity to sunlight. Avoid unnecessary
exposure to sunlight and also avoid tanning booths. Use sunscreen and
wear protective clothing when outside.

Avoid sudden position changes that can cause an abrupt decrease in
blood pressure. This includes rising quickly from a sitting or lying position. In addition, hot tubs, showers, and baths may worsen the symptoms
of dizziness.

**What are possible food and drug interactions associated with
this medication?**
If trifluoperazine is taken with certain other drugs, the effects of either
could be increased, decreased, or altered. It is especially important to
check with your doctor before combining trifluoperazine with the following: alcohol, antihistamines, antiseizure medication, atropine, barbiturates, beta blockers, blood thinners such as warfarin, cisapride,
diazepam, guanethidine, lithium, propranolol, metrizamide, paroxetine,
percocet, phenobarbital, sparfloxacin, thiazide diuretics.

What are the possible side effects of this medication?
Side effects cannot be anticipated. If any develop or change in intensity,
tell your doctor as soon as possible. Only your doctor can determine if it
is safe for you to continue taking this drug.

Side effects may include: blood disorders, convulsions, dry mouth,
headache, muscle stiffness or rigidity, nausea, restlessness, drowsiness,
dizziness, skin reactions, insomnia, fatigue, anorexia, muscle weakness,
lactation, blurred vision

Can I receive this medication if I am pregnant or breastfeeding?
The effects of trifluoperazine during pregnancy are unknown. Tell your
doctor immediately if you are pregnant or plan to become pregnant.

Because trifluoperazine passes into breast milk, women taking this drug must avoid breastfeeding.

What should I do if I miss a dose of this medication?
If you take 1 dose a day, take the dose you missed as soon as you remember. Then go back to your regular schedule. If you do not remember until the next day, skip the missed dose and go back to your regular schedule.

If you take more than 1 dose a day, take the dose you missed if it is within an hour or so of the scheduled time. If you do not remember until later, skip the missed dose and go back to your regular schedule. Do not take 2 doses at once.

How should I store this medication?
Store at room temperature, away from moisture and light.

TRIHEXYPHENIDYL HYDROCHLORIDE

What is this medication?
Trihexyphenidyl is used to treat symptoms of Parkinson's disease and tremors caused by other medical problems.

What is the most important information I should know about this medication?
Trihexyphenidyl may increase the risk of developing glaucoma. Tell your doctor immediately if you experience any eye problems or change in vision.

Who should not take this medication?
Do not take this medication if you are allergic to trihexyphenidyl or any of its components.

What should I tell my doctor before I take the first dose of this medication?
Tell your doctor about all prescription, over-the-counter, and herbal medications you are taking before beginning treatment with trihexyphenidyl. Also, talk to your doctor about your complete medical history, especially if you have heart problems, high blood pressure, liver or kidney disease, glaucoma, or vision problems.

What is the usual dosage?
The information below is based on the dosage guidelines your doctor uses. Depending on your condition and medical history, your doctor may prescribe a different regimen. Do not change the dosage or stop taking your medication without your doctor's approval.

Adults: The doctor will need to individualize the dose based on your condition and any other medications you are taking.

How should I take this medication?
Take this medication exactly as prescribed by your doctor.

What should I avoid while taking this medication?

Trihexyphenidyl may cause dizziness or blurred vision. Use caution when driving, operating machinery, or performing other hazardous activities until you know how this drug affects you.

Avoid combining trihexyphenidyl with alcohol, since this may increase drowsiness and dizziness.

Avoid becoming overheated. Trihexyphenidyl may cause decreased sweating. This could lead to heat stroke in hot weather or with vigorous exercise.

What are possible food and drug interactions associated with this medication?

If trihexyphenidyl is taken with certain other drugs, the effects of either could be increased, decreased, or altered. It is especially important to check with your doctor before combining this medication with any the following: fluvoxamine, fluoxetine, Levodopa, paroxetine, pindolol, propranolol, tranquilizers.

What are the possible side effects of this medication?

Side effects cannot be anticipated. If any develop or change in intensity, inform your doctor as soon as possible. Only your doctor can determine if it is safe for you to continue taking this drug.

Side effects may include: drowsiness, dizziness, mild nausea, nervousness, blurred vision, dry mouth, constipation

Can I receive this medication if I am pregnant or breastfeeding?

The effects of trihexyphenidyl during pregnancy and breastfeeding are unknown. Tell your doctor immediately if you are pregnant, plan to become pregnant, or are breastfeeding.

What should I do if I miss a dose of this medication?

Take the missed dose as soon as you remember. However, if it is almost time for the next dose, skip the missed dose and continue with your regular schedule. Do not take 2 doses at once.

How should I store this medication?

Store at room temperature in a tight container.

VALIUM

Generic name: Diazepam

What is this medication?

Valium is used to treat anxiety disorders, the symptoms of sudden alcohol withdrawal, muscle spasms, and seizures.

What is the most important information I should know about this medication?

Due to the sleepiness and tiredness Valium can cause, you should not drive or operate dangerous machinery until you know how this drug affects you.

If you are taking Valium as part of seizure therapy, you should not suddenly stop taking it because this may worsen or even cause seizures.

You should not drink alcohol or take other medications that can make you tired or drowsy while you are taking Valium.

Some studies have shown that Valium may increase the risk of birth defects during the first trimester. You should tell your doctor immediately if you are pregnant or plan to become pregnant while taking Valium.

Use this drug with caution if you have any type of kidney or liver problems. If you take Valium for a long time, your doctor will likely perform blood tests to check your liver function and also the number of disease fighting cells in your blood.

You should talk to your doctor before increasing your Valium dose or before stopping therapy. Suddenly stopping Valium may cause you to experience symptoms of withdrawal that include shaking, stomach and muscle cramps, vomiting, sweating, insomnia, and seizures.

You may develop a physical or mental dependence on Valium, especially if you take it for a long time or if you have a history of alcohol or drug abuse.

Who should not take this medication?

You should not take Valium if you are pregnant, if you have an eye disorder known as acute narrow-angle glaucoma, or if you are allergic to diazepam or any other ingredient in Valium.

You should not use Valium if you have severe breathing problems, liver disease, sleep apnea, or a condition known as myasthenia gravis.

What should I tell my doctor before I take the first dose of this medication?

Tell your doctor about all prescription, over-the-counter, and herbal medications you are taking before beginning treatment with Valium. Also, talk to your doctor about your complete medical history, especially if you have kidney or liver problems, acute narrow-angle glaucoma, or if you drink alcohol regularly. Also tell your doctor if you have a history of drug abuse, breathing problems, or mental disorders.

What is the usual dosage?

The information below is based on the dosage guidelines your doctor uses. Depending on your condition and medical history, your doctor may prescribe a different regimen. Do not change the dosage or stop taking your medication without your doctor's approval.

Anxiety Disorders, Temporary Symptoms of Anxiety, Muscle Spasms, and Seizure Disorders

Adults: The usual dosage is 2-10 milligrams (mg) taken 2-4 times a day.
Children: Valium can be given to children 6 months and older. The usual dosage is 1-2.5 mg given 3-4 times a day.

Sudden Alcohol Withdrawal

Adults: The starting dose is 10 mg taken 3-4 times during the first 24 hours. The dose is then reduced to 5 mg, taken 3-4 times daily as needed.

How should I take this medication?

Take Valium at the same time every day. It may be taken with or without food.

What should I avoid while taking this medication?

Do not drink alcohol or take other medications that can make you tired or drowsy while you are taking Valium.

Avoid suddenly stopping Valium therapy without first talking to your doctor. Do not take more than is prescribed without your doctor's approval.

What are possible food and drug interactions associated with this medication?

If Valium is taken with certain other drugs, the effects of either could be increased, decreased, or altered. It is especially important to check with your doctor before combining Valium with the following: antidepressants, barbiturates, cimetidine, monoamine oxidase inhibitors (MAOIs), narcotics, phenothiazines.

What are the possible side effects of this medication?

Side effects cannot be anticipated. If any develop or change in intensity, tell your doctor as soon as possible. Only your doctor can determine if it is safe for you to continue taking this drug.

Side effects may include: difficulty walking, drowsiness, tiredness, constipation, blurred vision

Can I receive this medication if I am pregnant or breastfeeding?

The effects of Valium during pregnancy and breastfeeding are unknown. Tell your doctor immediately if you are pregnant, plan to become pregnant, or are breastfeeding.

What should I do if I miss a dose of this medication?

Skip the dose you missed and return to your normal schedule.

How should I store this medication?

Store at room temperature, away from light.

VISTARIL

Generic name: Hydroxyzine hydrochloride

What is this medication?

Vistaril is used to treat anxiety, tension, and agitation caused by emotional stress. It is also prescribed as a sedative to alleviate anxiety and tension before or after certain medical procedures (eg, dental procedures or surgery). In addition, Vistaril is used to help control the following: nausea and vomiting (except during pregnancy), anxiety due to alcohol withdrawal, and extreme emotional distress associated with certain allergic conditions such as asthma, chronic hives, and severe itching.

What is the most important information I should know about this medication?

Vistaril should not be combined with other central nervous system depressants such as narcotics, barbiturates, or alcohol.

Who should not take this medication?

Vistaril should not be used during early pregnancy. Also, do not take Vistaril if you have ever had an allergic reaction to it.

What should I tell my doctor before I take the first dose of this medication?

Tell your doctor about all prescription, over-the-counter, and herbal medications you are taking before beginning treatment with Vistaril. Also talk to your doctor about your complete medical history, especially if you are pregnant, planning to become pregnant, or are breastfeeding.

What is the usual dosage?

The information below is based on the dosage guidelines your doctor uses. Depending on your condition and medical history, your doctor may prescribe a different regimen. Do not change the dosage or stop taking your medication without your doctor's approval.

Relief of Anxiety and Tension

Adults: 50-100 milligrams (mg) 4 times a day.
Children: Under 6 years old: 50 mg daily in divided doses. Over 6 years old: 50-100 mg daily in divided doses.

Relief of Itching Due to Allergic Reactions

Adults: 25 mg 3-4 times a day.
Children: Under 6 years old: 50 mg daily in divided doses. Over 6 years old: 50-100 mg daily in divided doses.

As a Sedative Before or After Surgery

Adults: 50-100 mg.
Children: The doctor will calculate an appropriate dose based on your child's weight.

How should I take this medication?

Take Vistaril exactly as prescribed by your doctor. It is usually taken in divided doses.

What should I avoid while taking this medication?

Avoid drinking alcohol or taking any other medications that may cause drowsiness or decrease your alertness.

This drug may cause drowsiness; be careful when engaging in activities that require alertness such as driving or operating heavy machinery.

What are possible food and drug interactions associated with this medication?

If Vistaril is taken with certain other drugs, the effects of either could be increased, decreased, or altered. It is especially important to check with your doctor before combining Vistaril with the following: barbiturates, other sedatives or nervous system depressants, narcotics, non-narcotic painkillers.

What are the possible side effects of this medication?

Side effects cannot be anticipated. If any develop or change in intensity, tell your doctor as soon as possible. Only your doctor can determine if it is safe for you to continue taking this drug.

Side effects may include: dry mouth, drowsiness, tremor, convulsions

Can I receive this medication if I am pregnant or breastfeeding?

Tell your doctor immediately if you are pregnant, planning to become pregnant, or are breastfeeding. Vistaril should not be used during early pregnancy. It is not known whether Vistaril is secreted in breast milk. Since many drugs do appear in breast milk, you should not take Vistaril if you are nursing.

What should I do if I miss a dose of this medication?

Take it as soon as you remember. If it is almost time for your next dose, skip the one you missed and return to your normal schedule.

How should I store this medication?

Store at room temperature away from heat, light, and moisture.

VIVACTIL

Generic name: Protriptyline hydrochloride

What is this medication?

Vivactil is a tricyclic antidepressant used to treat depression in people who are under close medical supervision. It is particularly suitable for those who are inactive and withdrawn.

What is the most important information I should know about this medication?

Antidepressants can increase the risk of suicidal thinking and behavior in children and teenagers. Adult and pediatric patients taking antidepressants should be watched closely for changes in moods or actions, especially when they first start therapy or when their dose is increased or decreased. Patients and their families should contact the doctor immediately if new symptoms develop or seem to get worse. Signs to watch for include anxiety, hostility, sleeplessness, restlessness, impulsive or dangerous behavior, and thoughts about suicide or dying.

Because Vivactil can affect blood sugar levels, the doctor may monitor your blood sugar or change the dose of any diabetes medication you are taking.

Tell your doctor or dentist that you take Vivactil before receiving any medical or dental care, emergency treatment, or surgery.

Do not abruptly stop taking Vivactil without talking to your doctor first. Suddenly stopping this medication may cause withdrawal symptoms such as headache, nausea, and tiredness.

Who should not take this medication?

Do not take monoamine oxidase inhibitors (MAOIs) within 2 weeks before or after treatment with Vivactil. In some cases, a serious, possibly fatal, reaction may occur. Examples of MAOIs include selegiline and the antidepressants phenelzine and tranylcypromine. Do not combine Vivactil with cisapride.

Vivactil should not be used during the recovery phase following a heart attack.

Do not use Vivactil if you are allergic to any of its ingredients.

What should I tell my doctor before I take the first dose of this medication?

Tell your doctor about all prescription, over-the-counter, and herbal medications you are taking before beginning treatment with Vivactil. Also, talk to your doctor about your complete medical history, especially if you have an overactive thyroid, glaucoma, heart problems, kidney or liver problems, diabetes, seizures, blood diseases, an enlarged prostate, difficulty urinating, and psychiatric disorders including bipolar disorder, schizophrenia, suicide attempts, or suicidal thoughts.

What is the usual dosage?

The information below is based on the dosage guidelines your doctor uses. Depending on your condition and medical history, your doctor may prescribe a different regimen. Do not change the dosage or stop taking your medication without your doctor's approval.

Adults: 15-40 milligrams (mg) a day, taken in divided doses 3-4 times a day. Your doctor may increase the daily dose to 60 mg; daily doses above 60 mg are not recommended.

Elderly and Adolescents: The usual starting dose is 5 mg 3 times a day with gradual increases if needed. In older patients, careful monitoring of the heart is necessary if the daily dose exceeds 20 mg.

How should I take this medication?

Take Vivactil at the same time every day, with or without food.

What should I avoid while taking this medication?

Do not drive or perform other possibly dangerous activities until you know how this drug affects you.

Do not drink alcohol while taking Vivactil, since this may increase the risk of side effects.

Vivactil may cause dizziness, lightheadedness, or fainting. Alcohol, hot weather, exercise, or fever may increase these effects. To prevent them, sit up or stand slowly, especially in the morning. Sit or lie down at the first sign of any of these side effects.

To prevent heatstroke while taking Vivactil, do not become overheated while doing physical activity outdoors.

Vivactil may increase sensitivity to the sun. Avoid exposure to the sun, sunlamps, or tanning booths until you know how this drug affects you. Always use sunscreen when you are outside.

What are possible food and drug interactions associated with this medication?

If Vivactil is taken with certain other drugs, the effects of either could be increased, decreased, or altered. It is especially important to check with your doctor before combining Vivactil with the following: other antidepressants, astemizole, antifungals such as fluconazole, barbiturates and other sedatives, cisapride, cimetidine, clonidine, duloxetine, guanethidine, MAOIs, quinolone antibiotics such as ciprofloxacin, dalfpristin and similar drugs, phenylephrine and similar drugs, terbinafine, tramadol.

What are the possible side effects of this medication?

Side effects cannot be anticipated. If any develop or change in intensity, tell your doctor as soon as possible. Only your doctor can determine if it is safe for you to continue taking this drug.

Side effects may include: agitation, dizziness, drowsiness, headache, impotence, sweating, tiredness, upset stomach, weight loss or gain, pupil dilation, sensitivity to sunlight, excitement, anxiety, blurred vision, confusion, constipation, diarrhea, nausea, seizures, trouble urinating, vomiting

Can I receive this medication if I am pregnant or breastfeeding?
The effects of Vivactil during pregnancy and breastfeeding are unknown. Tell your doctor immediately if you are pregnant, plan to become pregnant, or are breastfeeding.

What should I do if I miss a dose of this medication?
Take it as soon as you remember. If it is almost time for your next dose, skip the one you missed and go back to your regular schedule. Do not take two doses at once. If you take one dose daily at bedtime, do not take the missed dose the next morning.

How should I store this medication?
Store at room temperature away from heat, moisture, and light. Do not store in the bathroom.

VIVITROL
Generic name: Naltrexone

What is this medication?
Vivitrol is used to treat alcohol dependence in patients 18 years and older.

What is the most important information I should know about this medication?
Vivitrol may cause damage to your liver. If you already have liver problems, tell your doctor before beginning treatment with this drug. Call your doctor immediately if you develop pain around your stomach for more than a few days, light-colored bowel movements, dark urine, or yellowing of the whites of your eyes.

Vivitrol blocks the effects of opioid-containing medicines. You may not feel the same effects of opioid-containing medicines including ones for pain, cough, and diarrhea. You may not feel the same effects if you use heroin and other illegal (street) opioids. Do not take large amounts of opioid medicines to overcome the Vivitrol block. This can lead to serious injury, coma, or death.

Vivitrol has been associated with severe allergic pneumonia. Call your doctor if you develop shortness of breath, coughing, or wheezing.

Be aware that Vivitrol can cause depression and suicidal thoughts. If these symptoms occur, or if you have any changes in mood, notify your doctor immediately.

To benefit from Vivitrol, you need to stop drinking before starting treatment with this medication. To be effective, treatment with Vivitrol must be used along with other alcoholism recovery measures such as counseling.

Who should not take this medication?

If you are taking an opioid (such as heroin), are dependent on opioids, are in opiate withdrawal, or have tested positive for opiates in your urine, do not begin treatment with Vivitrol. This drug should not be used to treat opiate dependency.

Do not use Vivitrol if you have liver problems or if you are allergic to any of the drug's ingredients.

What should I tell my doctor before I take the first dose of this medication?

Tell your doctor about all prescription, over-the-counter, and herbal medications you are currently taking. Also, talk to your doctor about your complete medical history, especially if you have liver or kidney problems, bleeding problems, are pregnant or planning to become pregnant, have a history of drug abuse, or are opiate-dependent.

What is the usual dosage?

The information below is based on the dosage guidelines your doctor uses. Depending on your condition and medical history, your doctor may prescribe a different regimen. Do not change the dosage or stop taking your medication without your doctor's approval.

Adults: The recommended dose is 380 milligrams injected every 4 weeks by a doctor.

How should I take this medication?

Vivitrol should be injected by your doctor into your buttocks, alternating sides with each injection.

What should I avoid while taking this medication?

Vivitrol may make you feel dizzy. Do not engage in any potentially dangerous activities, such as driving a car, until you know how this drug affects you.

Avoid nursing or becoming pregnant; if you become pregnant while on Vivitrol, contact your doctor immediately.

What are possible food and drug interactions associated with this medication?

If Vivitrol is taken with certain other drugs, the effects of either could be increased, decreased, or altered. It is especially important to check with your doctor before combining Vivitrol with the following: antidiarrheal medication, antitussives, street drugs, opioid-containing medicines including ones for pain, cough, and diarrhea.

What are the possible side effects of this medication?

Side effects cannot be anticipated. If any develop or change in intensity, tell your doctor as soon as possible. Only your doctor can determine if it is safe for you to continue taking this drug.

Side effects may include: cramps, decreased appetite/anorexia, dizziness, dry mouth, fatigue, headache, injection-site reaction such as redness/swelling, nausea, stomach pain, suicidal thoughts, vomiting

Can I receive this medication if I am pregnant or breastfeeding?
The effects of Vivitrol during pregnancy and breastfeeding are unknown. Tell your doctor immediately if you are pregnant, plan to become pregnant, or are breastfeeding.

What should I do if a miss a dose of this medication?
If you miss a dose of Vivitrol, see your doctor immediately for an injection.

VYVANSE
Generic name: Lisdexamfetamine dimesylate

What is this medication?
Vyvanse is a central nervous system stimulant used for the treatment of attention-deficit/hyperactivity disorder (ADHD) in children 6-12 years old and adults.

What is the most important information I should know about this medication?
Because Vyvanse is an amphetamine stimulant, using it for a long period may lead to drug dependence. Misuse can lead to serious heart problems and sudden death.

Do not take Vyvanse if you are suffering from advanced heart disease or other heart-related problems, hardening of the arteries, moderate to severe high blood pressure, hyperthyroidism, glaucoma, or if you are allergic to amphetamines.

Do not use Vyvanse while in agitated states or if you have a history of drug abuse.

Vyvanse may worsen behavior and thought disorders if you have a history of other mental illnesses, such as bipolar disorder. Aggressive behavior or hostility is often observed in children and adolescents with ADHD.

Growth should be monitored during treatment with Vyvanse, and patients who are not growing or gaining weight as expected may need to temporarily stop their treatment.

Vyvanse may increase the risk of having a seizure, especially if you have a history of seizures. Vyvanse may also worsen symptoms related to Tourette's syndrome.

Amphetamines may impair your ability to engage in potentially hazardous activities such as driving or operating machinery.

Who should not take this medication?
Vyvanse should not be taken if you are suffering from advanced heart disease or other heart-related problems, hardening of the arteries, moder-

ate to severe high blood pressure, hyperthyroidism, glaucoma, or if you are allergic to amphetamines.

Vyvanse should not be taken if you are in agitated states or if you have a history of drug abuse.

Do not take this medicine if you have been using drugs known as monoamine oxidase inhibitors (MAOIs) within the past 14 days.

What should I tell my doctor before I take the first dose of this medication?

Tell your doctor about all prescription, over-the-counter, and herbal medications you are taking before beginning treatment with Vyvanse. Also, talk to your doctor about your complete medical history, especially if you have any heart conditions, an overactive thyroid, glaucoma, any psychiatric conditions, or if you have ever had a seizure.

What is the usual dosage?

The information below is based on the dosage guidelines your doctor uses. Depending on your condition and medical history, your doctor may prescribe a different regimen. Do not change the dosage or stop taking your medication without your doctor's approval.

Adults: Adults are recommended to receive 30 mg once daily in the morning. Doses may be increased by your doctor and should not exceed 70 mg per day.

Children: For children 6-12 years old, the recommended dose is 30 milligrams (mg) once daily in the morning. The doctor may want to increase the dose based on your child's condition.

How should I take this medication?

Take this medicine in the morning. Afternoon doses should be avoided because of the potential for insomnia (difficulty sleeping). You can take Vyvanse with or without food.

If you are unable to swallow the capsule, you may open it and dissolve the contents in a glass of water. Drink the entire glass; do not store it for later use. Do not take less than one capsule per day.

What should I avoid while taking this medication?

Use caution when driving or operating dangerous machinery while taking Vyvanse.

Avoid splitting the dose within a capsule; also avoid taking Vyvanse later in the day.

What are possible food and drug interactions associated with this medication?

If Vyvanse is taken with certain other drugs, the effects of either could be increased, decreased, or altered. It is especially important to check with your doctor before combining Vyvanse with the following: antidepressants including monoamine oxidase inhibitors (MAOIs), antipsychotic medication, lithium, blood pressure medication, seizure medication, narcotic painkillers.

What are the possible side effects of this medication?
Side effects cannot be anticipated. If any develop or change in intensity, tell your doctor as soon as possible. Only your doctor can determine if it is safe for you to continue taking this drug.

Side effects may include: upper belly pains, decreased appetite, dizziness, dry mouth, irritability, trouble sleeping, nausea and vomiting, weight loss, slowing of growth, seizures (especially in patients with a history of seizures), blurred vision

Can I receive this medication if I am pregnant or breastfeeding?
Talk with your doctor before taking this drug if you are pregnant, plan to become pregnant, or are breastfeeding. Amphetamines have been shown to cause birth defects in laboratory animals, but the effects in humans are unknown. Because amphetamines are secreted in breast milk, women should not breastfeed while using this drug.

What should I do if I miss a dose of this medication?
Do not take an extra dose to make up for the one you missed. Wait and take your next dose at the regular time.

How should I store this medication?
Store at room temperature.

WELLBUTRIN
Generic name: Bupropion hydrochloride

What is this medication?
Wellbutrin is used to treat major depression. Depression may be caused by an imbalance of brain chemicals called neurotransmitters. Wellbutrin helps balance the levels of two neurotransmitters called dopamine and norepinephrine.

What is the most important information I should know about this medication?
Antidepressants can increase the risk of suicidal thinking and behavior in children and teenagers. Adult and pediatric patients taking antidepressants should be watched closely for changes in moods or actions, especially when they first start therapy or when their dose is increased or decreased. Patients and their families should contact the doctor immediately if new symptoms develop or seem to get worse. Signs to watch for include anxiety, hostility, sleeplessness, restlessness, impulsive or dangerous behavior, and thoughts about suicide or dying.

Who should not take this medication?

Do not take Wellbutrin if you have a seizure disorder, anorexia or bulimia (eating disorders), or if you are going through alcohol recovery. Also, do not begin treatment with Wellbutrin if you are allergic to any of its ingredients.

Do not take monoamine oxidase inhibitors (MAOIs) within 2 weeks before or after treatment with this medication. In some cases a serious, possibly fatal, reaction may occur. Examples of MAOIs include selegiline and the antidepressants phenelzine and tranylcypromine.

Also, do not begin treatment with Wellbutrin if you are allergic to any of its ingredients.

What should I tell my doctor before I take the first dose of this medication?

Tell your doctor about all prescription, over-the-counter, and herbal medications you are taking before beginning treatment with Wellbutrin. Also, talk to your doctor about your complete medical history, especially if you have had seizure problems, eating disorders, or an addiction (eg, drug/alcohol problems).

What is the usual dosage?

The information below is based on the dosage guidelines your doctor uses. Depending on your condition and medical history, your doctor may prescribe a different regimen. Do not change the dosage or stop taking your medication without your doctor's approval.

Adults: The usual starting dose is 200 milligrams (mg) a day, taken as 100 mg twice a day. Depending on your response, the doctor may increase the dose to 300 mg a day, taken as 100 mg three times a day. The maximum daily dose for Wellbutrin is 450 mg. Taking doses greater than 450 mg a day may increase the risk of serious side effects, including seizures.

How should I take this medication?

Take Wellbutrin at the same time every day, at least 6 hours apart. You can take it with or without food.

What should I avoid while taking this medication?

Do not chew, cut, or crush Wellbutrin tablets.

What are possible food and drug interactions associated with this medication?

If Wellbutrin is taken with certain other drugs, the effects of either could be increased, decreased, or altered. It is especially important to check with your doctor before combining Wellbutrin with the following: amantadine, other antidepressants including MAOIs, antipsychotic medications, blood pressure medications known as beta blockers, levodopa, phenelzine, antiarrhythmics such as propafenone and flecainide.

What are the possible side effects of this medication?
Side effects cannot be anticipated. If any develop or change in intensity, tell your doctor as soon as possible. Only your doctor can determine if it is safe for you to continue taking this drug.

Side effects may include: abnormal behavior, agitation, headaches, nausea and vomiting, neurological problems, seizures, sleeping problems, skin problems such as rashes, stomach problems

Can I receive this medication if I am pregnant or breastfeeding?
The effects of Wellbutrin during pregnancy and breastfeeding are unknown. Tell your doctor immediately if you are pregnant, plan to become pregnant, or are breastfeeding.

What should I do if I miss a dose of this medication?
Do not double your next dose. Skip the dose you missed and return to your regular dosing schedule. This is very important because taking too much Wellbutrin can increase your risk of having a seizure.

How should I store this medication?
Store at room temperature, away from light and moisture.

WELLBUTRIN SR

Generic name: Bupropion hydrochloride, sustained-release

What is this medication?
Wellbutrin SR is used to treat major depression. Depression may be caused by an imbalance of brain chemicals called neurotransmitters. Wellbutrin SR helps balance the levels of two neurotransmitters called dopamine and norepinephrine.

What is the most important information I should know about this medication?
Antidepressants can increase the risk of suicidal thinking and behavior in children and teenagers. Adult and pediatric patients taking antidepressants should be watched closely for changes in moods or actions, especially when they first start therapy or when their dose is increased or decreased. Patients and their families should contact the doctor immediately if new symptoms develop or seem to get worse. Signs to watch for include anxiety, hostility, sleeplessness, restlessness, impulsive or dangerous behavior, and thoughts about suicide or dying.

Who should not take this medication?
Do not take Wellbutrin SR if you have a seizure disorder, anorexia or bulimia (eating disorders), or if you are going through alcohol recovery. In addition, you should not take Wellbutrin SR if you are taking Zyban or any other medicines that contain bupropion hydrochloride, such as

Wellbutrin or Wellbutrin XL, or if you have suddenly stopped taking sedatives.

Do not take monoamine oxidase inhibitors (MAOIs) within 2 weeks before or after treatment with this medication. In some cases a serious, possibly fatal, reaction may occur. Examples of MAOIs include selegiline and the antidepressants phenelzine and tranylcypromine.

Also, do not begin treatment with Wellbutrin SR if you are allergic to any of its ingredients.

What should I tell my doctor before I take the first dose of this medication?

Tell your doctor about all prescription, over-the-counter, and herbal medications you are taking before beginning treatment with Wellbutrin SR. Also, talk to your doctor about your complete medical history, especially if you have seizure problems, eating disorders, liver or kidney problems, or an addiction (eg, drug/alcohol problems).

What is the usual dosage?

The information below is based on the dosage guidelines your doctor uses. Depending on your condition and medical history, your doctor may prescribe a different regimen. Do not change the dosage or stop taking your medication without your doctor's approval.

Adults: The usual dose is 150 milligrams (mg) once a day in the morning. Depending on your response, the doctor may increase your dose to 300 mg a day, taken as 150 mg twice a day.

How should I take this medication?

You should take Wellbutrin SR at the same time every day, at least 8 hours apart. You can take it with or without food.

What should I avoid while taking this medication?

You should not drink a lot of alcohol while taking Wellbutrin SR. If you currently drink a lot of alcohol and suddenly stop, you should tell your doctor, since this may increase your risk of having a seizure. You should also not drive a car or operate heavy machinery until you know how this drug affects you.

What are possible food and drug interactions associated with this medication?

If Wellbutrin SR is taken with certain other drugs, the effects of either could be increased, decreased, or altered. It is especially important to check with your doctor before combining Wellbutrin SR with the following: alcohol, amantadine, other antidepressants including MAOIs, antipsychotics, blood pressure drugs known as beta blockers, carbamazepine, cimetidine, efavirenz, fluvoxamine, antiarrhythmics such as propafenone and flecainide, lamotrigine, levodopa, nelfinavir, nicotine patches, norfluoxetine, phenobarbital, phenytoin, ritonavir, steroids, theophylline.

What are the possible side effects of this medication?

Side effects cannot be anticipated. If any develop or change in intensity, tell your doctor as soon as possible. Only your doctor can determine if it is safe for you to continue taking this drug.

Side effects may include: headache, infection, stomach or chest pains, dry mouth, nausea, diarrhea, constipation, loss of appetite, vomiting, difficulty sleeping (insomnia), dizziness, agitation, tremor, anxiety, nervousness, irritability, sore throat, sinus inflammation, sweating, rash, ringing in the ears, blurred vision

Can I receive this medication if I am pregnant or breastfeeding?

The effects of Wellbutrin SR during pregnancy and breastfeeding are unknown. Tell your doctor immediately if you are pregnant, plan to become pregnant, or are breastfeeding.

What should I do if I miss a dose of this medication?

Do not double your next dose. Skip the dose you missed and return to your regular dosing schedule. This is very important because taking too much Wellbutrin SR can increase your risk of having a seizure.

How should I store this medication?

Store at room temperature, away from light and moisture.

WELLBUTRIN XL

Generic name: Bupropion hydrochloride, extended-release

What is this medication?

Wellbutrin XL is used to treat major depression and seasonal depression known as seasonal affective disorder (SAD). Depression may be caused by an imbalance of brain chemicals called neurotransmitters. Wellbutrin XL helps balance the levels of two neurotransmitters called dopamine and norepinephrine.

What is the most important information I should know about this medication?

Antidepressants can increase the risk of suicidal thinking and behavior in children and teenagers. Adult and pediatric patients taking antidepressants should be watched closely for changes in moods or actions, especially when they first start therapy or when their dose is increased or decreased. Patients and their families should contact the doctor immediately if new symptoms develop or seem to get worse. Signs to watch for include anxiety, hostility, sleeplessness, restlessness, impulsive or dangerous behavior, and thoughts about suicide or dying.

Who should not take this medication?

Do not take Wellbutrin XL if you have a seizure disorder, anorexia or bulimia (eating disorders), or if you are going through alcohol recovery. In addition, you should not take Wellbutrin XL if you are taking Zyban or any other medicines that contain bupropion hydrochloride, such as Wellbutrin or Wellbutrin SR, or if you have suddenly stopped taking sedatives.

Do not take monoamine oxidase inhibitors (MAOIs) within 2 weeks before or after treatment with this medication. In some cases a serious, possibly fatal, reaction may occur. Examples of MAOIs include selegiline and the antidepressants phenelzine and tranylcypromine.

Also, do not begin treatment with Wellbutrin XL if you are allergic to any of its ingredients.

What should I tell my doctor before I take the first dose of this medication?

Tell your doctor about all prescription, over-the-counter, and herbal medications you are taking before beginning treatment with Wellbutrin XL. Also, talk to your doctor about your complete medical history, especially if you have ever had a seizure, eating disorders, liver or kidney problems, or an addiction (eg, drug/alcohol problems).

What is the usual dosage?

The information below is based on the dosage guidelines your doctor uses. Depending on your condition and medical history, your doctor may prescribe a different regimen. Do not change the dosage or stop taking your medication without your doctor's approval.

Depression

Adults: The usual dose is 150 milligrams (mg) once a day in the morning. Depending on your response, the doctor may increase the dose to 300 mg once a day.

Seasonal Affective Disorder

Adults: The usual dose is 150 mg once a day in the morning, starting in autumn before the onset of depressive symptoms. Depending on your response, the doctor may increase the dose to 300 mg once a day. If you are taking 300 mg a day, your doctor may taper the dose to 150 mg a day for 2 weeks before telling you to stop taking Wellbutrin XL in early spring.

How should I take this medication?

Wellbutrin XL is a once-daily tablet. Take it at the same time every day at least 24 hours apart. You can take Wellbutrin XL with or without food.

What should I avoid while taking this medication?

You should not drink a lot of alcohol while taking Wellbutrin XL. If you currently drink a lot of alcohol and suddenly stop, you should tell your doctor, since this may increase your risk of having a seizure. You should also not drive a car or operate heavy machinery until you know how this drug affects you.

What are possible food and drug interactions associated with this medication?

If Wellbutrin XL is taken with certain other drugs, the effects of either could be increased, decreased, or altered. It is especially important to check with your doctor before combining Wellbutrin XL with the following: alcohol, amantadine, other antidepressants including MAOIs, antipsychotics, blood pressure drugs known as beta blockers, carbamazepine, cimetidine, efavirenz, fluvoxamine, antiarrhythmics such as propafenone and flecainide, lamotrigine, levodopa, nelfinavir, nicotine patches, norfluoxetine, phenobarbital, phenytoin, ritonavir, steroids, theophylline.

What are the possible side effects of this medication?

Side effects cannot be anticipated. If any develop or change in intensity, tell your doctor as soon as possible. Only your doctor can determine if it is safe for you to continue taking this drug.

Side effects may include: dry mouth, nausea, constipation, gas, headache, dizziness, tremor (shakiness), upper respiratory tract infection, nasal or throat irritation, inflammation of the sinuses, trouble sleeping (insomnia), anxiety, abnormal dreams, pain in the hands or feet, muscle pain, feeling jittery, decreased appetite, rash, ringing in the ears

Can I receive this medication if I am pregnant or breastfeeding?

The effects of Wellbutrin XL during pregnancy and breastfeeding are unknown. Tell your doctor immediately if you are pregnant, plan to become pregnant, or are breastfeeding.

What should I do if I miss a dose of this medication?

Do not double your next dose. Skip the dose you missed and return to your regular dosing schedule. This is very important because taking too much Wellbutrin XL can increase your risk of having a seizure.

How should I store this medication?

Store at room temperature, away from light and moisture.

XANAX

Generic name: Alprazolam

What is this medication?

Xanax is a medicine known as a benzodiazepine; it works by slowing down the movement of chemicals in the brain. Xanax is used to treat anxiety and panic disorders.

What is the most important information I should know about this medication?

If you take more than 4 milligrams (mg) of Xanax per day, you are at risk of extreme physical or mental dependence. You may also experience more severe withdrawal symptoms (including seizures) if you stop taking Xanax or if you lower the dose.

Even if you take Xanax for a short period of time, you may become mentally or physically dependent. Physical dependence could put you at risk for experiencing withdrawal symptoms if you stop taking Xanax. Withdrawal symptoms include seizures or a worsening of anxiety and associated symptoms.

Xanax binds to certain receptors in the brain that may cause you to become drowsy or sedated. Do not drive, operate machinery, or do anything else that could be dangerous until you know how this drug affects you.

You should not increase, decrease, or stop taking your Xanax doses without first talking to your doctor.

Avoid drinking alcohol or taking other medications that cause drowsiness (such as sedatives and tranquilizers) while taking Xanax. This medication will add to the effects of alcohol and other depressants.

Do not smoke while using Xanax. Cigarette smoking decreases blood levels of Xanax. Tell your doctor if you smoke or if you have recently stopped smoking.

Who should not take this medication?

You should not take Xanax if you are pregnant, plan to become pregnant, or are breastfeeding.

Do not use this medication if you have an eye condition called acute narrow-angle glaucoma. (If you have open-angle glaucoma, Xanax may be used if you are receiving appropriate therapy.)

Do not take Xanax if you are allergic to any of its ingredients. Also avoid this drug if you are currently taking the medications itraconazole or ketoconazole.

What should I tell my doctor before I take the first dose of this medication?

Tell your doctor about all prescription, over-the-counter, and herbal medications you are taking before beginning treatment with Xanax. Also, talk to your doctor about your complete medical history, especially if you have a history of alcohol abuse; liver, lung, or kidney problems; glaucoma; muscle problems; depression or suicidal tendencies; or if you have ever been physically or mentally dependent on a benzodiazepine medication.

What is the usual dosage?

The information below is based on the dosage guidelines your doctor uses. Depending on your condition and medical history, your doctor may prescribe a different regimen. Do not change the dosage or stop taking your medication without your doctor's approval.

Anxiety Disorders and Temporary Symptoms of Anxiety

Adults: The usual starting dose is 0.25-0.5 milligrams (mg), taken 3 times a day. You doctor may increase the dose up to a maximum of 4 mg per day, taken in divided doses (three to four times a day), depending on your condition. The risk of dependence may increase with more frequent doses and the length of treatment.

Panic Disorders

Adults: The usual dose is 1-10 mg per day, taken in divided doses. Treatment may be started with a dose of 0.5 mg 3 times daily and then adjusted based on your response.

How should I take this medication?

Xanax should be taken exactly as prescribed. You should not take more or stop the medication altogether without first talking to your doctor. Take Xanax at the same time every day, with or without food. If stomach upset occurs, take Xanax with food to reduce stomach irritation.

What should I avoid while taking this medication?

Do not increase, decrease, or stop taking Xanax without first talking to your doctor.

You should not drink alcohol while taking Xanax. You should also not drive a car or operate heavy machinery until you know how this drug affects you.

Avoid eating grapefruit or drinking grapefruit juice while you are being treated with Xanax.

What are possible food and drug interactions associated with this medication?

If Xanax is taken with certain other drugs, the effects of either could be increased, decreased, or altered. It is especially important to check with your doctor before combining Xanax with the following: alcohol, amiodarone, anticonvulsants, antihistamines, carbamazepine, cyclosporine, desipramine, diltiazem, ergotamine, fluoxetine, grapefruit juice, imipramine, isoniazid, itraconazole, ketoconazole, macrolide antibiotics such as erythromycin and clarithromycin, nicardipine, nifedipine, oral contraceptives, propoxyphene.

What are the possible side effects of this medication?

Side effects cannot be anticipated. If any develop or change in intensity, tell your doctor as soon as possible. Only your doctor can determine if it is safe for you to continue taking this drug.

Side effects may include: drowsiness, tiredness, fatigue, impaired coordination, irritability, memory impairment, dizziness, lightheadedness, headache, joint pain, trouble sleeping (insomnia), anxiety, abnormal involuntary movements, decreased or increased sexual drive, depression, confusion, muscle twitching, weakness, fainting, numbness, nausea, vomiting, diarrhea, increased or decreased salivation, stomach pain, upper respiratory tract infection, ringing in the ears, fast heartbeat, chest pain, blurred vision, rash, sweating, increased rate of breathing, change in appetite, weight loss or gain, menstrual disorders, trouble urinating, sexual dysfunction, water retention

Can I receive this medication if I am pregnant or breastfeeding?

No. Xanax should not be taken if you are pregnant or breastfeeding due to the possible harm it may cause to an unborn or nursing infant. Tell your doctor immediately if you are pregnant, plan to become pregnant, or are breastfeeding.

What should I do if I miss a dose of this medication?

If you miss a dose of Xanax and you are using it regularly, take it as soon as possible. If it is almost time for your next dose, skip the missed dose and go back to your regular dosing schedule. Do not take 2 doses at once.

How should I store this medication?

Store at room temperature away from heat, moisture, and light. Do not store in the bathroom.

XANAX XR

Generic name: Alprazolam, extended-release

What is this medication?

Xanax XR is a medicine known as a benzodiazepine; it works by slowing down the movement of chemicals in the brain. Xanax XR is used to treat panic disorders.

What is the most important information I should know about this medication?

If you take more than 4 milligrams (mg) of Xanax XR per day, you are at risk of extreme physical or mental dependence. You may also experience more severe withdrawal symptoms (including seizures) if you stop taking Xanax XR or if you lower the dose.

Even if you take Xanax XR for a short period of time, you may become mentally or physically dependent. Physical dependence could put you at risk for experiencing withdrawal symptoms if you stop taking Xanax XR. Withdrawal symptoms include seizures or a worsening of anxiety and associated symptoms.

Xanax XR binds to certain receptors in the brain that may cause you to become drowsy or sedated. Do not drive, operate machinery, or do anything else that could be dangerous until you know how you react to Xanax XR.

You should not increase, decrease, or stop taking your Xanax XR doses without first talking to your doctor.

Avoid drinking alcohol or taking other medications that cause drowsiness (such as sedatives and tranquilizers) while taking Xanax XR. This medication will add to the effects of alcohol and other depressants.

Do not smoke while using Xanax XR. Cigarette smoking decreases blood levels of Xanax XR. Tell your doctor if you smoke or if you have recently stopped smoking.

Who should not take this medication?
You should not take Xanax XR if you are pregnant, plan to become pregnant, or are breastfeeding.

Do not use this medication if you have an eye condition called acute narrow-angle glaucoma. (If you have open-angle glaucoma, Xanax XR may be used if you are receiving appropriate therapy.)

Do not take Xanax XR if you are allergic to any of its ingredients. Also avoid this drug if you are currently taking the medications itraconazole or ketoconazole.

What should I tell my doctor before I take the first dose of this medication?
Tell your doctor about all prescription, over-the-counter, and herbal medications you are taking before beginning treatment with Xanax XR. Also, talk to your doctor about your complete medical history, especially if you have a history of alcohol abuse; liver, lung, or kidney problems; glaucoma; muscle problems; depression or suicidal tendencies; or if you have ever been physically or mentally dependent on a benzodiazepine medication.

What is the usual dosage?
The information below is based on the dosage guidelines your doctor uses. Depending on your condition and medical history, your doctor may prescribe a different regimen. Do not change the dosage or stop taking your medication without your doctor's approval.

Adults: The recommended dose is 3-6 milligrams (mg) a day. Treatment may be started with a dose of 0.5-1 mg a day. Depending on your response, the dose may be increased at intervals of 3 to 4 days and in increments of no more than 1 mg per day.

How should I take this medication?
Take Xanax XR once a day, preferably in the morning. Take it exactly as prescribed. You should not take more or stop the medication altogether without first talking to your doctor.

You can take Xanax XR with or without food. If stomach upset occurs, take it with food to reduce stomach irritation. Swallow the tablets whole; do not break, crush, or chew them.

What should I avoid while taking this medication?
Do not increase, decrease, or stop taking Xanax XR without first talking to your doctor.

You should not drink alcohol while taking Xanax XR. You should also not drive a car or operate heavy machinery until you know how this drug affects you.

Avoid eating grapefruit or drinking grapefruit juice while you are being treated with Xanax XR.

What are possible food and drug interactions associated with this medication?

If Xanax XR is taken with certain other drugs, the effects of either could be increased, decreased, or altered. It is especially important to check with your doctor before combining Xanax XR with the following: alcohol, amiodarone, anticonvulsants, antihistamines, carbamazepine, cyclosporine, desipramine, diltiazem, ergotamine, fluoxetine, grapefruit juice, imipramine, isoniazid, itraconazole, ketoconazole, macrolide antibiotics such as erythromycin and clarithromycin, nicardipine, nifedipine, oral contraceptives, propoxyphene, rifampin, St. John's wort.

What are the possible side effects of this medication?

Side effects cannot be anticipated. If any develop or change in intensity, tell your doctor as soon as possible. Only your doctor can determine if it is safe for you to continue taking this drug.

Side effects may include: drowsiness, tiredness, constipation, fatigue, impaired coordination, irritability, memory impairment, dizziness, lightheadedness, headache, joint pain, trouble sleeping (insomnia), anxiety, abnormal involuntary movements, decreased or increased sexual drive, depression, confusion, muscle twitching weakness, fainting, numbness, nausea, vomiting, diarrhea, increased or decreased salivation, stomach pain, upper respiratory tract infection, ringing in the ears, fast heartbeat, chest pain, blurred vision, rash, sweating, increased rate of breathing, change in appetite, weight loss or gain, menstrual disorders, trouble urinating, sexual dysfunction, water retention

Can I receive this medication if I am pregnant or breastfeeding?

No. Xanax XR should not be taken if you are pregnant or breastfeeding due to the possible harm it may cause to an unborn or nursing infant. Tell your doctor immediately if you are pregnant, plan to become pregnant, or are breastfeeding.

What should I do if I miss a dose of this medication?

If you miss a dose of Xanax XR and you are using it regularly, take it as soon as possible. If it is almost time for your next dose, skip the missed dose and go back to your regular dosing schedule. Do not take 2 doses at once.

How should I store this medication?

Store at room temperature away from heat, moisture, and light. Do not store in the bathroom.

ZOLOFT

Generic name: Sertraline hydrochloride

What is this medication?

Zoloft is an antidepressant medication known as a selective serotonin reuptake inhibitor (SSRI). It is used to treat major depression, obsessive-compulsive disorder, panic disorder, post-traumatic stress disorder, pre-menstrual dysphoric disorder, and social anxiety disorder.

What is the most important information I should know about this medication?

Antidepressants can increase the risk of suicidal thinking and behavior in children and teenagers. Adult and pediatric patients taking antidepressants should be watched closely for changes in moods or actions, especially when they first start therapy or when their dose is increased or decreased. Patients and their families should contact the doctor immediately if new symptoms develop or seem to get worse. Signs to watch for include anxiety, hostility, sleeplessness, restlessness, impulsive or dangerous behavior, and thoughts about suicide or dying.

Zoloft is not recommended in children and adolescents, except for the treatment of obsessive-compulsive disorder.

Who should not take this medication?

Do not take monoamine oxidase inhibitors (MAOIs) within 2 weeks before or after treatment with this medication. In some cases a serious, possibly fatal, reaction may occur. Examples of MAOIs include selegiline and the antidepressants phenelzine and tranylcypromine.

What should I tell my doctor before I take the first dose of this medication?

Tell your doctor about all prescription, over-the-counter, and herbal medications you are taking before beginning treatment with Zoloft. Also, talk to your doctor about your complete medical history, especially if you have liver or kidney problems, seizure or bleeding disorders, or a history of suicide or mental illness.

What is the usual dosage?

The information below is based on the dosage guidelines your doctor uses. Depending on your condition and medical history, your doctor may prescribe a different regimen. Do not change the dosage or stop taking your medication without your doctor's approval.

Major Depression

Adults: The usual starting dose is 50 milligrams (mg) once a day. If needed, your dose may be increased to up to 200 mg once a day.

Obsessive-Compulsive Disorder

Adults: The usual starting dose is 50 mg once a day. If needed, your dose may be increased to up to 200 mg once a day.

Children: For children 6-12 years old, the usual starting dose is 25 mg once a day. For children 13-17 years old, the usual starting dose is 50 mg once a day. Your child's dose may be increased up to a maximum of 200 mg per day depending on his or her condition.

Panic Disorder, Post-traumatic Stress Disorder, and Social Anxiety Disorder

Adults: The usual starting dose is 25 mg once a day. After 1 week, your dose may be increased to 50 mg once a day. If needed, your dose may be increased to 200 mg once a day.

Premenstrual Dysphoric Disorder

Adults: The usual starting dose is 50 mg once a day. If needed, your dose may be increased to 150 mg once a day.

How should I take this medication?

Zoloft should be taken once a day in the morning or in the evening. Take it at the same time every day. Zoloft may be taken with or without food.

What should I avoid while taking this medication?

You should not drink alcohol while taking Zoloft. You should also not drive a car or operate heavy machinery until you know how this drug affects you.

What are possible food and drug interactions associated with this medication?

If Zoloft is taken with certain other drugs, the effects of either could be increased, decreased, or altered. It is especially important to check with your doctor before combining Zoloft with the following: alcohol, aspirin, cimetidine, diazepam, digitoxin, flecainide, lithium, other antidepressants, MAOIs, nonsteroidal anti-inflammatory drugs (NSAIDs), phenytoin, pimozide, propafenone, sumatriptan, tolbutamide, valproate, warfarin.

What are the possible side effects of this medication?

Side effects cannot be anticipated. If any develop or change in intensity, tell your doctor as soon as possible. Only your doctor can determine if it is safe for you to continue taking this drug.

Side effects may include: stomach pain, agitation, anxiety, changes in vision, constipation, decreased sexual drive, diarrhea, dizziness, dry mouth, fatigue, inability to sleep, increased sweating, loss of appetite/upset stomach, nausea, ejaculation problems, shakiness, tiredness

Can I receive this medication if I am pregnant or breastfeeding?

The effects of Zoloft during pregnancy and breastfeeding are unknown. Tell your doctor immediately if you are pregnant, plan to become pregnant, or are breastfeeding.

What should I do if I miss a dose of this medication?

Take it as soon as your remember. If it is almost time for your next scheduled dose, skip the dose you missed and return to your regular schedule. Do not double your doses.

How should I store this medication?

Store at room temperature.

ZYBAN

Generic name: Bupropion hydrochloride

What is this medication?

Zyban is a nicotine-free medication used to help people quit smoking.

What is the most important information I should know about this medication?

About 1 person in 1,000 suffers a seizure while taking Zyban. For this reason, people with epilepsy should never take this medication. Do not share Zyban with your friends. Only a doctor can decide whether it's safe for a particular individual to take this medication.

Zyban contains the same ingredient as the antidepressants Wellbutrin, Wellbutrin SR, and Wellbutrin XL. Antidepressants can increase the risk of suicidal thinking and behavior in children and teenagers. Adult and pediatric patients taking antidepressants should be watched closely for changes in moods or actions, especially when they first start therapy or when their dose is increased or decreased. Patients and their families should contact the doctor immediately if new symptoms develop or seem to get worse. Signs to watch for include anxiety, hostility, sleeplessness, restlessness, impulsive or dangerous behavior, and thoughts about suicide or dying.

Who should not take this medication?

Do not take Zyban if you have a seizure disorder, anorexia or bulimia (eating disorders), or if you are going through alcohol recovery. In addition, you should not take Zyban if you are taking any other medicines that contain bupropion hydrochloride, such as Wellbutrin, Wellbutrin SR, or Wellbutrin XL, or if you have suddenly stopped taking sedatives.

Do not take monoamine oxidase inhibitors (MAOIs) within 2 weeks before or after treatment with this medication. In some cases a serious, possibly fatal, reaction may occur. Examples of MAOIs include selegiline and the antidepressants phenelzine and tranylcypromine.

Also, do not begin treatment with Zyban if you are allergic to any of its ingredients.

What should I tell my doctor before I take the first dose of this medication?

Tell your doctor about all prescription, over-the-counter, and herbal medications you are taking before beginning treatment with Zyban. Also, talk to your doctor about your complete medical history, especially if you have ever had a seizure, eating disorders, liver or kidney problems, heart problems, high blood sugar, head injuries, or an addiction (eg, alcohol or drug abuse).

What is the usual dosage?

The information below is based on the dosage guidelines your doctor uses. Depending on your condition and medical history, your doctor may prescribe a different regimen. Do not change the dosage or stop taking your medication without your doctor's approval.

Adults: The recommended starting dose is 150 milligrams (mg) a day for the first 3 days. If needed, the doctor may increase your dose up to a maximum dose of 300 mg a day, given in two divided doses.

How should I take this medication?

Take Zyban exactly as prescribed by your doctor. Swallow the tablets whole; do not chew, divide, or crush them. Take the tablets at the same time each day, at least 8 hours apart.

What should I avoid while taking this medication?

Do not drink alcohol or smoke while taking Zyban. If you currently drink a lot of alcohol and suddenly stop, you should tell your doctor, since this may increase your risk of having a seizure. You should also not drive a car or operate heavy machinery until you know how this drug affects you.

What are possible food and drug interactions associated with this medication?

If Zyban is taken with certain other drugs, the effects of either could be increased, decreased, or altered. It is especially important to check with your doctor before combining Zyban with any the following: alcohol, amantadine, antidepressants, blood pressure medications called beta blockers, carbamazepine, cimetidine, cyclophosphamide, heart-stabilizing drugs, levodopa, major tranquilizers, MAOIs, orphenadrine, phenobarbital, phenytoin, steroids such as prednisone and hydrocortisone, theophylline, warfarin.

What are the possible side effects of this medication?

Side effects cannot be anticipated. If any develop or change in intensity, inform your doctor as soon as possible. Only your doctor can determine if it is safe for you to continue taking this drug.

Side effects include: dry mouth, difficulty sleeping

Can I receive this medication if I am pregnant or breastfeeding?

Zyban has not been tested in pregnant women. If you are pregnant or plan to become pregnant, do your best to quit smoking with the aid of counseling and support before taking Zyban. You should avoid smoking or taking nicotine in any other form while pregnant.

Zyban appears in breast milk and could affect a nursing infant. Ask your doctor whether it will be better to discontinue the medication or to stop breastfeeding.

What should I do if I miss a dose of this medication?

Do not double your next dose. Skip the dose you missed and return to your regular dosing schedule. This is very important because taking too much Zyban can increase your risk of having a seizure.

How should I store this medication?

Store at room temperature, away from light and moisture.

ZYPREXA/ZYPREXA ZYDIS/ZYPREXA INTRAMUSCULAR

Generic name: Olanzapine

What is this medication?

Zyprexa is used to treat schizophrenia, bipolar disorder, and agitation associated with these disorders.

What is the most important information I should know about this medication?

When you first start taking Zyprexa, you can develop very low blood pressure, increased heart rate, dizziness, and, in rare cases, a tendency to faint when first standing up. These problems are more likely to occur if you are dehydrated, have heart problems, or take blood pressure medications. To avoid such problems, your doctor may start with a low dose of Zyprexa and increase your dosage gradually.

Zyprexa and similar medications have been associated with an increased risk of developing high blood sugar, which on rare occasions has led to coma or death. See your doctor right away if you develop signs of high blood sugar, including dry mouth, unusual thirst, increased urination, and tiredness. If you have diabetes or have a high risk of developing it, see your doctor regularly for blood sugar testing.

Zyprexa should not be used to treat elderly patients who have dementia because the drug could increase the risk of stroke. In addition, Zyprexa has also been associated with swallowing and breathing problems in older people and those with Alzheimer's disease.

The safety and effectiveness of Zyprexa have not been studied in children.

Who should not take this medication?
Do not take Zyprexa if you are allergic to any of its ingredients.

What should I tell my doctor before I take the first dose of this medication?
Tell your doctor about all prescription, over-the-counter, and herbal medications you are taking before beginning treatment with Zyprexa. Also, talk to your doctor about your complete medical history, especially if you have liver or kidney disease or if you smoke.

What is the usual dosage?
The information below is based on the dosage guidelines your doctor uses. Depending on your condition and medical history, your doctor may prescribe a different regimen. Do not change the dosage or stop taking your medication without your doctor's approval.

Schizophrenia
Adults: The usual starting dose is 5-10 milligrams (mg) once a day. If you start at the lower dose, after a few days the doctor will increase it to 10 mg. After that, your dose will be increased no more than once a week, 5 mg at a time, up to a maximum of 20 mg a day. Once your condition is stabilized, your doctor may continue maintenance therapy at doses of 10-20 mg once a day.

Manic Episodes Associated with Bipolar Disorder
Adults: The usual starting dose is 10-15 mg once a day. If needed, your dose can be increased every 24 hours by 5 mg a day, up to a maximum daily dose of 20 mg. Once your condition is stabilized, your doctor may continue maintenance therapy at doses of 5- 20 mg once a day. If Zyprexa is being combined with lithium or valproate, the usual starting dose is 10 mg once a day.

How should I take this medication?
Take this medication exactly as prescribed by your doctor. Zyprexa comes in regular tablets, orally disintegrating tablets, and as an intramuscular injection. Regular Zyprexa tablets should be taken once a day with or without food.

Zyprexa Zydis is a tablet that will dissolve in your mouth. Immediately after opening the blister packet, use dry hands to remove the tablet and place it in your mouth. The tablet will dissolve quickly in your saliva so it can easily be swallowed with or without liquids.

Zyprexa Intramuscular is an injection that must be given by a doctor.

What should I avoid while taking this medication?

Avoid alcohol while taking Zyprexa. The combination can cause a sudden drop in blood pressure. Zyprexa sometimes causes drowsiness and can impair your judgment, thinking, and movements. Use caution while driving and don't operate dangerous machinery until you know how this drug affects you.

What are possible food and drug interactions associated with this medication?

If Zyprexa is taken with certain other drugs, the effects of either could be increased, decreased, or altered. It is especially important to check with your doctor before combining Zyprexa with any the following: blood pressure medications, benzodiazepines, carbamazepine, diazepam, drugs that boost the effect of dopamine such as Parkinson's medications, fluvoxamine, levodopa, omeprazole, rifampin.

What are the possible side effects of this medication?

Side effects cannot be anticipated. If any develop or change in intensity, inform your doctor as soon as possible. Only your doctor can determine if it is safe for you to continue taking this drug.

Side effects may include: agitation, change in personality, constipation, dizziness, dry mouth, increased appetite, indigestion, low blood pressure upon standing, sleepiness, tremor, weakness, weight gain

Can I receive this medication if I am pregnant or breastfeeding?

If you are pregnant or plan to become pregnant, inform your doctor immediately. Zyprexa should be used during pregnancy only if absolutely necessary. Zyprexa may appear in breast milk; do not breastfeed while taking this medication.

What should I do if I miss a dose of this medication?

Take it as soon as you remember. If it is almost time for your next dose, skip the one you missed and go back to your regular schedule. Do not take 2 doses at once.

How should I store this medication?

Store at room temperature, away from light and moisture.

Index